全国高等中医药院校中药学类专业双语规划教材
Bilingual Planned Textbooks for Chinese Materia Medica Majors in TCM Colleges and Universities

U0265555

# 中药分析学

# Traditional Chinese Medicine Analysis

（供中药学类及相关专业使用）

(For Chinese Materia Medica and other related majors)

主　编　王小平

副主编　冯素香　邵　晶　陈明刚　魏凤环

编　者　（以姓氏笔画为序）

王　瑞（山西中医药大学）　　王小平（陕西中医药大学）

冯素香（河南中医药大学）　　任　波（成都中医药大学）

汤　丹（广东药科大学）　　　杨兴鑫（云南中医药大学）

杨燕云（辽宁中医药大学）　　邹海艳（首都医科大学）

张云静（安徽中医药大学）　　陈明刚（哈尔滨医科大学）

邵　晶（甘肃中医药大学）　　单鸣秋（南京中医药大学）

赵惠茹（西安医学院）　　　　袁瑞娟（北京中医药大学）

曹玉嫔（广西中医药大学）　　谢允东（陕西中医药大学）

魏凤环（南方医科大学）

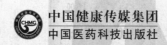

中国健康传媒集团

中国医药科技出版社

## 内 容 提 要

　　本教材为"全国高等中医药院校中药学类专业双语规划教材"之一。共分十章，主要介绍了中药分析学的概念、研究对象、意义和任务，中药分析的基本程序、特点，药品标准，中药的鉴别、检查、指纹图谱和特征图谱、含量测定，中药各类化学成分分析，不同类型中药质量分析的特点，生物样品内中药成分分析及中药质量标准的制定等内容。内容既体现中药分析的特点，又反映中药分析的发展趋势，实例具有代表性。本教材为书网融合教材，即纸质教材有机融合电子教材、教学配套资源（PPT、微课、习题）、数字化教学服务（在线教学、在线作业、在线考试），使教学资源更加多样化、立体化。

　　本教材可供全国高等中医药院校中药学类及相关专业教学使用，还可供从事中药质量检验、中药生产、中药新药研发等的专业技术人员参阅。

**图书在版编目（CIP）数据**

中药分析学：汉英对照 / 王小平主编 .—北京：中国医药科技出版社，2020.8
全国高等中医药院校中药学类专业双语规划教材
ISBN 978-7-5214-1877-4

Ⅰ.①中⋯　Ⅱ.①王⋯　Ⅲ.①中药材 - 药物分析 - 双语教学 - 中医学院 - 教材 - 汉、英　Ⅳ.① R284.1

中国版本图书馆 CIP 数据核字（2020）第 097260 号

**美术编辑**　陈君杞
**版式设计**　辰轩文化

出版　**中国健康传媒集团** | 中国医药科技出版社
地址　北京市海淀区文慧园北路甲 22 号
邮编　100082
电话　发行：010-62227427　邮购：010-62236938
网址　www.cmstp.com
规格　889×1194 mm $\frac{1}{16}$
印张　18¾
字数　482 千字
版次　2020 年 8 月第 1 版
印次　2020 年 8 月第 1 次印刷
印刷　三河市万龙印装有限公司
经销　全国各地新华书店
书号　ISBN 978-7-5214-1877-4
定价　**59.00** 元

获取新书信息、投稿、为图书纠错，请扫码联系我们。

# 出版说明

近些年随着世界范围的中医药热潮的涌动，来中国学习中医药学的留学生逐年增多，走出国门的中医药学人才也在增加。为了适应中医药国际交流与合作的需要，加快中医药国际化进程，提高来中国留学生和国际班学生的教学质量，满足双语教学的需要和中医药对外交流需求，培养优秀的国际化中医药人才，进一步推动中医药国际化进程，根据教育部、国家中医药管理局、国家药品监督管理局等部门的有关精神，在本套教材建设指导委员会主任委员成都中医药大学彭成教授等专家的指导和顶层设计下，中国医药科技出版社组织全国50余所高等中医药院校及附属医疗机构约420名专家、教师精心编撰了全国高等中医药院校中药学类专业双语规划教材，该套教材即将付梓出版。

本套教材共计23门，主要供全国高等中医药院校中药学类专业教学使用。本套教材定位清晰、特色鲜明，主要体现在以下方面。

## 一、立足双语教学实际，培养复合应用型人才

本套教材以高校双语教学课程建设要求为依据，以满足国内医药院校开展留学生教学和双语教学的需求为目标，突出中医药文化特色鲜明、中医药专业术语规范的特点，注重培养中医药技能、反映中医药传承和现代研究成果，旨在优化教育质量，培养优秀的国际化中医药人才，推进中医药对外交流。

本套教材建设围绕目前中医药院校本科教育教学改革方向对教材体系进行科学规划、合理设计，坚持以培养创新型和复合型人才为宗旨，以社会需求为导向，以培养适应中药开发、利用、管理、服务等各个领域需求的高素质应用型人才为目标的教材建设思路与原则。

## 二、遵循教材编写规律，整体优化，紧跟学科发展步伐

本套教材的编写遵循"三基、五性、三特定"的教材编写规律；以"必需、够用"为度；坚持与时俱进，注意吸收新技术和新方法，适当拓展知识面，为学生后续发展奠定必要的基础。实验教材密切结合主干教材内容，体现理实一体，注重培养学生实践技能训练的同时，按照教育部相关精神，增加设计性实验部分，以现实问题作为驱动力来培养学生自主获取和应用新知识的能力，从而培养学生独立思考能力、实验设计能力、实践操作能力和可持续发展能力，满足培养应用型和复合型人才的要求。强调全套教材内容的整体优化，并注重不同教材内容的联系与衔接，避免遗漏和不必要的交叉重复。

1

### 三、对接职业资格考试，"教考""理实"密切融合

本套教材的内容和结构设计紧密对接国家执业中药师职业资格考试大纲要求，实现教学与考试、理论与实践的密切融合，并且在教材编写过程中，吸收具有丰富实践经验的企业人员参与教材的编写，确保教材的内容密切结合应用，更加体现高等教育的实践性和开放性，为学生参加考试和实践工作打下坚实基础。

### 四、创新教材呈现形式，书网融合，使教与学更便捷更轻松

全套教材为书网融合教材，即纸质教材与数字教材、配套教学资源、题库系统、数字化教学服务有机融合。通过"一书一码"的强关联，为读者提供全免费增值服务。按教材封底的提示激活教材后，读者可通过 PC、手机阅读电子教材和配套课程资源（PPT、微课、视频等），并可在线进行同步练习，实时收到答案反馈和解析。同时，读者也可以直接扫描书中二维码，阅读与教材内容关联的课程资源，从而丰富学习体验，使学习更便捷。教师可通过 PC 在线创建课程，与学生互动，开展在线课程内容定制、布置和批改作业、在线组织考试、讨论与答疑等教学活动，学生通过 PC、手机均可实现在线作业、在线考试，提升学习效率，使教与学更轻松。此外，平台尚有数据分析、教学诊断等功能，可为教学研究与管理提供技术和数据支撑。需要特殊说明的是，有些专业基础课程，例如《药理学》等 9 种教材，起源于西方医学，因篇幅所限，在本次双语教材建设中纸质教材以英语为主，仅将专业词汇对照了中文翻译，同时在中国医药科技出版社数字平台"医药大学堂"上配套了中文电子教材供学生学习参考。

编写出版本套高质量教材，得到了全国知名专家的精心指导和各有关院校领导与编者的大力支持，在此一并表示衷心感谢。希望广大师生在教学中积极使用本套教材和提出宝贵意见，以便修订完善，共同打造精品教材，为促进我国高等中医药院校中药学类专业教育教学改革和人才培养做出积极贡献。

# 数字化教材编委会

**主　编**　王小平

**副主编**　冯素香　邵　晶　陈明刚　魏凤环

**编　者**（以姓氏笔画为序）

王　瑞（山西中医药大学）　　王小平（陕西中医药大学）

冯素香（河南中医药大学）　　任　波（成都中医药大学）

汤　丹（广东药科大学）　　　杨兴鑫（云南中医药大学）

杨燕云（辽宁中医药大学）　　邹海艳（首都医科大学）

张云静（安徽中医药大学）　　陈明刚（哈尔滨医科大学）

邵　晶（甘肃中医药大学）　　单鸣秋（南京中医药大学）

赵惠茹（西安医学院）　　　　袁瑞娟（北京中医药大学）

曹玉嫔（广西中医药大学）　　谢允东（陕西中医药大学）

魏凤环（南方医科大学）

# 前　言

本教材为"全国高等中医药院校中药学类专业双语规划教材"之一,是根据教育部相关文件精神、中药学类专业教学要求、课程特点及人才培养目标,结合最新执业药师考试大纲,紧扣2020年版《中国药典》编写而成。内容共分十章,主要包括中药分析学的概念、研究对象、意义和任务,中药分析的基本程序、特点,药品标准,中药的鉴别、检查、指纹图谱和特征图谱、含量测定,中药各类化学成分分析,各类中药质量分析的特点,生物样品内中药成分分析及中药质量标准的制定等。本教材的内容既体现中药分析的特点,又反映中药分析的发展趋势,各章实例均具有代表性。可供全国高等中医药院校中药学类及相关专业教学使用,还可供从事中药质量检验、中药生产、中药新药研发等的专业技术人员参阅。

本教材为书网融合教材,即纸质教材有机融合电子教材、教学配套资源(PPT、微课、习题)、数字化教学服务(在线教学、在线作业、在线考试),使教学资源更加多样化、立体化。

本教材的具体编写分工如下:王小平编写第一章;谢允东编写第二章;任波、邵晶编写第三章;杨燕云、曹玉嫔编写第四章;王瑞编写第五章;冯素香、袁瑞娟编写第六章;单鸣秋、赵惠茹编写第七章;汤丹、邹海艳编写第八章;魏凤环编写第九章;陈明刚、杨兴鑫、张云静编写第十章。

在编写本教材过程中得到了各编者所在单位的大力支持,在此表示衷心的感谢。由于编者水平有限,加之中药分析学的发展飞速,书中内容难免存在不足之处,敬请同行专家、学者及使用本教材的师生和广大读者提出宝贵意见和建议,以便修订时进一步完善。

编　者

2020 年 3 月

# Preface

This textbook is one of the "bilingual planning textbooks for traditional Chinese pharmacy majors in national colleges and universities of traditional Chinese medicine". It is based on the spirit of relevant documents of the Ministry of Education, teaching requirements of traditional Chinese pharmacy majors, course characteristics and talent training objectives, combined with the latest licensed pharmacist exam outline. It was compiled in accordance with the 2020 edition of "Chinese Pharmacopoeia". The content is divided into ten chapters, mainly including the concept, research objects, significance and tasks of traditional Chinese medicine analysis, basic procedures and characteristics of traditional Chinese medicine analysis, drug standards, identification, inspection, fingerprint and characteristic chromatogram of traditional Chinese medicine, content determination, various types Chemical composition analysis of traditional Chinese medicine, characteristics of various traditional Chinese medicine quality analysis, analysis of traditional Chinese medicine composition in biological samples and formulation of traditional Chinese medicine quality standards, etc. The content of this textbook not only reflects the characteristics of traditional Chinese medicine analysis, but also reflects the development trend of traditional Chinese medicine analysis. The examples in each chapter are representative. It can be used for the teaching of Chinese pharmacy majors and related majors in national colleges and universities of Chinese medicine. It can also be used by professional and technical personnel engaged in quality inspection of traditional Chinese medicine, production of traditional Chinese medicine, and research and development of new Chinese medicine.

This textbook is a combination of book and web textbooks, that is, organic integration of paper textbooks, electronic textbooks, teaching supporting resources (PPT, micro-classes, exercises), and digital teaching services (online teaching, online assignments, online exams), making teaching resources more diverse, Three-imensional.

The specific arrangement for this textbook is as follows: Xiaoping Wang wrote the first chapter; Yundong Xie wrote the second chapter; Bo Ren and Jing Shao wrote the third chapter; Yanyun Yang and Yubin Cao wrote the fourth chapter; Rui Wang wrote the fifth chapter; Suxiang Feng and Ruijuan Yuan wrote Chapter 6; Mingqiu Shan and Huiru Zhao wrote chapter 7; Dan Tang and Haiyan Zou wrote chapter 8; Fenghuan Wei wrote Chapter 9; Minggang Chen, Xingxin Yang and Yunjing Zhang wrote Chapter 10.

In the process of writing this textbook, I have received the strong support of the employer where the editors are, and I would like to express my heartfelt thanks. Due to the limited level of editors and the rapid development of Chinese medicine analysis, it is inevitable that there are deficiencies in the contents of the textbook. Please experts, scholars, teachers, students and readers who use this textbook to provide valuable comments and suggestions so that textbook can be further improved when revised.

**Editor**

March 2020

# 目录 | Contents

# 第一章　绪　论
# Chapter 1　Introduction

 **学习目标┊ Learning Goal**

知识要求：

**1. 掌握**　中药分析学的概念、研究对象、意义、基本程序及《中国药典》的凡例。

**2. 熟悉**　中药分析学的内容、任务和特点及《中国药典》的历史沿革。

**3. 了解**　中药分析学的历史、发展趋势和国外药典。

能力要求：

学会应用国家药品标准和中药分析的基本程序解决中药分析学中抽样。

**Knowledge Requirement**

**1. Master**　The concept, research object, significance, basic procedures of traditional Chinese medicine analysis and General Notices of *Chinese Pharmacopoeia*.

**2. Familiar**　The contents, tasks and characteristics of traditional Chinese medicine analysis, and the history of *Chinese Pharmacopoeia*.

**3. Understand**　The history and development trend of traditional Chinese medicine analysis.

**Ability Requirement**

Learn to apply national drug standards and basic procedures for analysis of traditional Chinese medicine to solve sampling in traditional Chinese medicine analysis.

## 第一节　概述
## 1.1　Overview

PPT

　　中药分析学是以中医药理论为指导，应用物理学、化学、生物学等分析技术与方法，研究中药的质量控制与评价方法的一门学科。中药分析学是中药学类及相关专业的专业核心课程之一，它不仅是一门研究中药质量控制与评价方法的学科，而且还为中药学等相关学科的研究与发展提供技术支撑，推动其发展和提高。

The analysis of traditional Chinese medicine is a subject which studies the quality control and evaluation methods of traditional Chinese medicine under the guidance of the theory of traditional Chinese medicine by the application of various analytical techniques and methods (physics, chemistry, biology, etc.). Traditional Chinese medicine analysis is one of the core curriculums of traditional Chinese medicine related majors. It is not only a subject that studies the methods of quality control and evaluation of traditional Chinese medicine, but also provides technical support for the research and development of traditional Chinese medicine and other related disciplines, promotes the development and improvement of traditional Chinese medicine related disciplines.

### 一、中药分析的意义和任务
### 1.1.1 Significance and Task of Traditional Chinese Medicine Analysis

中药分析的主要对象是中药材（饮片）、植物油脂和提取物、成方制剂和单味制剂等，均属于特殊商品，其质量的优劣不仅影响临床疗效，而且还关系到使用者的健康，甚至生命安危，所以中药质量控制不同于其他商品，应更加严格。中药分析的意义就在于确保临床用药的安全、有效及中药质量可控。

The main objects of traditional Chinese medicine analysis are Chinese crude drugs and decoction pieces, vegetable oil fat and extracts, single item preparations and multiple item preparations, all of which belong to special commodities. The quality not only affects the clinical efficacy, but also relates to the health of users, and even life safety. Therefore, the quality control of traditional Chinese medicine is different from other commodities and should be more stringent. The significance of traditional Chinese medicine analysis is to ensure the safety and effectiveness of clinical drug use, and the quality of traditional Chinese medicine can be controlled.

中药分析涉及药材（饮片）和提取物的生产，中药制剂的开发、生产等各个环节，主要任务包括：①建立符合中医药特点的质量评价模式；②建立系统化的中药质量标准体系；③建立体内、体外中药分析的双向评价模式；④中药标准物质研究；⑤新技术、新方法研究。

Traditional Chinese medicine analysis involves the production of medicinal materials (the prepared slices of Chinese crude drugs) and extracts, the research and the development, and production of traditional Chinese medicine preparations, its main tasks are as follows:① Establishing a quality evaluation model in line with characteristics of traditional Chinese medicine; ② Establishing the systematic quality standard system of traditional Chinese medicine; ③ Establishing the two-way evaluation model of traditional Chinese medicine analysis *in vitro* and *in vivo*; ④ Study on the standard substance of traditional Chinese medicine; ⑤ Research on new technologies and new methods.

### 二、中药分析的基本程序
### 1.1.2 Basic Procedures for the Analysis of Traditional Chinese Medicine

中药分析基本程序：抽样、供试品溶液的制备、供试品的分析（鉴别、检查、含量测定）、原始记录和检验报告。

Basic procedures for the analysis of traditional Chinese medicine: sampling, preparation of sample solution, analysis (identification, physic-chemical inspection, content determination), original record and inspection report.

（一）抽样

## 1. Sampling

随机抽样：保证总体中每个样品单位都有同等机会被抽中。强调抽样的代表性和覆盖面，适用于评价性抽验。

*Random sampling* Ensuring that every unit in the total sample has an equal chance of being selected. It emphasizes the representativeness and coverage of sampling, which is suitable for evaluative sampling.

偶遇抽样：研究者根据实际情况，为方便开展工作，选择偶然遇到的样品作为调查对象，或者仅仅选择那些离得最近的、最容易找到的样品作为调查对象。

*Accidental sampling* According to the actual situation, in order to facilitate the work, the researchers choose the accidental samples as the survey subjects, or only the closest and easy to find samples as the survey subjects.

针对性抽样：当发现某一批或者若干批药品质量可疑时，应当针对性抽样。其目的是尽可能从被抽样品中找到不合格药品。该抽样方法目的性强，强调的是如何选准不合格样品，而不强调其代表性，同时针对性抽样可减少抽验成本，以最小必要量的药品抽验，获取最大程度的药品质量监督效能。

*Targeted sampling* When it is found that the quality of a batch or more batches of drugs is suspicious, targeted sampling shall be taken. The aim is to find substandard drugs from the sampled samples as much as possible. The sampling method is purposeful and emphasizes how to select unqualified samples without emphasizing their representativeness, at the same time, targeted sampling can reduce the cost of sampling and obtain the maximum effectiveness of drug quality supervision with the minimum necessary quantity of drugs.

1. **中药材和饮片** 从同批药材和饮片包件中抽取供检验用样品的原则如下：药材总包件数不足 5 件的，逐件取样；5~99 件的，随机抽 5 件取样；100~1000 件，按 5% 的比例取样；超过 1000 件的，超过部分按 1% 的比例取样；贵重药材和饮片，不论包件多少均逐件取样。

(1) **Chinese Medicinal Materials and Prepared Slices** The principles of taking samples for inspection from the same batch of Chinese medicinal materials and prepared pieces are as follows: For less than 5 packages, sample each package. For 5-99 packages, sample 5 packages at random. For 100-1000 packages, sample 5% of the packages. For more than 1000 packages, sample 1% of the part in excess of 1000 packages. For precious Chinese medicinal materials and decoction pieces, sample each package, regardless of the number of packages.

每一包件的取样量：一般药材和饮片抽取 100~500g；粉末状药材和饮片抽取 25~50g；贵重药材和饮片抽取 5~10g。

The quantity of samples collected from each package: ordinary Chinese medicinal materials and decoction pieces, 100-500g. Powdered Chinese medicinal materials and decoction pieces, 25-50g. Precious Chinese medicinal materials and decoction pieces, 5-10g.

若抽取样品总量超过检验用量数倍时，可按四分法再取样，即将所有样品摊成正方形，依对角线划 "X"，使分为四等份，取用对角两份；再如上操作，反复数次，直至最后剩余量能满足供检验用样品量。

If the total quantity of samples exceeds several times of that required for the tests, take sample by quartering, i.e., spread the sample as a square, draw diagonal lines to divide the sample into four parts, and use samples from two parts in opposite positions. Keep this quartering repeatedly until the finally obtained sample is just sufficient for the tests.

**2. 中药提取物**　固体或者半固体提取物：一般应当从上、中、下、前、后、左、右等不同部位取样，可在同一抽样单元的不同部位取样，也可在不同抽样单元的不同部位取样。

**(2) Traditional Chinese Medicine Extract**　Solid or semi-solid: generally, samples should be taken from different parts (such as upper, middle, lower, front, back, left and right etc.) in same the sampling unit or different sampling units.

液体提取物：有结晶析出的液体，应当在不影响药品质量的情况下，使结晶溶解并混匀后取样。不易混匀的应在顶部、中部、底部分别抽样混匀后进行检验分析。

Liquid: If liquids with crystal precipitation, the crystals should be dissolved and mixed without affecting the quality of the drug, then sampling. If it is difficult to mix, it should be sampled at the top, middle and bottom respectively, then mixed for inspection and analysis.

**3. 中药制剂**　当药品包装为箱或袋，且数量较大时，可随机从大批样品中取出部分箱或袋，再从留取的箱或袋中用专用的取样工具从各个部位取出一定样品，以备检验。

**(3) Chinese Medicine Preparation**　When the Chinese medicinal preparation is packaged as a box or bag and large amount, firstly, some boxes or bags can be randomly taken out from a large number of samples, and then sampling using suitable sampling tool from various parts of the boxes or bags for inspection.

**4. 最终抽取的供检验用样品量**　一般不得少于检验所需用量的 3 倍，即 1/3 供实验室分析用，另 1/3 供复核用，其余 1/3 留样保存。

**(4) Sample Size**　The finally obtained sample for examination should be at least three times the quantity required for the tests, using 1/3 for laboratory analysis, 1/3 for conformance verification, and the remaining 1/3 as reserve specimen.

（二）供试溶液的制备

## 2. Preparation of Test Solution

中药分析大多情况下需要制备供试溶液（详见第二章）。中药多为固体，成分复杂，被测成分含量较低，大多需要提取、纯化、富集后才可分析。

In most cases, the test solution needs to be prepared for the analysis of traditional Chinese medicine (Chapter 2 for details). Most of the traditional Chinese medicines are solid, the components are complex, and the content of the tested components is low, so most of them need to be extracted, purified and enriched before analysis.

（三）供试品的分析

## 3. Analysis of Samples

主要包含鉴别（详见第三章）、检查（详见第四章）、含量测定（详见第六章）等。

Including identification (Chapter 3 for details), inspection (Chapter 4 for details), content determination (Chapter 6 for details) and so on.

（四）原始记录和检验报告

## 4. Original Record and Inspection Report

**1. 原始记录**　要求真实、完整、清晰、具体。使用专用记录本，原则上不得缺页或挖补，如有缺漏页，应详细说明原因；用钢笔或中性笔书写，一般不得涂改（若有写错时，应在原数据上划单线或双线，然后在旁边改正重写并签名确认）；使用规范的专业术语，计量单位采用国际标准计量单位，有效数字的取舍应符合实验要求；即使实验失败也要有详细记录，并记录失败的原因。记录内容包括品名、来源、批号、数量、规格、包装、日期，方法及依据，检验中观察到的现象、数据、结果、结论等。

**(1) Original Record** True, complete, clear and specific. In principle, The dedicated record book shall not be missing pages or mended, and if there is a missing page, the reason should be explained in detail; writing with a pen or neutral pen, original record generally shall not be altered (if there is a mistake in writing, the original data should be marked with a single or double lines, then correct and rewrite next to it and sign to confirm it); language adopts the professional term of the standard term, the unit of measurement adopts the international standard unit of measurement, and the choice of valid numbers should meet the requirements of the experiment. Record contents include product name, source, batch number, quantity, specification, sampling method, appearance, packaging, date, purpose, method and basis of inspection, phenomena observed in the inspection, data, results, conclusions, etc.

2. 检验报告 文字简洁，内容完整，结论明确。主要内容有取样日期、报告日期，品名、批号、规格、数量、来源、包装，检验目的、项目、依据、结果、结论。

**(2) Inspection Report** The text is concise, the content is complete, and the conclusion is clear. Main contents include sampling date, report date, product name, batch number, specification, quantity, source, packaging, inspection purpose, item, basis, result, conclusion.

### 三、中药分析的特点
### 1.1.3 Characteristics of Traditional Chinese Medicine Analysis

中药因其所含成分复杂、含量差异大、杂质多，且大多是复方制剂，使得中药分析具有明显不同于化学药物分析的特点。

The analysis of traditional Chinese medicine has distinct characteristics different from that of chemical medicine, because traditional Chinese medicine contains complex components, large differences in content, many impurities, and most are compound preparations.

### （一）以中医药理论为指导
### 1. Under the Guidance of the Theory of Traditional Chinese Medicine

中药制剂多为复方，所含药味众多，有的十几种或者几十种药味，在进行质量分析时，我们不能做到对每味药进行分析，此时，根据中医组方原则，分析出组方中的君、臣、佐、使药味，为了保证中药制剂的有效性和安全性，首选方中君、臣药和毒剧药。药味确定后，还不能直接分析，由于每味中药所含化学成分众多，因此，需要选择药理活性和该制剂功能主治相一致的成分为指标评价中药制剂的质量。

Most of the traditional Chinese medicine preparations are compound prescriptions with multiplex Chinese medicinal materials or prepared slices. In the quality analysis, we can′t analyze each Chinese medicinal materials. At this time, according to the formulating principle of Chinese medicine to divide sovereign medicine, minister medicine, assistant medicine and courier herb in the prescription. In order to ensure the effectiveness and safety of the preparation of traditional Chinese medicine, sovereign medicine, minister medicine and poison drama medicine are preferred for analysis. After the determination of Chinese medicine materials for analysis, it can′t be analyzed directly. Because there are many chemical components in each Chinese medicine materials, it is necessary to select the components whose pharmacological activity is consistent with the function of the preparation as an index to evaluate the quality of traditional Chinese medicine preparation.

（二）化学成分的复杂多样性

## 2. Complexity and Diversity of Chemical Composition

中药所含化学成分十分复杂，主要体现在以下三个方面：①中药中可能含有一类结构、性质极其相似的化学成分，如黄连中的巴马汀、小檗碱、黄连碱和表小檗碱等生物碱类成分等。②中药中可能会含有不同类别的化合物，如三黄片中含有黄酮类、生物碱类和蒽醌类成分等。③复方配伍和制剂过程中，有些成分相互影响及新物质的生成。如当黄连与甘草、金银花等中药配伍时，黄连中的小檗碱和甘草中的甘草酸及金银花中的绿原酸等有机酸形成难溶于水的复合物而沉淀析出，既影响酸性或者碱性成分的含量又有新物质的产生。

The chemical components of traditional Chinese medicine are very complex, mainly reflected in the following three aspects: ① traditional Chinese medicine may contain a kind of chemical components with very similar structure and properties, such as alkaloids (palmatine, berberine, coptisine and epiberberine) in Coptidis Rhizoma. ② There may be different kinds of compounds in traditional Chinese medicine, such as flavonoids, alkaloids and anthraquinones in Sanhuang tablets, etc. ③ In the process of compound compatibility and preparation, some components influence each other and the formation of new substances. For example, when the Coptidis Rhizoma is compatible with traditional Chinese medicines such as Nardostachyos Radix et Rhizoma and Lonicerae Japonicae Flos, berberine in Coptidis Rhizoma and the organic acids such as glycyrrhizic acid in Nardostachyos Radix et Rhizoma and chlorogenic acid in Lonicerae Japonicae Flos form substances insoluble in water and precipitate out, which affects the content of alkaline component and acidic component, and produces new substances at the same time.

（三）杂质来源的多途径性

## 3. The Multi-path of the Sources of Impurities

中药的杂质来源远比化学药物多，如药材中非药用部位及带入的泥土沙石；药材产地水源、土壤、空气等生长环境的污染；农药化肥的滥用；贮藏不当发生的霉变、走油、泛糖、虫蛀等均可引入杂质。

There are more sources of impurities in traditional Chinese medicine than chemical drugs, such as the non-medicinal parts of medicinal materials, the soil and sand brought in, the pollution of growing environment such as water source, soil and air, and the abuse of pesticides and fertilizers. Impurities can be introduced through improper storage, such as mildew and rot, floating oil, floating sugar, rotten due to insect bites and so on.

（四）质量影响因素的多样性

## 4. Diversity of Factors Affecting Quality

影响中药质量的因素多种多样，如药材的来源、产地、采收时间、药用部位等；饮片的炮制、加工过程等；制剂的生产过程、辅料等；中药的包装、贮藏等。

There are a variety of factors affecting the quality of traditional Chinese medicine, such as the variety, origin, harvest time, medicinal parts and so on in Chinese medicinal materials, the processing of prepared slices, the production process and excipients of the preparation, and the packaging and storage of traditional Chinese medicine.

（五）有效成分的非单一性

## 5. Non-Uniqueness of Active Ingredients

中药产生的疗效不是某个单一化学成分作用的结果，而是多种成分通过多条途径，作用于机体的多个靶点，通过修复、调整等多种方式调动机体的某些机能而发挥的综合疗效。因此，仅用一种有效成分的存在与否或含量高低来评价其质量是不恰当的。

The curative effect of traditional Chinese medicine is not the result of a single chemical component, but a comprehensive effect of multiple components acting on multiple targets of the body or repair, adjustment some functions of the body through multiple ways. Therefore, it is not appropriate to evaluate the quality of traditional Chinese medicine by an active component only existence or content.

### 四、中药分析的历史与发展趋势
### 1.1.4 History and Development Trend of the Traditional Chinese Medicine Analysis

伴随中药发现，就有了中药的质量评价。随着中药事业和分析技术的不断发展，人们对中药质量评价方法经历了由主观到客观，由简单浅显到深入全面的过程。

With the discovery of traditional Chinese medicine, there is the quality evaluation. With the continuous development of traditional Chinese medicine and analytical technology, the quality evaluation method of traditional Chinese medicine has experienced a process from subjective to objective, from simple to comprehensive.

### （一）中药分析的历史
### 1. The History of Traditional Chinese Medicine Analysis

中药分析大致经历了以下三个阶段：① 性状鉴别阶段，以外观性状（形状、大小、颜色）、气味、质地、断面等特征，部分药材亦辅以火试法和水试法为判断质量的依据；② 显微鉴别阶段，该方法作为药材、饮片及含粉末中药制剂的重要鉴别手段；③ 理化分析的综合评价阶段，中药分析引入 UV、IR 等光谱技术与 PC、TLC、HPLC、GC 及色谱－质谱联用等色谱技术，建立针对化学成分的定性、定量质量评价模式。

The analysis of traditional Chinese medicine can be divided into three stages.① External characteristic identification, judging quality of Chinese medicinal materials by appearance traits (shape, size, color), odor, taste, texture, cross-section and so on, some medicinal materials are judged by fire test and water test; ② Microscopic identification, this method is used as an important way for identification of medicinal materials, the prepared slices, traditional Chinese medicine preparations with medicinal materials powder; ③ Physical and chemical analysis, the analysis of traditional Chinese medicine widely introduced UV, IR and other spectral techniques and PC, TLC, HPLC, GC and chromatography-mass spectrometry analysis techniques to establish qualitative and quantitative standards of traditional Chinese medicine.

### （二）中药分析的发展趋势
### 2. The Development Trend of Traditional Chinese Medicine Analysis

随着相关学科的发展，中药分析呈现如下的发展趋势：建立能控制中药有效性的质量标准体系；强化现代方法技术及中药的安全性评价；建立个体化的质量标准；建立多指标、整体性的中药质量评价模式；加强中药在线检测和体内分析。

With the development of related disciplines, the traditional Chinese medicine analysis shows the following development trend:① Establishing a quality standard system of controlling the effectiveness of traditional Chinese medicine; ② Strengthening the application of modern methods and techniques in the analysis of traditional Chinese medicine; ③ Strengthen the safety evaluation of traditional Chinese medicine; ④ Establish individualized quality standards establish individualized quality standards; ⑤ Establish a multi-index and holistic quality evaluation model of traditional chinese medicine;

医药大学堂
WWW.YIYAODXT.COM

⑥ Strengthen traditional Chinese medicine online testing and *in vivo* analysis.

## 第二节　药品标准
## 1.2　Drug Standards

药品是特殊的商品，其质量的优劣不仅影响临床疗效，还关系到使用者的健康乃至生命安危。因此，药品必须有严格的可控制和评价其质量的标准。

Medicine is a special commodity, its quality not only affects the clinical efficacy, but also is related to the health of users and even life and safety. Therefore, drugs must have strict standards, which can control and evaluate their quality.

### 一、药品标准的概念与分类
### 1.2.1　Concept and Classification of Drug Standards

药品标准是指根据药物来源、制药工艺等生产及贮存过程中的各个环节所制定的、用以检测药品质量是否达到用药要求并衡量其是否稳定均一的技术规定，是药品的生产、流通、使用及检验、监督管理部门共同遵循的法定依据。

Drug standards refer to the technical regulations formulated according to the source of drugs, pharmaceutical technology and other links in the process of production and storage, which are used to detect whether the quality of drugs meets the requirements of drug use and to measure whether they are stable and uniform. It is the legal basis followed by the production, circulation, use, inspection, supervision and management departments of drugs.

按照成熟程度，药品标准分为国家标准、地方标准和其他标准。根据药品标准的属性又分为强制性标准和推荐性标准。强制性标准是指在一定范围内，通过法律、行政法规等强制性手段加以实施的标准，具有法律属性，一经颁布，必须贯彻执行。推荐性标准通常无法定约束力，属于非强制性或自愿性标准。

According to the mature degree of drug standards, they are divided into national standards, local standards and other standards. According to the attribute of drug standards, they can be divided into mandatory standard and recommended standard. Mandatory standards are abided within a certain range through laws, rules, administrative regulations and other compulsory means, which have legal attributes and must be implemented once promulgated. Recommended standards are usually non-legally binding and belong to non-mandatory or voluntary standards.

### 二、国家药品标准
### 1.2.2　National Drug Standards

国家药品标准，是指国家为保证药品质量所制定的用以检测药品质量是否达到用药要求并衡量其是否稳定均一的技术规定，包括质量指标、检验方法以及生产工艺等的技术要求。国家药品标准包括《中华人民共和国药典》，局（部）颁标准。

The national drug standard refers to the technical regulations formulated by the state to ensure the drug quality, which is used in order to test whether the drug quality meets the drug use requirements and measure its stability and uniformity, including the technical requirements of quality indicators, inspection methods and production processes. National drug standards include *the Pharmacopoeia of the people's Republic of China* (ChP), the standards of traditional Chinese medicine approved by the National Medical Products Administration (NMPA) or the National Health Commission of the People's Republic of China.

（一）《中国药典》

## 1. Chinese Pharmacopoeia

《中华人民共和国药典》简称《中国药典》，由国家药品监督管理部门组织国家药典委员会，依据《中华人民共和国药品管理法》组织制定和颁布实施，具有国家法律效力，是我国记载药品标准、规格的法典，一经颁布实施，作为药品生产、检验、供应与使用的依据，其同品种的上版标准或原国家标准即同时停止使用。

*The Pharmacopoeia of the people's Republic of China* is referred to as the *Chinese Pharmacopoeia*. Chinese Pharmacopoeia Commission is organized by the National Medical Products Administration to formulate, promulgate and implement *the Pharmacopoeia of the people's Republic of China* in accordance with the "Drug Administration Law of the people's Republic of China". Where the Pharmacopoeia is issued for enforcement, as the basis for the production, inspection, supply and use of drugs, the same drug standard of the previous Pharmacopoeia or the original national drug standard shall not be used.

1.《中国药典》历史沿革　自 1949 年中华人民共和国成立后，已出版发行了 1953 年版、1963 年版、1977 年版、1985 年版、1990 年版、1995 年版、2000 年版、2005 年版、2010 年版、2015 年版和 2020 年版共 11 个版次的《中国药典》。自 1985 年版开始每 5 年修订改版一次。1988 年 10 月，第一部英文版《中国药典》（1985 年版）出版发行。《中国药典》自 2015 年版开始分为四部。一部收载中药，二部收载化学药品等，三部收载生物制品，四部收载通用技术要求和药用辅料。

**(1) The Historical Evolution of *Chinese Pharmacopoeia***　After the founding of the people's Republic of China in 1949, the *Chinese Pharmacopoeia* has been published in 11 editions: 1953 edition, 1963 edition, 1977 edition, 1985 edition, 1990 edition, 1995 edition, 2000 edition, 2005 edition, 2010 edition, 2015 edition and 2020 edition. Since the 1985 edition, it is revised and published every 5 years. In October 1988, the first English version of *Chinese Pharmacopoeia* (1985 edition) was published. Since the *Chinese Pharmacopoeia* 2015 edition has comprised four volumes. The Volume Ⅰ contains traditional Chinese medicines, the Volume Ⅱ contains chemical drugs, the Volume Ⅲ contains biologics, and the Volume Ⅳ contains general chapters and pharmaceutical excipients.

2. 2020 年版《中国药典》发展的特点

**(2) Characteristics of *Chinese Pharmacopoeia* 2020 Edition**

a. **收载品种增加**　历版《中国药典》收载品种统计见表 1-1。

① **The Number of Included Products has been Increased**　Statistical Tables of the number of monographs contained in the original *Chinese Pharmacopoeia* is shown in Table 1-1.

表 1-1 历版《中国药典》收载品种

Table 1-1　The number of monographs contained in the original Chinese Pharmacopoeia

| 版次<br>(Edition) | 收载总数<br>(Total Number) | 一部 (Volume Ⅰ) | | 二部 (Volume Ⅱ) | | 三部 (Volume Ⅲ) | | 四部 (Volume Ⅳ) | |
|---|---|---|---|---|---|---|---|---|---|
| | | 正文<br>(Monographs) | 附录<br>(Appendices) | 正文<br>(Monographs) | 附录<br>(Appendices) | 正文<br>(Monographs) | 附录<br>(Appendices) | 通则<br>(General Chapters) | 辅料<br>(Pharmaceutical Excipients) |
| 1953 | 531 | | | | | | | | |
| 1963 | 1310 | 643 | | 667 | | | | | |
| 1977 | 1925 | 1152 | | 773 | | | | | |
| 1985 | 1489 | 713 | | 776 | | | | | |
| 1990 | 1751 | 784 | | 967 | | | | | |
| 1995 | 2375 | 920 | | 1455 | | | | | |
| 2000 | 2691 | 992 | | 1699 | | | | | |
| 2005 | 3217 | 1146 | 98 | 1970 | 137 | 101 | 134 | | |
| 2010 | 4567 | 2165 | 112 | 2271 | 152 | 131 | 149 | | |
| 2015 | 5608 | 2598 | | 2603 | | 137 | | 317 | 270 |
| 2020 | 5911 | 2711 | | 2712 | | 153 | | 361 | 335 |

b. **强化标准的专属性和特征性** 穿心莲，一测多评法同时测定 4 个主要成分。银杏叶提取物，供试品指纹图谱中应呈现 17 个与对照提取物指纹图谱相对应的色谱峰。冠脉宁胶囊，建立液相色谱条件同时测定丹参中的丹酚酸 B 和葛根中的葛根素的含量测定方法。

② **Strengthen the specificity and character of the standard** Andrographis Herba, one test and multiple evaluation methods simultaneously determine 4 main components. Ginkgo biloba extract, the fingerprint of the test product should show 17 chromatographic peaks corresponding to the fingerprint of the control extract. Guanxinning capsules, established liquid chromatography conditions for simultaneous determination of salvianolic acid B in Salvia miltiorrhizae and puerarin in Pueraria lobata.

c. **药品安全性进一步提高** 完善了"药材和饮片检定通则""药用辅料通则"和"中药有害残留物限量制定指导原则"等通则。现行版《中国药典》一部修订了人参、西洋参等 11 个中药大品种重金属和农药残留标准，对蜂房、土鳖虫等 4 味易受黄曲霉毒素感染药材及饮片增加了"黄曲霉毒素"检查项目和限度标准；对 500 余个植物类药材提出重金属有害物质和农药残留的通用要求。

③ **Drug Safety Assurance has been Further Improved** This edition of pharmacopoeia has improved "General Principle for Inspection of Crude Drugs and Decoction Pieces", and "General Requirements for Pharmaceutical Excipients"; and "Guidelines for Establishment Limit for Harmful Residue of Traditional Chinese Medicine" etc. This edition of pharmacopoeia (Volume Ⅰ) has revised limit standards of heavy metals and pesticide residues in 11 traditional Chinese medicine, such as Ginseng Radix et Rhizoma and Panacis Quinquefolii Radix, and newly included the inspection item and limit of "aflatoxin" for 4 Chinese medicinal materials including Eupolyphaga Steleophaga and Vespae Nidus. The general requirements of heavy metals harmful substances and pesticide residues are mentioned in more than 500 traditional Chinese medicine materials.

d. **药品有效性控制进一步完善** 对检测方法进行了全面增修订。药典一部中，强化标准的专属性和整体性，重点开展了基于中医临床疗效的生物评价和测定方法研究。如在穿心莲标准中引入一测多评；银杏叶提取物的标准中建立了特征图谱；增加地黄苷 D 作为熟地黄的含量测定指标；增加特女贞苷为女贞子含量测定指标，红景天苷为酒女贞子含量测定指标。

④ **Drug Efficacy Control has been Further Improved** Testing methods have been revised and added in a comprehensive manner. Volume Ⅰ has strengthened the specificity and integrity of the standard and focused on the research of biological evaluation and measurement methods based on the clinical efficacy of traditional Chinese medicine. The quantitative analysis of multi-components by single marker has been used in standards of Andrographis Herba. Characteristic spectrums has been established in standards of Ginkgo Leaves Extract, added the assay of rehmannioside D in Rehmanniae Radix Praeparata, added the assay of specnuezhenide in Ligustri Lucidi Fructus, added the assay of rhodopsin in Liquor Ligustri Lucidi Fructus.

3.《中国药典》的结构与内容 2020 年版《中国药典》由一部、二部、三部和四部组成，其中一部、二部和三部均由凡例、正文、索引三部分构成；四部包括制剂通则、通用检测方法、标准物质、试剂试药、指导原则和药用辅料等。

(3) **The Structure and Content of *Chinese Pharmacopoeia*** 2020 edition of *Chinese Pharmacopoeia* comprises Volume Ⅰ, Volume Ⅱ, Volume Ⅲ and Volume Ⅳ, and Volume Ⅰ, Volume Ⅱ, Volume Ⅲ are all composed of General Notices, Monographs and Index, Volume Ⅳ contains general requirements of preparations, general testing methods, standard substances, reagents, guidelines and

pharmaceutical excipients.

**凡例** 凡例是正确使用《中国药典》进行药品质量检定的基本原则，是对《中国药典》正文、通则及与质量检定有关的共性问题的统一规定。凡例与通则对未载入《中国药典》的其他药品标准具同等效力。

**General Notices** General Notices serve as the basic principles for the proper interpretation and application of the *Chinese Pharmacopoeia* in quality control. It applies to any monographs, general chapters and general statements related to quality control of drugs so as to obviate replication in this compendium. The General Notices and the General Chapters in the current edition of *Chinese Pharmacopoeia* are also official for other standards of drugs in addition to those contained in *Chinese Pharmacopoeia*.

**正文** 《中国药典》各品种项下收载的内容统称为标准正文，正文系根据药物自身的理化与生物学特性，按照批准的来源、处方、制法、贮藏、运输等条件所制定的、用以检测药品质量是否达到用药要求并衡量其质量是否稳定均一的技术规定。

**Monographs** Full test under individual article in the *Chinese Pharmacopoeia* is monograph. The monographs are established based on physic chemical characteristics and biological properties of the drugs, formulation and processing, manufacturing techniques as well as conditions for storage and transportation that are authorized officially, and are the technical requirements in order to determine if quality of drugs is for medical use. stable and homogenous.

**索引** 《中国药典》的索引包括中文索引、汉语拼音索引、拉丁名索引、拉丁学名索引。

**Index** The index of *Chinese Pharmacopoeia* includes Chinese index, Chinese phonetic alphabet index, Latin name index and Latin scientific name index.

**通则** 通则主要收载制剂通则、通用检测方法和指导原则。制剂通则系按照药物剂型分类，针对剂型特点所规定的基本技术要求；通用检测方法系各正文品种进行相同检查项目的检测时所应采用的统一的设备、程序、方法及限度等；指导原则系为执行药典、考察药品质量、起草与复核药品标准等所制定的指导性规定。

**General Chapters** General Requirements for Preparations, General Testing methods and guidelines are compiled in General Chapters. General Requirements for Preparations classified on the basis of different preparations are basic technical requirements depending on the characteristic of preparations. General testing methods are established for those same tests specified in monographs concerned using same apparatus, procedures, methods and limits. The Guidelines stated in General Chapters are not considered as official requirements but used as statements in principles applied to the implementation of Pharmacopoeia, monitoring of drug quality and revising or verifying of drug standards.

4.《中国药典》凡例中有关项目与要求

(4) Specifications of General Notices in *Chinese Pharmacopoeia*

【贮藏】项下的规定，系为避免污染和降解而对药品贮藏与保管的基本要求，一般以下列名词术语表示，见表1-2。

*Storage* refers to the basic conditions for storage and preservation of a drug in order to avoid contamination or degradation, which is stated by the following terms, as shown in Table 1-2.

表 1-2 贮藏的名词术语

| 名词术语 | 释义 |
|---|---|
| 遮光 | 系指用不透光的容器包装，例如棕色容器或黑纸包裹的无色透明、半透明容器 |
| 避光 | 系指避免日光直射 |
| 密闭 | 系指将容器密闭，以防止尘土及异物进入 |
| 密封 | 系指将容器密封，以防止风化、吸潮、挥发或异物进入 |
| 熔封或严封 | 系指将容器熔封或用适宜的材料严封，以防止空气与水分的侵入并防止污染 |
| 阴凉处 | 系指不超过 20℃ |
| 凉暗处 | 系指避光并不超过 20℃ |
| 冷处 | 系指 2~10℃ |
| 常温 | 系指 10~30℃ |

Table 1-2 The terms of storage

| Terms | Indicating |
|---|---|
| *Protected from light* | a drug should be kept in light resistant container such as amber colored container, or a colourless transparent or semitransparent container wrapped with black paper; |
| *Protected from sunlight* | avoiding the direct illumination by sunlight; |
| *Well closed* | container is able to protect the contents from extraneous matters or lose of contents on normal handling condition; |
| *Tightly closed* | container should be able to protect the contents from efflorescence, deliquescence, volatilization or interference of extraneous matters; |
| *Hermetically sealed or Tightly sealed* | container is sealed on fusion or sealed tightly with suitable material to protect against contamination and from permeability of air and moisture; |
| *Cool place* | the storage temperature is not exceeding 20℃; |
| *Cool and dark place* | container is kept in the dark place, protected from light and the ambient temperature is not exceeding 20℃; |
| Cold place | container is kept at ambient temperature of 2-10℃; |
| *Normal temperature* | container is kept at ambient temperature of 10-30℃. |

除另有规定外，【贮藏】项未规定贮存温度的一般系指常温。

Unless specified otherwise, the storage temperature not specified in item "storage" generally refers to the normal temperature.

**计量** 温度以摄氏度（℃）表示。水浴温度除另有规定外，均指 98~100℃；热水系指 70~80℃；微温或温水系指 40~50℃；室温（常温）系指 10~30℃；冷水系指 2~10℃；冰浴系指约 0℃；放冷系指放冷至室温。

**Units of Measurement** The temperature are expressed in terms of centigrade in this edition of Pharmacopoeia. Unless specified otherwise, the temperature of a *Water bath* is 98-100℃; *Hot water* refers to that at a temperature of 70-80℃; *Slightly warm or warm water* refers to that at a temperature of 40-50℃; *Room temperature* refers to that at a temperature of 10-30℃; Cold water refers to that at a temperature of 2-10℃; *Ice bath* refers to the bath temperature kept at about 0℃; *Allow to cool* refers to that the object is cooled to room temperature.

符号"%"表示百分比，系指重量的比例；但溶液的百分比，除另有规定外，系指溶液100ml中含有溶质若干克；乙醇的百分比，系指在20℃时容量的比例。

The symbol used for the expression of percentage is %, usually by weight, but the percentage of solutions, unless specified otherwise, refers to the number of grams of solute in 100ml of the solution. The percentage of ethanol refers to percentage by volume at 20℃.

液体的滴，系指在20℃时，以1.0ml水为20滴进行换算。

The drop of a liquid refers to that 1.0ml of water is equivalent to 20 drops at the temperature of 20℃.

溶液后标示的"（1→10）"，系指固体溶质1.0g或液体溶质1.0ml加溶剂使成10ml的溶液；未指明用何种溶剂时，均系指水溶液；两种或两种以上液体的混合物，名称间用半字线"-"隔开，其后括号内所示的"："符号，系指各液体混合时的体积（重量）比例。

The expression "(1→10)" stated under the solution refers to a solution of 10ml produced by adding a sufficient quantity of solvent to dissolve 1.0g or 1.0ml of a solute. It is understood to be aqueous solution, if the solvent is not specified. In case of two or more solvents are used as a mixture, a hyphen is inserted between different solvents indicated by names and the parenthesis followed expresses the proportion of each solvent by volume in the mixture.

乙醇未指明浓度时，均系指95%（ml/ml）的乙醇。

Ethanol refers to that of 95% (ml/ml) in strength, unless specified otherwise.

粉末分等如下：

Powders are graded as follows:

最粗粉　指能全部通过一号筛，但混有能通过三号筛不超过20%的粉末；

*Very coarse*　All particles pass through No.1 sieve, not more than 20% pass through No. 3 sieve;

粗粉　指能全部通过二号筛，但混有能通过四号筛不超过40%的粉末；

*Coarse*　All particles pass through No. 2 sieve, not more than 40% pass through No. 4 sieve;

中粉　指能全部通过四号筛，但混有能通过五号筛不超过60%的粉末；

*Medium*　All particles pass through No. 4 sieve, not more than 60% pass through No.5 sieve;

细粉　指能全部通过五号筛，并含能通过六号筛不少于95%的粉末；

*Fine*　All particles pass through No. 5 sieve, not less than 95% pass through No. 6 sieve;

最细粉　指能全部通过六号筛，并含能通过七号筛不少于95%的粉末；

*Very fine*　All particles pass through No. 6 sieve, not less than 95% pass through No. 7 sieve;

极细粉　指能全部通过八号筛，并含能通过九号筛不少于95%的粉末。

*Ultra fine*　All particles pass through No. 8 sieve, not less than 95% pass through No. 9 sieve.

**精确度**　供试品与试药等"称重"或"量取"的量，均以阿拉伯数码表示，其精确度可根据数值的有效数位来确定，如称取"0.1g"系指称取重量可为0.06~0.14g；称取"2g"系指称取重量可为1.5~2.5g；称取"2.0g"系指称取重量可为1.95~2.05g；称取"2.00g"，系指称取重量可为1.995~2.005g。

**Precision and Accuracy**　The quantity obtained by weighing or measuring the substance being examined and reagent being used is expressed in Arabic figures. The required precision is expressed by the significant numerical place. For example, the measurement of "0.1g" by weight refers to that 0.06-0.14g of the substance, may be weighed; for "2g", 1.5-2.5g of the substance may be weighed; for "2.0g", it refers to that 1.95- 2.05g of the substance may be weighed; for "2.00g", it refers to that 1.995-2.005g of the substance may be weighed.

"精密称定"系指称取重量应准确至所取重量的千分之一;"称定"系指称取重量应准确至所取重量的百分之一;"精密量取"系指量取体积的准确度应符合国家标准中对该体积移液管的精密度要求;"量取"系指可用量筒或按照量取体积的有效数位选用量具。取用量为"约"若干时,系指取用量不得超过规定量的 ±10% 。

*Weigh accurately* indicates that the precision of measurement should be made to an accuracy of 0.1%; *Weigh* indicates that an accuracy being made to 1%. *Measure accurately* indicates the accuracy of the volume being measured complies with the national standard of pipet being used for the measurement of required volume; *Measure* indicates that the measuring cylinder or other measuring apparatus being used complies with requirements for the measurement of volume to the significant numerical place. The word *about* states that the measuring quantity should not exceed ± 10% of the specified quantity.

恒重,除另有规定外,系指供试品连续两次干燥或炽灼后称重的差异在 0.3mg 以下的重量;干燥至恒重的第二次及以后各次称重均应在规定条件下继续干燥 1 小时后进行;炽灼至恒重的第二次称重应在继续炽灼 30 分钟后进行。

*Constant weight*, unless specified otherwise, refers to that the drying or ignition of a substance or material in two consecutive weighing do not differ by more than 0.3mg. The second and subsequent weighing are made after an additional hour of drying each time under the similar condition. The second weighing of the substance or material made to constant weight by ignition is made after 30 minutes under similar condition.

### （二）局（部）版标准

### 2. Standards of Traditional Chinese Medicine Approved by NMPA and the National Health Commission of the People's Republic of China

《部颁标准》由国家药典委员会编纂出版,国家卫健委颁布执行。1986 年以来,原卫生部先后颁布了进口药材标准、卫生部颁药品标准（中药材第一册）,中药成方制剂部颁标准（1~20 册）、化学药品部颁标准（1~6 册）。1998 年国家药品监督管理局成立,新药标准改为由国家药品监督管理局负责,2003 年更名为国家食品药品监督管理局,由国家食品药品监督管理局批准的新药标准称国家食品药品监督管理局标准（简称《局颁标准》）,先后颁布局颁国家中成药标准汇编、中药标准（1~14 册）、化学药品标准（1~16 册）、局颁新药转正标准（1~76 册）。2007 年 10 月 1 日起,我国批准的新药,为"药品注册标准"。

The drug standards of Ministry of Health of the People's Republic of China (referred to as ministerial standards), which were compiled by the Chinese Pharmacopoeia Committee and approved by the National Health Commission of the People's Republic of China. Since 1986, Ministry of Health of the People's Republic of China has successively promulgated the standards for imported medicinal materials, the Pharmaceutical Standards of Ministry of Health of the People's Republic of China (Volume Ⅰ), the standards of Chinese medicine prescription issued by Ministry of Health of the People's Republic of China (1-20 volumes), and the standards of Chemical medicine issued by Ministry of Health of the People's Republic of China (1-6 volumes). National Medical Products Administration was established in 1998, and the new drug standard was approved by the National Medical Products Administration. In 2003, the National Medical Products Administration was renamed the China Food and Drug Administration. The new drug standards approved by the China Food and Drug Administration is called the China Food and Drug Administration Standards (abbreviated as "Standards approved CFDA"). It has successively promulgated the compilation of Chinese patent medicine standards, traditional Chinese medicine standards (1-14 volumes), chemical medicine standards (1-16 volumes), and new drug standards issued by CFDA (1-76 volumes). since

October 1, 2007, the new drugs approved by our country are the Drug Registration Standard.

### 三、地方药品标准
### 1.2.3　Local Drug Standards

地方药品标准由地方（省、自治区、直辖市）药品监督管理部门批准发布，在某一地区范围内的标准。主要包括药材标准、饮片标准、饮片炮制规范及批准给特定医院的院内制剂。是国家药品标准体系的重要补充，但必须按照《中国药典》规定的内容制定并及时修订。

Local standards are approved, promulgated and unified within a certain area by the local drug and food administration (provinces, autonomous regions and municipalities directly under the Central Government). It mainly includes the standard of medicinal materials, the standard of prepared slices, the standard of processing prepared slices and the hospital preparations approved to specific hospitals. It is an important supplement to the national drug standard system, but it must be formulated and revised in time in accordance with the provisions of the *Chinese Pharmacopoeia*.

### 四、其他药品标准
### 1.2.4　Other Drug Standards

企业标准是国家标准、行业标准的补充标准，在企业内部适用。已有国家标准的，国家鼓励企业制订严于国家标准或行业标准的企标，鼓励采用国际标准或国外先进标准。

Enterprise standard is the supplementary standard of national standard and industry standard, which is applicable within the enterprise. If there are already national standards, the state encourages enterprises to formulate enterprise standards that are stricter than national standards or industry standards, and encourages the adoption of international standards or advanced foreign standards.

行业标准包括国家中医药管理局组织制定的标准及行业协会、商会、产业技术联盟按照市场需要制定发布的社会团体标准。

The industry standards include the standards formulated by the National Administration of Traditional Chinese Medicine and the standards of social groups formulated and issued by industry associations, chambers of commerce and industrial technology alliances in accordance with the needs of the market.

### 五、主要国外药典简介
### 1.2.5　Brief Introduction of Major Foreign Pharmacopoeia

目前全世界已有多个国家和地区编制出版药典，对我国药品研发、生产和质量控制具有参考价值的主要有《美国药典》《英国药典》《欧洲药典》《日本药局方》和《国际药典》。

At present, many countries and regions in the world have compiled and published Pharmacopoeia. The main reference values for drug research and development, production and quality control in China are *United States Pharmacopoeia, British Pharmacopoeia, European Pharmacopoeia, Japanese Pharmacopoeia* and *International Pharmacopoeia*.

（一）《美国药典》

### 1. The United States Pharmacopoeia
美国药典是美国政府对药品质量标准和检定方法作出的技术规定，也是药品生产、使用、管

理、检验的法律依据，包括《美国药典》（USP）和国家处方集（NF），合并出版称《美国药典 –
国家处方集》（USP-NF），USP-NF 是唯一由美国食品药品管理局（FDA）强制执行的法定标准。
从 2002 年开始每年一版。目前最新版为 USP43-NF38，2019 年 11 月 1 日出版，2020 年 5 月 1 日
起正式生效。有印刷版、U 盘版和互联网在线版。《美国药典》正文药品名录分别按法定药名字
母顺序排列，各药品条目大都列有药名、结构式、分子式、CAS 登记号、成分和含量说明、包装
和贮藏规格、鉴定方法、干燥失重、炽灼残渣、检测方法等常规项目。每版 USP 均有食品补充
剂，收载一定数量的传统植物药。2013 年 5 月 USP 草药卷（HMC）正式发布。主要提供草药制
剂中各单味药及其相关提取物或制剂的标准。

The *United States Pharmacopoeia* (USP) is a technical regulation made by the United States
government on drug quality standards and testing methods, and it is also the legal basis for drug
production, use, management and inspection, includes USP and National Formulary (NF), USP and NF
jointly published, called "United States Pharmacopoeia-National Formulary" (USP-NF). USP-NF is the
only statutory standard enforced by the US Food and Drug Administration (FDA). Since 2002, it was
published once a year. At present, the latest edition of USP43-NF38, is published on November 1, 2019,
and will come into effect on May 1, 2020. There are printed version of U disk and Internet online version.
The list of drugs in monographs of the *United States Pharmacopoeia* is arranged in alphabetical order
according to the legal drug names, and most of the drug entries include drug names, structural formulas,
molecular formulas, CAS registration numbers, descriptions of ingredients and contents, packaging and
storage specifications, identification methods, loss on drying, residue on ignition, detection methods
and other conventional items. Each edition of USP contains food supplements, which contain a certain
number of traditional plant medicines. USP Herbal Medicine Volume was officially released in May 2013.
It mainly provides the standard of each single medicine and its related extract or preparation in USP
Herbal Medicines Compendium.

（二）《英国药典》

## 2. British Pharmacopoeia

《英国药典》（BP）是英国药品委员会的正式出版物，是英国制药标准的重要来源。自 1816
年《伦敦药典》开始，后出版《爱丁堡药典》和《爱尔兰药典》，1864 年合并为 BP。BP 和《欧
洲药典》收载品种相同者，药品标准内容完全一致，BP 在品种名称下标明其在《欧洲药典》中
的收载位置。最新的版本为 2020 版（BP2020）。2019 年 8 月出版，2020 年 1 月生效，共 6 卷。
BP 收载的草药，首先规定其来源（种名、药用部位及科名）及质量要求（主要成分的含量限
度），有的品种还指明产地与采收；其质量控制项目包括定义（来源与有效成分含量）、特性（气
味及性状与显微特征）、鉴别（性状、粉末显微特征、化学反应与 TLC）、检查（外来物、干燥失
重、总灰分与酸不溶性灰分）、含量测定、贮藏、作用与用途、制剂等。BP 不仅在英国使用，加
拿大、澳大利亚及印度等英联邦国家也采用。

The *British Pharmacopoeia* (BP) is an official publication of the British Pharmacopoeia Commission
and an important source of British pharmaceutical standards. From the beginning of the *London
Pharmacopoeia* in 1816, the *Edinburgh Pharmacopoeia* and the *Irish Pharmacopoeia* were published
and merged into BP in 1864. If the variety is the same in BP and the *European Pharmacopoeia*, the
content of the drug standard is complete. BP indicates its position in the *European Pharmacopoeia* under
the variety name. The latest version is version 2020 (BP 2020). Published in August 2019 and effective
in January 2020, a total of 6 volumes. The herbs contained in BP first specify their source (species name,
medicinal part and family name) and quality requirements (content of main components, quantity limit),

and some varieties also specify the origin and harvest. Its quality control items include definition (including source and active ingredient content), characteristics (including odor, taste, description and microscopic characteristics), identification (including description, powder microscopic characteristics, chemical reactions and TLC), inspection (including foreign substances, loss on drying, total ash and acid-insoluble ash), content determination, storage, function and use, preparations, etc. BP is used not only in the UK, but also in Commonwealth of Nations such as Canada, Australia, New Zealand, Sri Lanka and India.

### （三）《欧洲药典》
### 3. European Pharmacopoeia

《欧洲药典》（EP）由欧洲药品质量管理局组织出版，是全球最具影响力的药典之一，有英文和法文两种法定文本。1977 年出版第一版《欧洲药典》。从 1980 年到 1996 年期间，每年将增修订的项目与新增品种出一本活页本，汇集为第二版《欧洲药典》各分册，未经修订的仍按照第一版执行。1997 年出版第三版《欧洲药典》合订本，并在随后的每一年出版一部增补本。2001 年 7 月，第四版《欧洲药典》出版，并于 2002 年 1 月生效。自 2004 年开始，EP 的出版周期为每三年修订一次。最新的版本为 2020 版（EP10）。2019 年 7 月出版，2020 年 1 月生效。EP 收载的草药及其制剂质量标准一般包括定义、鉴别、检查项和含量测定 4 个方面，其中检查项中根据项目不同分别选择外来杂质、干燥失重、总灰分、酸不溶性灰分等内容。

The *European Pharmacopoeia* (EP), published by the European Directorate for the Quality of Medicines (EDQM), is one of the most influential Pharmacopoeia in the world, with two official texts in English and French. Ph. Eur. The first edition of the *European Pharmacopoeia* was published in 1977. From 1980 to 1996, a loose-leaf edition of the revised items and new varieties was compiled into the second edition of the *European Pharmacopoeia,* and the unrevised ones were still implemented in accordance with the first edition. The third edition of the *European Pharmacopoeia* was published in 1997 and a supplement was published every year. In July 2001, the fourth edition of the *European Pharmacopoeia* was published and entered into force in January 2002. Since 2004, the publication cycle of EP has been revised every three years. The latest version is version 2020 (EP10). Published in July 2019 and became effective in January 2020. The quality standards of herbs and their preparations contained in EP generally include definition, identification, inspection items and content determination, in which foreign impurities, loss on drying, total ash and acid insoluble ash are selected according to different items.

### （四）《日本药局方》
### 4. Japanese Pharmacopoeia

日本药局方由日本药局方编集委员会编撰，厚生省颁布执行。第一版于 1886 年 6 月出版，1887 年 7 月实施。现在每 5 年修订出版一次，有日文和英文两种文本。最新版是第 18 版于 2021 年 4 月发行并执行。主要结构内容包括：凡例，原料通则，制剂通则，通用试验方法、步骤和仪器，正文、索引（日文索引、拉丁文索引）等。分两部出版，第一部收载化学原料药及其基础制剂，第二部主要收载生药（包括药材、粉末生药、复方散剂、提取物、酊剂、糖浆、精油、油脂），家庭药制剂和制剂原料。收载的生药质量标准一般包括品名（英义名、拉丁名和日文名）、来源、成分含量限度、性状、鉴别、纯度（外来有机物、重金属、砷盐及有害元素、农药残留等）、干燥失重、炽灼残渣、总灰分、酸不溶性灰分、含量测定、包装、贮藏等。

The *Japanese Pharmacopoeia* (JP) is compiled by Committee on JP and promulgated by Ministry of Health, Labour and Welfare. The first edition of JP was published in June 1886 and implemented in July 1887. Now it is revised and published every five years, and there are two versions in Japanese and

English. The latest version is the 18th edition of JP, which was released and implemented in April 2021. The main structure of JP includes: General Notices, General Requirements of raw materials, General Requirements of Preparations, General Testing methods, procedures and instruments, text, index (Japanese index, Latin index) and so on. It is published in two parts, the first part contains chemical raw materials and their basic preparations, and the second part mainly contains crude drugs (including medicinal materials, powder crude drugs, compound powders, extracts, tinctures, syrup, essential oil, oil fat), family medicine preparations and preparation raw materials. The quality standards of crude drugs contained in JP generally include product name (English name, Latin name and Japanese name), source, component content limit, discription, identification, purity (exotic organic matter, heavy metal, arsenic and harmful elements, pesticide residues, etc.), loss on drying, residue on ignition, total ash, acid insoluble ash, content determination, packaging, storage, etc.

（五）《国际药典》

### 5. International Pharmacopoeia

《国际药典》（Ph. Int.）由联合国世界卫生组织（WHO）与成员国药品监督管理部门协调，并由 WHO 药典专家委员会编撰出版，WHO 成员国免费使用。旨在实现原辅料和制剂的质量标准的全球协调统一，对药品进行全面质量控制和保障。Ph. Int. 第一版于 1951 年和 1955 年分两卷用英、法、西班牙文出版；第二版于 1967 年用英、法、俄、西班牙文出版。自 1979 年第三版 Ph. Int. 收载的药品均选自 WHO 的《基本药物目录》，近年来则关注于公众健康问题的一线药物及 WHO 疾病项目推荐的基本药物，如疟疾、结核、艾滋病治疗药物及儿科药物。收载药物的剂型以口服制剂为主，目前主要有片剂、口服液体制剂及胶囊剂。未来《国际药典》收载品种将优先考虑妇女儿童用药、三抗类药物（抗疟疾、抗结核、抗病毒）及热带病用药。现行版 Ph. Int. 为第五版，于 2015 年出版，同步发行网络版和光盘版。《国际药典》由凡例、正文品种、分析方法、对照红外光谱集、试剂、试液、滴定液及补充信息组成。正文品种分原料药、辅料、制剂和放射药品。

The *International Pharmacopoeia* (Ph. Int) is coordinated by the World Health Organization and the department of drug supervision and administration of the member states, and is compiled and published by  WHO Pharmacopoeia Committee and used by WHO member states free of charge. The aim is to achieve the global harmonization of the quality standards of excipients and preparations, and to carry out overall quality control and assurance of drugs. Ph. Int. The first edition was published in English, French and Spanish in two volumes in 1951 and 1955, and the second edition was published in English, French, Russian and Spanish in 1967. The medicines collected from the third edition of Ph. Int in 1979 are selected from the WHO Essential Medicines List, first-line drugs focusing on public health issues and essential drugs recommended by the WHO disease program in recent years, such as malaria, tuberculosis, AIDS treatments and paediatrics. The main dosage forms of loaded drugs are oral preparations, which mainly include tablets, oral liquid preparations and capsules at present. In the future, the varieties contained in the *International Pharmacopoeia* will give priority to drugs for women and children, triad drugs (anti-malaria, anti-tuberculosis, anti-virus) and tropical diseases. Current Ph. Int. It is the fifth edition, published in 2015, and released online and CD-ROM simultaneously. The *International Pharmacopoeia* consists of general notices, monographs, analytical methods, control infrared spectra, reagents, testing solutions, titration solutions and supplementary information. Monographs is divided into raw materials, excipients, preparations and radiopharmaceuticals.

# 岗 位 对 接
# Post Docking

本章为中药学、中药制药和中药资源专业学生必须掌握的内容，为成为合格的中药学服务人员奠定坚实的基础。

This task must be mastered by students majoring in traditional Chinese medicine, traditional Chinese medicine pharmacy and traditional Chinese medicine resources, and lay a solid foundation for becoming qualified Chinese medicine service personnel.

本章内容对应岗位包括中药师、中药调剂员、销售代表、QC、QA、产品经理、执业中药师、质量管理员等相关工种。

The corresponding positions of this task include traditional Chinese medicine pharmacist, traditional Chinese medicine dispenser, sales representative, QC, QA, product manager, licensed Chinese medicine pharmacist, quality manager and so on.

上述从事中药学服务及药品质量监督管理相关所有岗位的从业人员均需要掌握中药分析的基本程序、《中国药典》的凡例等，能熟记中药分析学的意义、特点等，学会应用国家药品标准开展中药学服务工作。

The above-mentioned practitioners in all positions related to traditional Chinese medicine service and drug quality supervision and management need to master the characteristics of traditional Chinese medicine analysis, the contents of national drug standards, and be able to memorize the significance and basic procedures of traditional Chinese medicine analysis, and learn to apply national drug standards to carry out traditional Chinese medicine services.

# 重 点 小 结
# Summary of Key Points

中药分析是以中医药理论为指导，应用各种分析技术与方法（物理、化学、生物学等），研究中药材（饮片）、植物油脂和提取物、成方制剂和单味制剂的质量控制与评价方法，确保临床用药的安全、有效，及中药质量可控。中药因其化学成分复杂、多样，需要在中医药理论的指导下选择分析指标；质量影响因素多，有效成分不唯一，杂质来源途径广，使得中药分析不同于化学药分析。

The analysis of traditional Chinese medicine is a subject which studies the quality control and evaluation methods of traditional Chinese medicine under the guidance of the theory of traditional Chinese medicine by the application of various analytical techniques and methods. The analysis of traditional Chinese medicine ensures the safety and effectiveness of clinical drug use, and the quality of traditional Chinese medicine can be controlled. The analysis of traditional Chinese medicine has distinct characteristics different from that of chemical medicine, because traditional Chinese medicine contains complex components, detection indicators are selected under the guidance of the theory of traditional Chinese medicine, non-uniqueness of active ingredients the multi-path of the sources of impurities, and diversity of factors affecting quality.

自新中国成立，已出版发行 11 个版次的《中国药典》，自 1985 年版开始每 5 年修订改版一次。《中国药典》自 2015 年版开始分为四部，一部收载中药；二部收载化学药品；三部收载生物制品；四部收载通则和药用辅料等。凡例与通则对未载入《中国药典》但经国务院药品监督管理部门颁布的其他中药标准具同等效力。

After the founding of the people＇s Republic of China in 1949, the Chinese Pharmacopoeia has been published in 11 editions. Since the 1985 edition, it is revised and published every 5 years. Since the Chinese Pharmacopoeia 2015 edition has comprised four volumes.

The Volume Ⅰ contains traditional Chinese medicines, the Volume Ⅱ contains chemical drugs, the Volume Ⅲ contains biologics, and the Volume Ⅳ contains general chapters and pharmaceutical excipients.

题库

# 目 标 检 测

## 一、选择题

### （一）单项选择题

1. 中药分析的任务是
   A. 对中药的原料进行质量分析
   B. 对中药的提取物进行质量分析
   C. 对中药制剂进行质量分析
   D. 对中药的各个环节进行质量分析

2. 中药分析的意义是
   A. 保证中药有效成分的含量
   B. 保证中药质量稳定、疗效可靠和使用安全
   C. 保证中药有毒有害成分合格
   D. 保证中药质量符合质量标准规定

3. 中药制剂分析的特点是
   A. 制剂工艺的复杂性
   B. 化学成分的多样性和复杂性
   C. 中药材炮制的重要性
   D. 多由大复方组成

4. 中医药理论在中药分析中的作用是
   A. 指导合理用药
   B. 指导合理撰写说明书
   C. 指导制定合理的质量分析方案
   D. 指导检测贵重药材

5. 中药分析的主要对象是
   A. 中药制剂中的有效成分
   B. 有毒有害元素
   C. 中药制剂中的微量成分
   D. 中药制剂中的无机成分

6. 中药分析与化学药分析的主要区别是
   A. 中药被测成分含量较高
   B. 影响中药含量测定的因素较少
   C. 中药被测成分含量较低、干扰较多
   D. 中药成分简单

7. 中药质量标准应全面保证
   A. 中药质量稳定和疗效可靠
   B. 中药质量稳定和使用安全
   C. 中药质量稳定、疗效可靠和使用安全
   D. 中药疗效可靠和使用安全

8. 中药的质量分析是指
   A. 对中药的定性鉴别
   B. 对中药的鉴别、检查和含量测定等方面的评价
   C. 对中药的检查

医药大学堂
www.YIYAODXT.com

D. 对中药的含量测定

9.《中国药典》规定，室温（常温）系指

    A. 0~10℃         B. 10~20℃         C. 10~30℃         D. 20~30℃

10.《中国药典》规定，热水温度是指

    A. 70~80℃         B. 60~80℃         C. 65~85℃         D. 50-60℃

11.《中国药典》规定，温水温度是指

    A. 20~40℃         B. 30~50℃         C. 40~50℃         D. 50~60℃

12.《中国药典》凡例中关于称重的精确度要求正确的是

    A. 称取 2g，指称取量可为 1.8~2.2g

    B. 称取 2.0g，指称取量可为 1.95~2.05g

    C. 称取 2.00g，指称取量可为 1.99~2.01g

    D. 称取 0.1g，指称取量可为 0.09~0.11g

13. 下列说法错误的是

    A. 精密称定指称取重量应准确至所取重量的千分之一

    B. 称取指称取重量应准确至所取重量的百分之一

    C. 精密量取系指量取体积的准确度应符合国家标准对体积移液管的精度要求

    D. 取用量为"约"系指取用量不得超过规定量的 ±5%

（二）多项选择题

1. 中药分析的任务包括

    A. 对中药材进行质量分析         B. 对中药制剂进行质量分析

    C. 对中药提取物进行质量分析         D. 对有毒有害成分进行质量控制

    E. 中药成分的体内分析

2. 中药分析的特点有

    A. 以中医药理论为指导         B. 化学成分的多样性与复杂性

    C. 中药质量的差异性和不稳定性         D. 中药杂质来源的多样性

    E. 中药有效成分的非单一性

3. 中药分析的发展趋势有

    A. 建立能控制中药有效性的分析体系         B. 分析方法向微量化、快速化发展

    C. 有毒有害成分的检测         D. 个体化质量标准研究

    E. 中药物质基础及标准物质研究

4. 中药制剂中化学成分的复杂性包括

    A. 含有多种类型的有机和无机化合物         B. 含有多种类型的同系物

    C. 含有结构性质相似的同系物         D. 在制剂工艺过程中产生新的物质

    E. 药用辅料的多样性

5. 影响中药质量的因素有

    A. 原料药材的品种、规格不同         B. 原料药材的产地不同

    C. 原料药材的采收季节不同         D. 原料药材的产地加工方法不同

    E. 饮片的炮制方法不同

6. 中药分析研究的内容有

    A. 中药质量评价研究         B. 中药分析新技术、新方法的研究

    C. 中药质量控制体系研究         D. 体内中药分析研究

    E. 中药标准物质研究

7. 我国药品质量标准体系包括
   A. 国家标准　　　　　　　B. 企业标准　　　　　　　C. 地方标准
   D. 临床研究用药品质量标准　E. 推荐性标准
8. 药品的质量特性包括
   A. 真实性　　　　　　　　B. 有效性　　　　　　　　C. 安全性
   D. 稳定性　　　　　　　　E. 均一性
9. 我国现行国家药品标准包括
   A.《中国药典》　　　　　　B.《英国药典》　　　　　　C. 局颁标准
   D. 药品注册标准　　　　　E. 某省药材标准品
10. 下列属于质量标准正文中内容的有
   A. 名称　　　　　　　　　B. 检查　　　　　　　　　C. 性状
   D. 鉴别　　　　　　　　　E. 含量测定

**二、思考题**

中药分析与化学药物分析有何异同？

# 第二章　供试品溶液的制备
# Chapter 2　Preparation of Test Solution

 **学习目标 | Learning Goal**

知识要求：

1．**掌握**　中药分析中供试样品粉碎、提取、纯化与富集方法。

2．**熟悉**　中药分析中样品的消解方法。

3．**了解**　中药分析中样品的衍生化方法。

能力要求：

学会应用粉碎、提取、纯化与富集的方法制备中药分析中供试品溶液。

**Knowledge Requirement**

**1. Master**　Methods of crushing, extraction, purification and enrichment of samples for testing in the analysis of traditional Chinese medicine.

**2. Familiar**　The digestion methods of samples in the analysis of traditional Chinese medicine.

**3. Understand**　The derivatization methods of samples in the analysis of traditional Chinese medicine.

**Ability Requirement**

Learn to apply the methods of crushing, extraction, purification and enrichment of test samples to solve the preparation of test solution in traditional Chinese medicine analysis.

中药成分复杂，分析前大都需要对其进行提取、净化、富集等不同程度的处理，以便制成便于分析的试样。供试品制备的总体原则是最大限度地保留待测组分，并尽可能多的除去干扰性成分。

The components of traditional Chinese medicine are complex, and most of them need to be extracted, purified, enriched and so on before analysis, in order to make the sample for analysis. The general principle for the preparation of test samples is to retain the components to be tested as much as possible and to remove as many interfering components as possible.

# 第一节　样品的粉碎与提取
## 2.1　Crushing and Extraction of Samples

PPT

### 一、样品的粉碎
### 2.1.1　Crushing of Sample

中药材、饮片及中药制剂等固体样品，分析之前大多需要粉碎。粉碎的目的：①保证分析样品的均匀性，使其具有代表性；②使样品中的被测组分更快、更充分地被提取出来。常用的粉碎设备：粉碎机、铜冲、研钵、各种食品料理机、匀浆仪等。

Most of the solid samples such as traditional Chinese medicine, prepared slices and traditional Chinese medicine preparations need to be crushed before analysis. The purpose of crushing: ① to ensure the uniformity of the analytical sample and make it representative; ② to extract the tested components from the sample more quickly and fully. Commonly used crushing equipment: dry Chinese medicinal material multi-function grinder, copper tamping pot, mortar and pestle, all kinds of food processor, homogenizer and so on.

样品粉碎的注意事项：①样品粉碎时，粒度大小合适；②粉碎过程中应尽量避免设备或其他因素对样品的污染；③粉碎过程中防止粉尘飞散或挥发性待测成分的损失；④过筛时，通不过筛孔的样品要反复粉碎或研磨，使其全部通过筛网，以确保样品的均匀性和代表性。

Points for attention in sample crushing: ① when the sample is crushed, the sample powder particle size is appropriate; ② the pollution of the sample caused by equipment or other unclean factors should be avoided as far as possible; ③ the dust or the loss of volatile components to be tested should be prevented loss during the grinding process; ④ when the sample is screened, the sample that cannot pass through the sieve hole should be crushed or ground repeatedly to make it all pass through the sieve mesh to ensure the uniformity and representativeness of the sample.

### 二、样品的提取
### 2.1.2　Sample Extraction

中药多为固体，大都不能直接进行分析，需要进行提取等处理。固体中药样品的提取方法众多，经典的提取方法按照原理不同可分为溶剂提取法、水蒸气蒸馏法、升华法等。

Most of the traditional Chinese medicines are solid, which can't be analyzed directly and need to be extracted and treated. There are many methods to extract solid traditional Chinese medicine. According to different principles, the classical extraction methods can be divided into solvent extraction, steam distillation, sublimation and so on.

#### （一）溶剂提取法
#### 1. Solvent Extraction Method

1. **溶剂的选择**　遵循"相似相溶"的原则。同时提取溶剂应具备以下三点要求：①对被测成分的溶解度大，对杂质溶解度小；②不能与被测成分或者共存成分发生化学反应；③溶剂价格低廉，使用安全、环保。常用的提取溶剂有：水、甲醇、乙醇、丙酮、三氯甲烷、乙酸乙酯、石油醚、乙醚等。

**(1) Selection of Solvents** On the basis of the theory of similarity and intermiscibility. At the same time, the extraction solvent should have the following three requirements: ① the solubility of the tested components is large, but the solubility of impurities is small; ② the chemical reaction can't occur with the tested components or coexisting components; ③ the solvent is cheap, safe and environmentally friendly. The commonly used extraction solvents are water, methanol, ethanol, acetone, chloroform, ethyl acetate, petroleum ether, ethyl ether and so on.

2. **常用的提取方法** 常用的溶剂提取方法有浸渍法、回流提取法、连续回流提取法和超声提取法等。

**(2) Common Extraction Methods** The commonly used solvent extraction methods of traditional Chinese medicine include impregnation method, reflux extraction method, continuous reflux extraction method and ultrasound extraction method and so on.

（1）浸渍法 根据浸渍时的温度分为冷浸（10~30℃）、温浸（30~60℃）和热浸（70~80℃）。浸泡期间应注意经常振摇。浸渍法的优点：操作简单，适于热不稳定的样品，且提取杂质少。缺点：费时、费溶剂、提取不充分，较少用于含量测定。如川芎茶调散中川芎的鉴别，其供试品溶液的制备方法如下：取本品 3g，置锥形瓶中，加石油醚（60~90℃）20ml，密塞，时时振摇，浸渍 4 小时，滤过，滤液浓缩至 1ml，即得。

① *Impregnation Method* According to the temperature of impregnation, it can be divided into cold dipping (10-30℃), warm dipping (30-60℃) and hot dipping (70-80℃). During soaking, you should pay attention to shaking frequently. The advantages of the impregnation method are as follows: easy to operate, suitable for thermally unstable samples, and less impurities are extracted. Disadvantages: time-consuming, solvent-consuming, inadequate extraction, less used for content determination. For example, for the identification of Chuanxiong Rhizoma in Chuanxiong Chatiao Powder, the preparation method of the test solution is as follows: take 3g of this product to a conical flask with stopper, add 20ml petroleum ether (60-90℃), stopper tightly and shake constantly, impregnate for 4 hours, filter, the filtrate is concentrated to 1ml, as the test solution.

（2）回流提取法 回流提取法是将样品粉末置烧瓶中，加一定量的有机溶剂，水浴加热使其微沸，进行提取。该法适用于固体样品的提取。在进行定量分析时，可多次更换溶剂提取，直至待测组分提取完全，合并提取液供分析用。对热不稳定或有挥发性组分不宜采用此法。如乙肝养阴活血颗粒中齐墩果酸的鉴别，其供试品溶液的制备方法如下：取本品 30g 或 15g（无蔗糖），研细，加三氯甲烷 40ml，置水浴上加热回流 1 小时，滤过，滤液蒸干，残渣加甲醇 1ml 使溶解，即得。

② *Reflux Extraction Method* The reflux extraction method is to put the sample powder in a flask, add a certain organic solvent, and heat it in a water bath to make it slightly boiled, and then extract it. This method is suitable for the extraction of solid samples. In the quantitative analysis, the solvent extraction can be changed many times until the components to be tested are extracted completely, and the extract is combined for analysis. This method is not suitable for thermally instable or volatile components. For example, for the identification of oleanolic acid in Yigan Yangyin Huoxue Granules, the preparation method of the test solution is as follows: to 30g or 15g (without sucrose) powder add 40ml chloroform, reflux extraction in a water bath for an hour, filter, steam dry the filtrate, and dissolve the residue with 1ml methanol, as the test solution.

（3）连续回流提取法 连续回流提取法适用于热稳定性好的待测成分的提取。如大山楂丸中熊果酸含量测定，其供试品溶液的制备方法如下：取重量差异项下的本品，剪碎、混匀，取约3g，精密称定，加水30ml，60℃水浴温热，使充分溶散，加硅藻土2g，搅匀，滤过，残渣用水30ml洗涤，100℃烘干，连同滤纸一并置于索氏提取器中，加乙醚适量，加热回流提取4小时，提取液回收溶剂至干，残渣用石油醚（30~60℃）浸泡2次（每次约2分钟），每次5ml，倾去石油醚液，残渣加无水乙醇－三氯甲烷（3∶2）的混合溶液适量，微热使溶解，转移至5ml量瓶中，用上述混合溶液稀释至刻度，摇匀，即得。

③ *Continuous Reflux Extraction Method* Continuous reflux extraction is a continuous extraction method using Soxhlet extractor. It is suitable for the extraction of components with good thermal stability. For example, the content of ursolic acid in the Dashanzha Pills is determined, the preparation method of the test solution is as follows: take the product under the test weight of variation, cut and mix it well, take about 3g, weigh it precisely, add 30ml of water, warm in a water bath at 60℃, fully dissolve, add 2g diatomite, stir well, filter, wash the residue with water 30ml, dry at 100℃, put it in the Soxhlet extractor together with filter paper, add appropriate amount of ethyl ether, reflux extraction for 4 hours. The solvent was recovered from the extract to dry, and the residue was soaked in petroleum ether (30-60℃) twice (about 2 minutes each time), 5ml each time, and the petroleum ether solution was poured out. The residue was dissolved with a mixture of anhydrous ethanol and chloroform (3∶2), dissolved by slight heat, transferred to a 5ml volumetric flask, add the above mixed solution to volume, shake well, as the test solution.

（4）超声提取法 超声波有助溶的作用，大大缩短了提取时间，是较为常用的一种提取方法。如二丁颗粒中秦皮乙素的含量测定，其供试品溶液的制备方法：取本品研细，取约2.5g或0.3g（无蔗糖），精密称定，置于具塞锥形瓶中，精密加入甲醇25ml，称定重量，超声处理（功率250W，频率50kHz）30分钟，放冷，再称定重量，用甲醇补足减失的重量，摇匀，滤过，取续滤液，即得。

④ *Ultrasonic Extraction* Ultrasonic extraction is a commonly used extraction method because of its solubilization and short extraction time. For example, the content of aesculetin in Erding Granules is determined, and the preparation method of the test solution is as follows: take this product for grinding and subdivision, about 2.5g or 0.3g (no sucrose), weigh accurately, placed in a conical flask with stopper, add exactly 25ml methanol and weigh, ultrasonicate (power 250W, frequency 50kHz) for 30 minutes, cool and weigh again, replenish the loss of the solvent with methanol, shake well, filter and use the successive continuous filtrate as the test solution.

（二）水蒸气蒸馏法

## 2. Steam Distillation Method

水蒸气蒸馏法是指将含有挥发性成分的样品与水共蒸馏，加热使挥发性成分随水蒸气蒸馏而出，经冷凝、分取挥发性成分。此法适用于具有挥发性、能随水蒸气蒸馏而不被破坏、遇水稳定且难溶或不溶于水的成分的提取。例如，中药中的挥发油，小分子的生物碱（麻黄碱、烟碱、槟榔碱）和小分子的酚类（丹皮酚）等。为了使挥发性成分分取完全，可配合盐析。如正骨水中挥发油的含量测定，其供试品溶液的制备方法如下：精密量取本品10ml，置于分液漏斗中，加饱和氯化钠溶液100ml，振摇1~2分钟，放置1~2小时，分取上层液，移入圆底烧瓶中，分液漏斗用热水洗涤数次，洗液并入圆底烧瓶中，照挥发油测定法（《中国药典》四部通则2204甲法）测定，读取挥发油量，计算样品中挥发油的含量（％）。

Steam distillation means that the samples containing volatile components are co-distilled with water, heated so that the volatile components are distilled with steam, and the volatile components are condensed and separated. This method is suitable for the extraction of components that are volatile, can't be destroyed with steam distillation, are stable in the presence of water, and are insoluble in water. For example, volatile oil in traditional Chinese medicine, small molecular alkaloids (ephedrine, nicotine, arecoline) and small molecular phenols (paeonol). In order to separate the volatile components completely, it can be combined with salting-out. For example, for the determination of the content of volatile oil in Zhenggu Tincture, the preparation method of the test solution is as follows: take 10ml of this product, place it in the separating funnel, add 100ml of saturated sodium chloride solution, shake for 1-2 minutes, standing for 1-2 hours, separate the upper liquid, move it into the round bottom flask, wash the separating funnel with hot water for several times, merge the washing solution into the round bottom flask, and determine the volatile oil according to the determination of volatile oil (2204 Determination of Volatile Oil in Volume Ⅳ Method of the 2020 edition of *Chinese Pharmacopoeia*). Read the amount of volatile oil and calculate the content of volatile oil in the sample (%).

（三）升华法
### 3. Sublimation

固体物质加热直接变成气体，遇冷又凝结为固体的现象称之为升华。利用某些成分具有升华性质的特点，使其与其他成分分离，再进行分析。如游离的羟基蒽醌、咖啡因、斑蝥素、冰片等成分。如牛黄解毒胶囊中冰片的鉴别，其供试品溶液的制备方法如下：取本品内容物适量（相当于饮片约 1.7g），进行微量升华，所得白色升华物，加甲醇 0.2ml 使溶解，即得。

The phenomenon that solid matter directly turns into gas when heated and then condenses into solid when cold is called sublimation. Take advantage of the sublimation of some components to separate them from other components and then analyze them. Such as free hydroxyanthraquinone, caffeine, cantharidin, borneol and other ingredients. For example, for the identification of the borneol in Niuhuang Jiedu Capsule, the preparation method of the test solution is as follows: take an appropriate amount of the contents of this product (equivalent to about 1.7g of decoction pieces) and perform sublimation. The white sublimate obtained is dissolved with 0.2ml of methanol as the test solution.

此外，还有超临界流体萃取法、半仿生提取、酶法提取等现代提取方法也有应用。

In addition, modern extraction methods such as supercritical fluid extraction (SFE), semi-bionic extraction and enzymatic extraction are also used.

### 三、分析目的与样品提取
### 2.1.3  The Purpose of Analysis and Sample Extraction

样品提取时除了根据待测成分的理化性质和样品组成选择合适的提取方法外，还要根据分析目的合理设计提取步骤。分析目的不同对样品提取的要求也不同。

In addition to selecting the appropriate extraction method according to the physical and chemical properties of the components to be tested and the composition of the sample, the extraction steps should be designed reasonably according to the purpose of analysis. Different analytical purposes have different requirements for sample extraction.

（一）供鉴别用样品的提取
### 1. Extraction of Samples for Identification

中药鉴别可采用显微、理化等手段进行定性分析。显微鉴别无需制备供试溶液，其他的理化鉴别则需要制备供试溶液。由于鉴别的目的是鉴定中药材和饮片的真伪或者判别中药制剂中某味药是否存在，所以用于鉴别的供试溶液制备不强调量（包括取样量和加入溶剂的体积等）的精确度，制备方法力求简便、易操作。如三黄片中大黄、黄芩的鉴别，其供试品溶液的制备如下：取本品 5 片，除去包衣，研细，取 0.25g 加甲醇 5ml，超声处理 5 分钟，滤过，即得。

The identification of traditional Chinese medicine is qualitative analysis by microscopic identification, physicochemical identification and other methods. Microscopic identification does not need to prepare the test solution, other physical and chemical identification needs to prepare the test solution. Because the purpose of identification is to identify the authenticity of traditional Chinese medicine and slices or to distinguish whether a certain Chinese medicine exists in the preparation of traditional Chinese medicine, the accuracy of the preparation of the sample solution (including the amount of sampling and the volume of solvent added, etc.) is not emphasized in the preparation of the test solution. The preparation method is simple and easy to operate. For example, for the identification of Rhei Radix et Rhizoma and Scutellariae Radix in Sanhuang tablets, the preparation of the test solution is as follows: take 5 tablets of this product, remove the coating, grind it, add 0.25g to methanol 5ml, ultrasonicate for 5 minutes, filter, and the filtrate is used as the test solution.

（二）供检查用样品的提取

## 2. Extraction of Samples for Inspection

中药中杂质种类多，有重金属、砷盐、灰分等无机杂质；也有黄曲霉毒素、农药残留、马兜铃酸、乌头碱、土大黄苷等有机杂质。对于无机杂质检查，样品的处理常用消化法，以干法或湿法消解植物组织或有机物，使无机杂质释放出来。对有机杂质的检查，可根据杂质检查方法，来选择样品的提取方法，如果杂质的检查用含量测定的方法，则按含量测定供试溶液制备方法的精确度要求制备供试溶液，如农药残留量、黄曲霉毒素的测定等；如果仅是限量检查，则按鉴别用供试溶液的制备方法要求制备供试溶液，如三黄片中土大黄苷的检查（限量检查），其供试品溶液的制备如下：取本品小片 2 片或大片 1 片，糖衣片除去糖衣，研细，加甲醇 15ml，加热回流 30 分钟，放冷，滤过，即得。

There are many kinds of impurities in traditional Chinese medicine, including heavy metals, arsenic, ash and other inorganic impurities, as well as aflatoxin, pesticide residues, aristolochic acid, aconitine, rhaponticin and other organic impurities. For the inspection of inorganic impurities, the sample treatment is often digested by dry or wet method to digest plant tissue or organic matter, so that inorganic impurities are released. For the inspection of organic impurities, the extraction method of the sample can be selected according to the requirements of the inspection. If the impurities are examined by the method of content determination, the sample solution is prepared according to the accuracy of the preparation of the sample solution by content determination, such as determination of pesticide residue, aflatoxins, etc. If it is only a limit test, the test solution is prepared according to the preparation method of the test solution for identification. For example, the examination of rhaponiticin in Sanhuang tablets, the preparation of the test solution is as follows: take 2 or 1 large tablets of this product, sugar-coated tablets to remove sugar coating, fine, add methanol 15ml, heat and reflux for 30 minutes, allow to cool, filter, the filtrate is used as the test solution.

（三）供含量测定用样品的提取

## 3. Extraction of Samples for Assay

含量测定时，样品的提取特别强调待测成分要提取完全，另外，含量测定的样品提取过程中还应注意对取样量、加入溶剂体积或者供试溶液总体积精确度的要求。样品的取样量需要精密称定，如果是用部分测定法，用准确度符合国家标准要求的移液管精密加入提取溶剂，提取前称重，提取后补重；如果用全部测定法，提取完后，洗涤滤纸和滤渣，洗液并入滤液，最终定容到相应的体积。如小儿百寿丸中木香烃内酯的含量测定（部分测定），其供试品溶液制备方法如下：取本品 10 丸，剪碎，混匀，取约 3g，精密称定，精密加入甲醇 50ml，密塞，称定重量，超声处理（功率 200W，频率 40kHz）45 分钟，放冷，再称定重量，用甲醇补足减失的重量，摇匀，滤过，取续滤液，即得。

小儿百部止咳糖浆中黄芩苷的含量测定（全部测定），其供试品溶液的制备方法如下：精密量取本品 2ml，置 100ml 量瓶中，用水溶解并稀释至刻度，摇匀，精密量取 10ml，置 50ml 量瓶中，加 65% 甲醇至刻度，摇匀，滤过，取续滤液，即得。

In the content determination, the extraction of the sample especially emphasizes that the components to be tested should be extracted completely. In addition, attention should be paid to the accuracy of the sample quantity, the added solvent volume or the total volume of the sample solution in the process of sample extraction. The sampling quantity of the sample needs to be accurately weighed, if the partial determination method is used, the extraction solvent is exactly added with the pipette whose accuracy meets the requirements of the national standard, weigh before extraction, and replenish the lost weight after extraction; if the full determination method is used, after extraction, wash the filter paper and filter residue, and the washing solution is incorporated into the filtrate, and finally add solvent to volume. For example, content determination of costunolide in Xiao´er Baishou Pill, the preparation method of the test solution is as follows: take 10 pills of this product, cut into pieces, mix well, take about 3g, weigh accurately, add exactly methanol 50ml, stopper tightly, weigh, ultrasonicate (power 200W, frequency 40kHz) for 45 minutes, cool, weigh again, replenish the lost weight with methanol, shake well, filter, use successive filtrate as the test solution.

Determination of baicalin in Xiao' er Baibu Zhike Syrups. the preparation method the test solution is as follows: take 2ml of the product accurately, put it in a 100ml volumetric flask, dissolve it with water and dilute to volume, shake well, take accurately 10ml of above solution, put it in a 50ml volumetric flask, add 65% methanol to volume, shake well, filter, use successive filtrate as the test solution.

## 第二节　样品的纯化与富集
## 2.2　Purification and Enrichment of Samples

### 一、样品的纯化
### 2.2.1　Purification of Sample

样品是否需要纯化，纯化到什么程度，取决于所选分析方法的专属性、分离能力和检测系统耐受杂质的程度。样品纯化的原则是除去干扰杂质，又不损失被测成分或尽可能少的损失被测成分。纯化方法的选择主要依据被测成分和杂质性质、存在形式、浓度范围上的差异，同时结合所采用的分析对象和方法。常用的纯化方法如下：

Whether the sample needs to be purified and to what extent it is purified depends on the specificity, the separation ability of the selected analytical method, and the tolerance of the detection system to impurities. The principle of sample purification is to remove interfering impurities without losing the tested components or losing as few tested components as possible. The selection of purification methods is mainly based on the differences in the properties, existing forms and concentration ranges of the tested components and impurities, as well as the analytical objects and methods used. The common purification methods are as follows:

（一）沉淀法

### 1. Precipitation Method

沉淀法是基于某试剂与被测成分（或杂质）生成沉淀，分离沉淀或保留溶液以达到纯化精制的目的；或是加入某试剂大大降低了被测成分（或杂质）在原溶液中的溶解度，使被测成分（或杂质）沉淀析出，分离沉淀或保留溶液以达到纯化精制的目的。采用沉淀法纯化样品时，须注意：当大量杂质以沉淀的形式除去时，①过量的试剂对被测组分的测定有干扰，则应设法除去；②被测成分不应产生共沉淀而损失。如果被测成分形成沉淀，沉淀经分离，重新溶解后分析或直接用重量法分析。

The precipitation method is based on the formation of precipitation between a reagent and the tested component (or impurity), separating precipitation or retaining the solution to achieve the purpose of purification, or the addition of a reagent greatly reduces the solubility of the tested component (or impurity) in the original solution, make the tested components (or impurities) precipitate, separating precipitation or retaining the solution to achieve the purpose of purification. When using the precipitation method to purify the sample, it should be noted that when a large number of impurities are removed in the form of precipitation, ① the excess reagent interferes with the determination of the tested components should try to be removed; ② the tested components should not be lost in the form of coprecipitation. If the tested components form precipitation, the precipitation can be separated and re-dissolved or directly analyzed by gravimetric method.

（二）液－液萃取法

### 2. Liquid-Liquid Extraction Method

液－液萃取法是利用样品中各组分在两种互不相溶的溶剂中分配系数的不同而达到分离纯化的目的。当样品中组分比较多时，可选用几种溶剂，由低极性到高极性分步进行萃取。对弱酸或弱碱性成分的萃取，需要调节水相的 pH，使弱酸、弱碱性成分主要以非离子化的游离形式存在，以提高其在有机溶剂中的溶解度，有利于萃取。在萃取过程中也常利用盐析作用（正骨水中挥发油的含量测定），有利于被测组分进入有机相，提高提取率。当样品中的组分是强酸或强碱时（如生物碱类），可采用离子对萃取法（如小儿宝泰康颗粒中生物碱含量测定）；酒剂、酊剂等含乙醇量比较高的液体制剂，在萃取前应先挥去乙醇。

The method of liquid-liquid extraction (LLE) method is to achieve the purpose of separation and purification by making use of the different partition coefficients of each component of the sample in two immiscible solvents. When there are many components in the sample, several solvents can be selected for step-by-step extraction from low polarity to high polarity. For the extraction of weak acid or weak basic components, it is necessary to adjust the pH of aqueous phase so that weak acid or weak basic components mainly exist in non-ionized free state, so as to improve their solubility in organic solvents and facilitate extraction. Salting-out is also often used in the extraction process, which is beneficial for the tested components to enter the organic phase and improve the extraction rate. Such as the assay of volatile oil in Zhenggu Tinctures. When the components in the sample are strong acids or alkaloids (such as alkaloids), ion pair extraction can be used (such as determination of total alkaloids in Xiao'er Baotaikang Granules). Alcohol should be removed before extraction in Medicinal Wines and Tincture.

萃取效率的高低取决于分配系数、萃取过程中两相之间的接触情况及萃取次数等。萃取次数取决于分析的目的和方法学验证。该方法的优点是仪器设备简便。缺点是操作较为繁琐，易出现乳化现象。如果出现乳化现象，则影响定量分析的结果。

The extraction efficiency depends on the distribution coefficient, the contact between the two phases in the extraction process and the extraction times. The times of extraction depends on the purpose of the analysis and validation of an analytical method. The advantage of this method is that the instrument is simple and convenient. The disadvantage is that the operation is more tedious and easily emulsify. If emulsification occurs, it will affect the results of quantitative analysis.

（三）色谱法

## 3. Chromatography Method

色谱法是中药分析中常用的样品纯化方法，根据样品中各成分与固定相和流动相相互作用不同而分离。色谱法包括柱色谱法、薄层色谱法和纸色谱法等，其中以柱色谱法用于纯化较为常用。柱色谱法中常用的填料有：硅胶、中性氧化铝、大孔树脂、聚酰胺、离子交换树脂等。如七制香附丸中白芍的鉴别，选用中性氧化铝纯化；四君子颗粒中党参的鉴别，用 D101 型大孔树脂纯化；地榆槐角丸中炒槐米的鉴别，用聚酰胺；妇康宁片中人参的鉴别，用 732-Na 型强酸性阳离子交换树脂。

Chromatography method is a commonly used sample purification method in the traditional Chinese medicine analysis. Chromatography method is based on the different interaction of individual components between two phases (the stationary phases and the mobile phase). Chromatography method may be classified into paper chromatography method, thin layer chromatography method, and column chromatography method etc., among which column chromatography method is commonly used for purification. Silica gel, neutral aluminum oxide, macroporous resin, polyamide powder, ion exchange resin are commonly used as the stationary phases in column chromatography method. For example, the identification of Paeoniae Radix Alba in Qizhi Xiangfu pill, neutral aluminum oxide was used as the stationary phases; The identification of Codonopsis Radix in Sijunzi granules, D101 macroporous resin was used as the stationary phases; the identification of Sophorae Flos (stir-fry) in Diyu Huaijiao pills, polyamide powder was used as the stationary phases, and the identification of Ginseng in Fukangning tablets, 732-Na strongly acidic cation exchange resin was used as the stationary phases

柱色谱法填料的选择：①保留测定组分在柱上，杂质不保留；②均保留，但程度不同；③保留杂质于柱上，待测成分不保留。在上述三种情况中，第二种情况居多，也就是待测成分与杂质的保留程度不同，一种是杂质弱保留而待测成分强保留，另一种是杂质强保留，而待测成分弱保留。

The selection of fillers in column chromatographic method: ① retain the determined components on the column and the impurities are not retained; ② retained all, but to different degrees; ③ the impurities are retained on the column, and the measured components are not retained. In the above three cases, the second case is mostly. The retention degree of the tested components and impurities is different, one is the weak retention of impurities and the strong retention of tested components, the other is the strong retention of impurities and the weak retention of tested components.

固相萃取（solid-phase extraction，SPE）是以液相色谱的分离原理为基础建立起来的分离纯化方法，在生物样品的制备方面日益受到重视并逐步发展起来。

Solid phase extraction (SPE) is a separation and purification method based on the separation principle of liquid chromatography, which has been paid more and more attention to and gradually developed in the preparation of biological samples.

SPE 小柱由柱管、筛板和固定相三部分组成。其中最重要的部分是固定相，它的选择取决于分析物质、样品基质和样品溶剂的极性，主要依据"相似相溶"的原理选择。常见的固定相是键合相硅胶，以十八烷基键合硅胶（简称 C18）最为常用，其次有辛基硅烷键合硅胶、苯基键合硅胶、氨基键合硅胶和氰基键合硅胶。常见规格 100g、200g、500g、1000g，以 100g 最为常用。一般操作程序为：①柱的活化，用甲醇冲洗以润湿键合相和除去杂质，再用水洗去柱中的甲醇；②上样，上样量一般为固定相质量的 1%~3%；③淋洗，用水清洗除去弱保留的亲水成分。④洗脱，用甲醇或甲醇－水洗脱强保留的待测组分。

The SPE column consists of three parts: column tube, sieve plate and the stationary phases. The most important part is the stationary phase, which is selected depended on the polarity of the analytical substance, sample matrix and sample solvent according to the theory of "similarity and intermiscibility". The common stationary phase is chemically bonded silica gel, and octadecyl silane bonded silica gel (C18) is the most commonly used, followed by octylsilane bonded silica gel, phenyl bonded silica gel, amino group bonded silica gel and cyano group bonded silica gel. The common specifications are 100, 200, 500 and 1000g, and 100g is the most commonly used. The general operating procedure is as follows: ① the activation of the column, rinsing with methanol to wet the bonded phase and remove impurities, and then washing the methanol in the column with water; ② upper sample, the mass of the sample is generally 1%-3% of the mass of the stationary phases; ③ rinsing, removing the weakly retained hydrophilic components with water; ④ elution, eluting strong retention of the tested components with methanol or methanol-water.

### （四）盐析法

### 4. Salting-out Method

盐析法是在样品的水提取液中加入无机盐至一定浓度或达到饱和状态，使待测成分在水中的溶解度降低而析出。NaCl、$Na_2SO_4$ 是常用的无机盐。

In the salting-out method, inorganic salts are added to the water extract of the sample to a certain concentration or to a saturated state, so that the solubility of the tested components in water is reduced and precipitated. NaCl and $Na_2SO_4$ are commonly used inorganic salt.

### （五）微萃取法

### 5. Microextraction Method

微萃取法可以分为固相微萃取（SPME）和液相微萃取（LPME）两种。SPME 是在 SPE 的基础上发展起来的一种集萃取、富集、进样功能于一体的新型样品前处理方法。其原理是待测成分在萃取涂层（萃取头）与样品之间的吸附或溶解－解吸附平衡时，待测成分在固定相上有较高的分配系数，从而可以将其定量萃取出来。目前 SPME 已实现了与气相和液相色谱的联用。LPME 是一个基于分析物在样品及小体积的有机溶剂（或受体）之间平衡分配的过程。根据萃取形式，可分为单滴微萃取、多孔中空纤维液相微萃取和分散液相微萃取。

Microextraction can be divided into solid phase microextraction (SPME) and liquid phase microextraction (LPME). SPME is a new sample pretreatment method developed on the basis of SPE, which integrates the functions of extraction, enrichment and sample injection. The principle is that the test components reach equilibrium in the adsorption or dissolution-desorption equilibrium between the extraction coating and the sample, the tested component has a higher distribution coefficient on the stationary phase, so it can be extracted quantitatively. At present, SPME has been coupled with gas chromatography and liquid chromatography. LPME is a process based on the equilibrium distribution of analytes between a sample and a small volume of organic solvents (or receptors). According to the extraction form, it can be divided into single drop microextraction, porous hollow fiber liquid microextraction and dispersed liquid microextraction.

### 二、样品的富集浓缩
### 2.2.2　Sample Enrichment and Concentration

中药经提取、纯化后，如待测成分浓度低于分析方法的检测灵敏度，或者所使用的溶剂不符合分析方法的要求，无法直接测定，此时均需要对样品溶液进行浓缩或者蒸干。常见的浓缩方法如下：

After extraction and purification of traditional Chinese medicine, if the concentration of the tested components is lower than the sensitivity of the analytical method, or if the solvent used does not meet the requirements of the analytical method, it can´t be determined directly, then the sample solution needs to be concentrated or evaporated to dry. Common concentrations methods are as follows:

1. 水浴蒸发法　将提取液置于蒸发皿中，水浴蒸干，残渣加适宜溶剂溶解。适合于热稳定性好的非挥发性成分。中药分析的薄层色谱鉴别在供试溶液的制备中水浴蒸发最为常用，一般情况下水浴蒸干后残渣加适当溶剂 1ml 使溶解，即得供试品溶液。如益母草膏中盐酸水苏碱的鉴别。

**(1) Water Bath Evaporation Method**　Put the extract in an evaporation dish, steam dry in a water bath, and dissolve the residue with suitable solvent. Suitable for non-volatile components with good thermal stability. In the TLC identification of traditional Chinese medicine, water bath evaporation is the most commonly used in the preparation of the test solution. In general, the residue is dissolved by adding appropriate solvent 1ml after remove original solvent to dryness in the water bath to get the test solution. Such as the identification of stachydrine hydrochloride in Yimucao extract preparation.

2. 自然挥散法　适用于小体积提取液，且溶剂的挥发性强，如乙醚提取液可以在室温下自然挥干。如麝香祛痛搽剂中麝香酮的鉴别。

**(2) Natural Evaporation Method**　It is suitable for small volume extract and the solvent is highly volatile, for example, ethyl ether extract solution can evaporate naturally at room temperature. Such as the identification of muscone in Shexiang Qutong liniment.

3. 减压蒸发法　此法具有温度低、浓缩速度快、溶剂可回收的优点，适宜热不稳定的样品。是残留分析中最常用的浓缩方法。如农药残留量测定时供试品溶液的浓缩等。

**(3) Vacuum Evaporation Method**　This method has the advantages of low temperature, fast concentration and solvent recovery, and is suitable for thermally unstable samples. It is the most commonly used concentration method in residue analysis. For example, the concentration of test solution in the determination of pesticide residues.

4. 气流吹蒸法　利用空气或者氮气流加速溶剂的蒸发，一般在加热条件下进行。常用的是氮气流吹蒸法，氮气可以防止被测成分的氧化。主要用于生物样品的浓缩。

**(4) Gas Blowing and Heating Method**　The evaporation of solvents is accelerated by air or nitrogen flow, usually under heating conditions. The commonly used method is nitrogen blowing and steaming, and nitrogen can prevent the oxidation of the tested components. It is mainly used for the concentration of biological samples.

5. 冷冻干燥法　将待干燥物快速冻结后，再在高真空条件下将其中的冰升华为蒸气的干燥方法。冰的升华过程是吸热过程，整个过程保持低温冻结状态，有利于保留一些生物样品（如蛋白质）的活性。提取液多为水溶液，主要用于热不稳定的生物样品。优点是：干燥后的物料保持原来的化学组成和物理性质（如多孔结构、胶体性质等）；热量消耗比其他浓缩方法少。缺点是费用较高。

**(5) Freeze Drying Method**　The drying method in which the ice is sublimated into steam under the condition of high vacuum after the drying material is frozen quickly. The sublimation process of ice is an endothermic process, and the whole process remains frozen at low temperature, which is helpful to retain the activity of some biological samples (such as proteins). The extract is mostly aqueous solution, which is mainly used for thermally unstable biological samples. The advantages are as follows: the dried material maintains the original chemical composition and physical properties (such as porous structure, colloid properties, etc.), and the heat consumption is less than other concentration methods. The disadvantage is that the cost is high.

## 第三节　样品的消解与衍生化
## 2.3　Digestion and Derivation of Samples

### 一、样品的消解
### 2.3.1　Digestion of Samples

测定中药中的无机元素，由于大量有机物的存在，常常会络合无机元素，所以需要破坏中药中的有机物，使被络合的无机物转化为可测的游离态。因此，检查中药中重金属、砷盐或其他有害元素时，必须采用合适的方法破坏药物中的有机物。常用的破坏方法有湿法消化、干法消化、高压消解、微波消解等。

For the determination of inorganic elements in traditional Chinese medicine, inorganic elements are often complexed with a large amount of organic matter, so it is necessary to destroy the organic matter in traditional Chinese medicine and transform the complexed inorganic matter into a measurable free state. Therefore, when examining heavy metals, arsenic or other harmful elements in traditional Chinese medicine, appropriate methods must be adopted to destroy the organic matter in the medicine. The commonly used destruction methods are wet digestion, dry digestion, high pressure digestion, microwave digestion and so on.

（一）湿法消化

#### 1. Wet Digestion
湿法消化也称酸消化法，用不同酸或混合酸与过氧化氢或其他氧化剂混合液，加热使待测元素转化为可测定形态的方法。常见的湿法消化方法如下：

Wet digestion, also known as acid digestion, uses mixture solvent of different acids or mixed acids with hydrogen peroxide or other oxidants to convert the state of the elements to be determined by heating. Common wet digestion methods are as follows:

**1. 硝酸 – 高氯酸法**　破坏能力强，反应较激烈，适用于血、尿、组织等生物样品的破坏以及含动、植物药的中药制剂的破坏，破坏后的无机金属离子均为高价态，但对含氮杂环类有机物破坏不够完全。破坏时，切勿将容器中的溶液蒸干，以免发生爆炸。

**(1) Nitric Acid-Perchloric Acid Method** The destructive ability is strong and the reaction is fierce. It is suitable for the destruction of biological samples such as blood, urine and tissue, as well as the destruction of traditional Chinese medicine containing animal and plant drugs. The destroyed inorganic metal ions are all in high valence state, but the destruction of nitrogen-containing heterocyclic organic compounds is not complete. When damaged, do not steam the solution in the container to avoid explosion.

2. 硝酸－硫酸法　适用于大多数有机物的破坏，破坏后的无机金属离子均为高价态。当药物中金属离子与硫酸能形成不溶性硫酸盐时，不宜采用此法破坏。

**(2) Nitric Acid-Sulfuric Acid Method** It is suitable for the destruction of most organic compounds, and the inorganic metal ions after destruction are in high valence state. When the metal ions in the medicine and sulfuric acid can form insoluble sulfate, it is not suitable to be destroyed by this method.

3. 硫酸－硫酸盐法　硫酸钾或无水硫酸钠为常用的硫酸盐，目的是提高硫酸的沸点，加速样品的破坏，促使样品破坏更加完全，同时防止硫酸在加热过程中过早分解为 $SO_3$ 而损失。破坏后所得金属离子多为低价态，常用于含砷、锑的药物的破坏，破坏后可得到三价砷或锑。

**(3) Sulfuric Acid-Sulfate Method** Potassium sulfate or anhydrous sodium sulfate is a commonly used sulfate. The purpose of adding the above salt is to increase the boiling point of sulfuric acid, accelerate the destruction of the sample, promote the destruction of the sample more completely, and prevent the loss of sulfuric acid from decomposing into $SO_3$ prematurely in the process of heating. Most of the metal ions obtained after destruction are in low valence state, which are often used for the destruction of drugs containing arsenic and antimony, and trivalent arsenic or antimony can be obtained after destruction.

湿法消化需要的仪器，一般为硅玻璃或硼玻璃材质的凯氏瓶（直火加热）或聚四氟乙烯消化罐（烘箱中加热）。所用试剂为优级纯，水为去离子水或高纯水；同时应按相同条件进行空白实验校正。操作应在通风橱内进行。

The instruments needed for wet digestion are usually KJELDAHL′S bottles made of silicon glass or boron glass (heated directly) or polytetrafluoroethylene digestion tanks (heated in the oven). The reagent used is high-grade pure, and the water is deionized water or high-purity water; at the same time, blank experimental correction should be carried out according to the same conditions. The operation should be carried out in the fume cupboard.

优点：有机物分解速度快，所用时间短；加热温度低，可减少金属挥发逸散的损失。缺点：常产生大量有害气体；消化初期，易产生大量泡沫外溢；试剂用量较大，空白值偏高。

The advantages of wet digestion: the decomposition speed of organic matter is fast, the time is short, and the low heating temperature can reduce the loss of metal volatilization. Disadvantages: a large number of harmful gases often occur; it is easy to produce a large number of foam spillover in the initial stage of digestion; the amount of reagent is large, and the blank value is on the high side.

（二）干法消化

## 2. Dry Digestion

将适量样品置瓷坩埚、镍坩埚或铂坩埚中，常加少量无水 $Na_2CO_3$ 或轻质 $MgO$ 等以助灰化，混匀后，先小火加热使样品完全炭化，然后放入马弗炉中炽灼使完全灰化。灰分放至室温，加入稍过量的稀盐酸－水（1∶3）或硝酸－水（1∶3）溶液，振摇，若溶液有颜色或有不溶物，说明灰化不完全，可将溶液水浴蒸干，小火炭化后，再行炽灼灰化。

Put an appropriate amount of samples into porcelain crucibles, nickel crucibles or platinum crucibles, and often add a small amount of anhydrous $Na_2CO_3$ or light MgO to help incineration, after mixing, the samples are completely charred by low heat, and then ignited in muffle furnace until the incineratation is complete. After ash cooling, add a little too much dilute hydrochloric acid-water (1∶3) or nitric acid-water (1∶3) solution, shake, if the solution has color or insoluble matter, indicating that incineration is not complete, the solution can be steamed dry in water bath, carbonized over low heat, and then ignited.

干法消化应注意以下几个问题：①加热炽灼时，控制炽灼温度，特别是易挥发的金属元素（如进行中药中重金属、砷盐的检查时，炽灼的温度应控制在500~600℃），以免挥发影响测定结果。②要完全灰化，否则影响测定结果。③为了防止待测元素的挥发，可加入灰化辅助剂（硝酸镁）。

The following problems should be paid attention to in dry digestion: ① when heating and ignite, the ignite temperature should be controlled, especially the volatile metal elements (such as the inspection heavy metals and arsenic in traditional Chinese medicine, the temperature should be controlled at 500-600℃), so as not to affect the determination results. ② It should be completely incinerated, otherwise it will affect the determination results. ③ In order to prevent the volatilization of the tested elements, auxiliaries (magnesium nitrate) can be added.

优点：空白值低；能处理较多的样品，可富集被测组分，降低检测限；有机物分解彻底，操作简单。缺点：所用时间长；因温度高易造成易挥发元素的损失。

The advantages of dry digestion: low blank value; dealing with more samples, enriching tested components, reducing the detection limit; organic matter is decomposed thoroughly, and the operation is simple. Disadvantages: it takes a long time; it is easy to cause the loss of volatile elements due to high temperature.

（三）高压消解

### 3. High Pressure Digestion

高压消解是一种在高温、高压下进行的湿法消解过程，即把样品和消解液（通常为混合酸或混合酸＋氧化剂）置于合适的容器中，再将容器装在保护套中，在密闭情况下进行分解。优点：无须消耗大量酸，降低了空白值，将复杂基体完全溶解，避免挥发性待测元素的损失。

High pressure digestion is a wet digestion process carried out at high temperature and high pressure. The sample and digestion solution (usually mixed acid or mixed acid - oxidant) are placed in a suitable container, and then the container is packed in a protective sleeve and decompose organic matter in the closed container. The advantage is that it does not need to consume a large amount of acid, reduces the determination blank, completely dissolves the complex matrix, and avoids the loss of volatile elements to be tested.

（四）微波消解

### 4. Microwave Digestion

微波消解是利用微波的穿透性和激活反应能力加热密闭容器内的试剂和样品的方法。微波消解的消化罐完全密闭，罐内压力增加，反应温度提高，大大缩短样品的消解时间，同时反应条件可控，制样精度高，且不需催化剂及升温剂，对环境的污染少，是样品消解的首选方法。

Microwave digestion is a method of heating reagents and samples in closed containers by using the penetration and activation ability of microwave. The digestion tank of microwave digestion is completely closed, the pressure in the tank increases and the reaction temperature increases, which greatly shortens the digestion time of the sample. At the same time, the reaction condition is controllable, the sample preparation precision is high, and it does not need catalyst and temperature rising agent, and has less pollution to the environment. It is the preferred method for sample digestion.

## 二、样品的衍生化
## 2.3.2 Derivation of Samples

中药分析中有些成分极性大，挥发性低或对检测器不够灵敏，使用常规的含量测定方法难以有效测定，需要先将样品进行衍生化反应，生成适合检测器要求的衍生物后再行测定。如中药中脂肪酸。含脂肪酸的中药有鱼腥草、板蓝根、五味子、苦杏仁、核桃仁等，研究表明，不饱和脂肪酸具有明显降低血清胆固醇、降血压作用，可以有效的降低冠状动脉硬化性心脏病及脑卒中等疾病的发病率；软脂酸、硬脂酸能够诱导人肝癌 HepG2 细胞的凋亡，起到抗肿瘤效果。但是脂肪酸沸点高、极性强，是一种热敏性物质，在高温下易发生聚合、脱酸、裂解等反应，直接分析比较困难，经衍生化后生成较易挥发、极性偏弱的衍生物后，则可以选择气相色谱（GC）进行分析。

In the analysis of traditional Chinese medicine, some components have high polarity, low volatility or insensitive to the detector, so it is difficult to determine effectively by using conventional content determination methods, so it is necessary to carry out derivatization reaction of the sample to produce derivatives suitable for the requirements of the detector before determination, such as fatty acids. Traditional Chinese medicine containing fatty acids include Houttuyniae Herba, Isatidis Radix, Schisandrae Shinensis Fructus, Corydalis Bungeanae Herba, Juglandis Semen and so on. Studies have shown that unsaturated fatty acids can significantly reduce serum cholesterol and blood pressure, and can effectively reduce the incidence of coronary heart disease and stroke; palmitic acid and stearic acid can induce apoptosis of human liver cancer HepG2 cells and play anti-tumor effect. However, fatty acid has high boiling point and strong polarity, is a kind of thermosensitive substance, which is easy to polymerize, deacidify and pyrolyze at high temperature, so it is difficult to analyze directly, after derivatization, it can be analyzed by gas chromatography (GC).

适用于 GC 的衍生化反应有：硅烷化，常用三甲基硅烷化试剂，可取代化学成分中极性基团的活泼氢原子，使生成三甲基硅烷化衍生物。适用于含 R-OH、R-COOH、R-NH-R′ 等极性基团化合物的衍生化。酰化，适用于含有 R-OH、R-NH$_2$、R-NH-R′ 等极性基团化学成分的衍生化。烷基化，适用于含有 R-OH、R-COOH、R-NH-R′ 等极性基团化学成分的衍生化。不对称衍生化等方法，其中以硅烷化法的应用最为广泛。

The derivatization reactions suitable for GC are silanization, trimethylsilylation reagents are commonly used, which can replace the active hydrogen atoms of polar groups in chemical components to form trimethylsilanized derivatives. It is suitable for the derivatization of compounds containing polar groups such as R-OH, R-COOH, R-NH-R′. Acylation is suitable for the derivatization of chemical components containing polar groups such as R-OH, R-NH$_2$, R-NH-R′. Alkylation is suitable for the derivatization of polar groups such as R-OH, R-COOH, R-NH-R′. The asymmetric derivatization and other methods are also used. Among which silanization is the most widely used.

此外还有适用于光谱分析和光谱检测器的紫外衍生化、荧光衍生化。如中药中黄曲霉素的检查采用柱后衍生化后，采用 HPLC 法 – 荧光检测器检测。

In addition, there are ultraviolet derivatization and fluorescence derivatization which are suitable for spectral analysis and spectral detector. For example, aflatoxins in traditional Chinese medicine was detected by HPLC-fluorescence detector after post-column derivatization.

# 岗 位 对 接
# Post Docking

本章为中药学、中药制药和中药资源专业学生必须掌握的内容，为成为合格的中药学服务人员奠定坚实的基础。

This task must be mastered by students majoring in traditional Chinese medicine, traditional Chinese medicine pharmaceutical and traditional Chinese medicine resources, and lay a solid foundation for becoming qualified Chinese medicine service personnel.

本章内容对应岗位包括中药师、QC、QA、执业中药师、质量管理员等相关工种。

The corresponding positions of this task include traditional Chinese medicine pharmacist, QC, QA, licensed Chinese medicine pharmacist, quality manager and other related jobs.

上述从事中药质量服务及药品质量监督相关所有岗位的从业人员均需要掌握中药分析供试品溶液的制备方法等，学会应用本章内容开展中药学服务工作。

The above employees engaged in all positions related to traditional Chinese medicine quality service and drug quality supervision need to master the preparation method of traditional Chinese medicine analysis solution, and learn to apply this task to carry out traditional Chinese medicine service.

# 重 点 小 结
# Summary of Key Points

中药多为固体，在分析前大多需要制备供试品溶液，中药分析中供试品溶液的制备包括粉碎、提取、纯化与富集、消解和衍生化等。根据分析的对象和所选的分析方法，选择供试品溶液的制备。

Traditional Chinese medicines are mostly solid, and test solution is usually prepared before analysis. The preparation methods of test solution in traditional Chinese medicine analysis includes crushing, extraction, purification and enrichment, digestion and derivatization. According to the analysis object and the selected analysis method, the preparation methods of test solution is selected.

# 目 标 检 测

一、选择题

（一）单项选择题

1. 在中药分析中，关于样品的粉碎目的错误的是
   A. 保证均匀性                B. 使样品提取更快
   C. 使样品提取更充分        D. 使样品提取更美观
2. 关于提取溶剂的选择，应遵循的原则是
   A. 价格低      B. 易挥发      C. 相似相溶      D. 易发生反应
3. 以下不属于溶剂提取法的是
   A. 水蒸气蒸馏法    B. 浸渍法      C. 回流提取法      D. 超声辅助提取法

题库

4. 固相萃取法的操作程序不包括

    A. 活化        B. 点样        C. 淋洗        D. 洗脱

5. 常见湿法消化方法不包括

    A. 硝酸 – 高氯酸法        B. 硝酸 – 硫酸法

    C. 硫酸 – 硫酸盐法        D. 硫酸 - 盐酸法

**（二）多项选择题**

1. 在中药分析中，样品的提取方法按照原理不同可分为

    A. 溶剂提取法        B. 水蒸气蒸馏法        C. 升华法

    D. SFE        E. 半仿生提取

2. 溶剂提取法中浸渍法的缺点有

    A. 费时        B. 费溶剂        C. 操作复杂

    D. 提取不充分        E. 提取杂质多

3. 中药分析中的分析目的有

    A. 鉴别样品        B. 检查样品        C. 样品含量测定

    D. 微生物检查        E. 水分测定

4. 中药分析中常用的样品纯化方法有

    A. 沉淀法        B. 液 - 液萃取法        C. 色谱法

    D. 盐析法        E. 微萃取法

5. 中药分析中关于样品的衍生化，适用于 GC 的衍生化反应有

    A. 硅烷化        B. 酰化        C. 烷基化

    D. 不对称衍生化        E. 羟基化

## 二、思考题

样品的消解法中湿法消化与干法消化的优缺点分别是什么？

# 第三章 中药的鉴别
# Chapter 3 Identification of Chinese Medicine

 **学习目标｜Learning Goal**

**知识要求：**

**1. 掌握** 中药的色谱鉴别法。

**2. 熟悉** 中药的显微鉴别法、化学反应鉴别法和光谱鉴别法。

**3. 了解** 中药的性状鉴别和色谱－质谱联用鉴别法。

**能力要求：**

学会应用中药的性状鉴别、显微鉴别和理化鉴别方法解决中药的真伪鉴别。

**Knowledge Requirement**

**1. Master** The chromatographic identification methods of traditional Chinese medicine.

**2. Familiar** Microscopic identification methods, chemical reaction identification methods and spectral identification methods of traditional Chinese medicine.

**3. Understand** Trait identification methods and chromatography-mass spectrometry identification methods of traditional Chinese medicine.

**Ability Requirement**

Learn to apply methods trait identification, microscopic identification, physical and chemical identification of traditional Chinese medicine to identify the authenticity of traditional Chinese medicine

中药的鉴别是利用中药材、中药饮片或中药制剂的形态组织学特征及其所含化学成分的结构特征、理化特性、光谱特征或色谱特征及某些物理常数进行定性分析，做出真伪的判断，是中药质量控制与评价的重要组成部分，是分析环节的首要任务。中药的鉴别主要包括性状鉴别、显微鉴别、理化鉴别和生物鉴别等方法。

The identification of Chinese medicine is the qualitative analysis based on the morphological and histological characteristics of Chinese medicinal materials, Chinese medicine decoction pieces or Chinese medicine preparations and the structural characteristics, physical and chemical characteristics, spectral characteristics or chromatographic characteristics of chemical components and certain physical constants, to identify the authenticity of traditional Chinese medicine. It is an important work for quality control and evaluation of Chinese medicine, is the first task in traditional Chinese medicine analysis. The identification of traditional Chinese medicine mainly includes trait identification, microscopic identification, physical and chemical identification, and biological identification and other methods.

中药的鉴别采用的鉴别方法是根据待检测的目标药物的性质特点确定的，具有一定的专属性，只能证实待检测的药物是否为其包装标识所描述的药物，而不具备对未知药物进行真伪鉴别的能力。

The identification of traditional Chinese medicine is to verify whether the drug to be tested is the drug described in its package label. Because the identification method adopted is determined according to the characteristics of the target drug to be tested. It has certain specificity, but can't identify the unknown drug.

## 第一节　性状鉴别

## 3.1　Trait Identification

PPT

性状鉴别是对中药的形状、形态、色泽、气和味等外观性状，用眼观、手摸、鼻闻、口尝、水试和火试等方法，鉴别其真伪。性状鉴别也叫"直观鉴定法"。具有操作简单、快速的特点，在中药材（饮片）的真伪鉴别中占有十分重要的地位。

Trait identification can identify the authenticity of traditional Chinese medicine based on the appearance, shape, color, odor and taste of Chinese medicine by simple methods such as eye view, hand touch, nose smell, taste, water test and fire test. It is also called "visual identification method". with the characteristics of simple and fast operation, this method especially, it plays an important role in the identification of Chinese medicinal materials, Chinese medicine decoction pieces.

### 一、性状鉴别的内容
### 3.1.1　Content of Trait Identification

中药材、中药饮片、中药提取物及中药制剂的外观性状和外在的性质明显不同，鉴别内容及所用方法也有所不同。

The appearance and external properties of Chinese medicinal materials, Chinese medicine decoction pieces, Chinese medicine extract and Chinese medicinal preparations are obviously different, the contents and methods of identification are also different.

（一）中药材和中药饮片
1. Chinese Medicinal Materials and Chinese Medicine Decoction Pieces

中药材和中药饮片的性状鉴别属于经验鉴别，即通过感观等途径，观察其外观性状特征来鉴别其真伪。性状鉴别的内容主要包括形状、大小、色泽、表面、断面、质地、气和味等内容。此外，中药饮片还需注意净度、粉碎粒度等质量评价指标。

The identification of Chinese medicinal materials and Chinese medicinal decoction pieces belongs to empirical identification, that is, through the way of perception, observe its appearance characteristics to identify its authenticity. Including shape, size, color, surface, section, texture, odor and taste. In addition, attention should be paid to the quality evaluation indexes such as the clarity and particle size of Chinese medicine decoction pieces.

《中国药典》中收载有典型样品性状特征描述的，可参照鉴别；条件允许时应与对照药材作比较。需要注意的是中药的外部形态也可因产地、加工炮制方法的不同而有一些改变，有些药材的野生品和栽培品有较大差异，新鲜药材与干燥药材也有区别，因此可结合显微及理化的方法予以鉴定。

Refer to the description of the characteristics of typical samples contained in the *Chinese Pharmacopoeia* can be identified by reference; comparison should be made with reference materials when conditions permit. It should be noted that the external form of traditional Chinese medicine may also vary depending on the origin and processing methods. Some wild and cultivated herbs are quite different. Fresh and dried herbs are also different. Combining microscopy and physical and chemical methods to identify.

（二）中药提取物

### 2. Chinese Medicine Extracts

中药提取物除了需要依据形状、颜色、气味等性状特征外，还可通过测定某些物理常数作为鉴别的依据。物理常数包括相对密度、馏程、熔点、凝点、旋光度或比旋度、折光率、黏度、吸收系数、碘值、皂化值和酸值等。

In addition to the characteristics of shape, color, odor, taste and other characteristics of Chinese medicine extracts, some physical constants are often used as the basis for identification. Physical constants include relative density, distillation range, melting point, freezing point, optical rotation or specific rotation, refractive index, viscosity, absorption coefficient, iodine value, saponification value and acid value.

（三）中药制剂

### 3. Chinese Medicine Preparations

中药制剂的性状是指除去包装后，对药品颜色和外表的感官描述，主要内容包括颜色、形态、大小、形状、气、味、表面特征、质地等。一种制剂的性状往往与所投原料的质量及制剂的生产工艺有关，原料质量保证、制剂工艺稳定，则成品的性状应该基本一致，但药品内在质量发生变化时往往也会引起其外观性状的改变，故中药制剂的性状鉴别能初步反映其质量状况。此外制剂的某些物理常数也可以作为性状鉴别的指标，如熔点、溶解度、相对密度、折光率等。

The trait of Chinese medicine preparations refers to the sensory description of the color and appearance of the medicine after removing the pack. The main contents include the appearance of the preparation and the color, morphology, size, shape, odor, taste, surface characteristics, texture, etc. of the preparation. The appearance of a preparation are often related to the quality of the raw materials and the production process. When the quality of the raw materials is guaranteed and the preparation process is stable, the appearance of the finished product should be basically identical. But the internal quality of a medicine changes, its appearance is often changed. Therefore, the trait identification of the traditional Chinese medicine preparation can initially reflect its quality. In addition, certain physical constants of the preparation can also be used as indicators of trait identification, such as melting point, solubility, relative density, refractive index, etc.

## 二、常用的性状描述
### 3.1.2 Common Trait Descriptions

（一）中药材和中药饮片的性状描述

### 1. Common Trait Descriptions of Chinese Medicinal Materials and Chinese Medicine Decoction Pieces

中药材经过栽培或迁移后性状发生变异，但质量仍符合药用要求，要对栽培药材性状进行描述。饮片在加工过程中经过切制或加入不同辅料，炮制药材的形状、大小、颜色甚至气味可能改变，故饮片鉴别时应结合完整药材的特征，如横切面、表面和气味进行识别。

After cultivation or migration, the appearance of Chinese medicinal materials is changed, but the quality still meets the medicinal requirements. The appearance of the cultivated Chinese medicinal materials should be described. The processed pieces are cut or added with different auxiliary materials during processing, the shape, size, colour and even odor and taste of the processed materials may change. Therefore, the identification of the decoction pieces should be based on the characteristics of the complete Chinese medicinal materials, such as cross-section, surface, odor and taste.

黄柏药材：本品呈板片状或浅槽状，长宽不一，厚1~6mm。外表面黄色或黄棕色，平坦或具纵沟纹，有的可见皮孔痕及残存的灰褐色粗皮；内表面暗黄色或淡棕色，具细密的纵棱纹。体轻，质硬，断面纤维性，呈裂片状分层，深黄色。气微，味极苦，嚼之有黏性。黄柏饮片：本品呈丝条状。外表面黄褐色或黄棕色。内表面暗黄色或淡棕色，具纵棱纹。切面纤维性，呈裂片状分层，深黄色。味极苦。

Phellodendri Chinensis Cortex: This product is plate-like or shallow groove-shaped, with different length and width, thickness 1-6mm. The outer surface is yellow or yellow-brown, flat or with longitudinal grooves, and some pore marks and residual gray-brown rough skin are visible; the inner surface is dark yellow or light brown with fine longitudinal ribs. Light body, hard, fibrous in section, layered in lobes, dark yellow. Slightly qi, bitter taste, sticky to chew. Cork decoction pieces: This product is silk-like. The outer surface is yellow-brown or yellow-brown. The inner surface is dark yellow or light brown with longitudinal ribs. The cut surface is fibrous, with lobes and layers, dark yellow. The taste is extremely bitter.

### （二）中药提取物的性状描述
### 2. Common Trait Descriptions of Chinese Medicine Extracts

中药提取物是指从中药材或饮片及其他药用植物中制得的挥发油和油脂、粗提物、有效部位、组分提取物和有效成分。其中，挥发油和油脂是指压榨或提取制成的油状提取物；粗提物是指以水或醇作为溶剂提取制成的流浸膏、浸膏或浸膏粉；有效部位、组分提取物是指含有一类或数类成分的有效部位或组分，其含量应达到50%以上；有效成分提取物是指有效成分含量达到90%以上的提取物。

Chinese medicine extracts refer to volatile oils and fats, crude extracts, effective parts, component extracts and active ingredients prepared from Chinese medicinal materials or decoction pieces and other medicinal plants. Among them, volatile oils and fats refer to oily extracts made by pressing or extraction; crude extracts refer to flow extracts, extracts or extract powders made by extraction with water or alcohol as solvents; effective parts, component extracts refer to the effective parts or components containing one or several types of ingredients, and its content should reach more than 50%; The active ingredient extract refers to the extract with the active ingredient content of more than 90%.

薄荷素油：本品为无色或淡黄色的澄清液体；有特殊清凉香气，味初辛、后凉。存放日久，色渐变深。本品与乙醇、三氯甲烷或乙醚能任意混溶。相对密度应为0.888~0.908。旋光度应为 –17°~–24°。折光率为1.456~1.466。

Peppermint Oil: This product is colorless or light yellow clear liquid; it has a special cool aroma, and has a cool and early taste. Long-term storage, deep color gradient. This product is miscible with ethanol, chloroform or ethyl ether. The relative density should be 0.888-0.908. The optical rotation should be –17°--24°. The refractive index is 1.456-1.466.

（三）中药制剂的性状描述

## 3. Common Trait Descriptions of Chinese Medicine Preparations

不同剂型的药品性状鉴别的主要特征不同，一般按照《中国药典》制剂通则项下对应剂型的要求及质量标准相关内容进行检验。

The main characteristics of trait identification are different in different formulation drugs, and the inspection is generally performed in accordance with general requirements of preparations and quality standards in the *Chinese Pharmacopoeia*.

（1）片剂　外观应完整光洁，色泽均匀，有适宜的硬度，无松片、裂片等现象。表面应无色斑或发霉等；断面各成分颜色应分布均匀，无杂质。包衣片除去包衣后的片芯也应符合质量标准的相关要求。如十一味参芪片：本品为糖衣或薄膜衣片，除去包衣后显棕褐色，气芳香，味微苦。

(1) Tablets　the appearance should be complete and smooth, uniform color and luster, suitable hardness, no loose tablets, cracks and other phenomena. The surface without stains or mold; the color of the components on the section should be evenly distributed and free of impurities. The core of the coated tablet after coating should also meet the relevant requirements of the quality standard. Such as Shiyiwei Shenqi Tablets: This product is sugar-coated or film-coated tablets. After removing the coating, brown, fragrant, slightly bitter.

（2）丸剂　外观应圆整，大小、色泽均匀，无粘连现象。蜜丸应细腻滋润，软硬适中。蜡丸表面应光滑无裂纹，丸内不得有蜡点和颗粒。滴丸剂表面无冷凝液黏附。若包糖衣或者薄膜衣，应描述去除包衣后丸芯的颜色及气味；若包药物衣（朱砂、氧化铁等），应先描述包衣的颜色，再描述去除包衣以后的颜色及气味。如梅花点舌丸：本品为朱红色的包衣水丸，除去包衣后，显棕黄色至棕色；气香，味苦、麻舌。

(2) Pills　The appearance should be round, size and the color should be uniform, no adhesion phenomenon. Honey pills should be delicate and moist, moderately soft and hard. The surface of the wax pills should be smooth and free of cracks, and there should be no wax drops or granules inside the pills. Cooling medium on the surface of dropping pills should be removed after preparation. If pills with sugarcoat or film-coated, the core color, odor and taste after removing the coating should be described; If pills with drug coating (cinnabar, iron oxide, etc.), the coating color should be described first, and then the core color, odor and taste after removing the coating should be described. Such as Meihua Dianshe Pills: This product is a vermilion-colored coated water pill. After removing the coating, it is brownish yellow to brown; it is fragrant, bitter and numb.

（3）注射剂　溶液型注射剂应澄明；乳状液型注射剂应稳定，不得有相分离现象；静脉用乳状液型注射液中乳滴的粒度 90% 应在 1μm 以下，不得有大于 5μm 的乳滴。

(3) Injection　Agueous solution for injections should be clear; emulsion for injections should be stable without phase separation; over 90% of the globules in the emulsion for intravenous injections should be less than 1μm, and none is greater than 5μm.

（4）糖浆剂　应为澄清的水溶液，在贮存期间不得有发霉、酸败、产生气体或其他变质现象，允许有少量摇之易散的沉淀。如小儿止咳糖浆：本品为红棕色的半透明黏稠液体；味甜。

(4) Syrup　It should be a clear aqueous solution. During the storage period, there must be no mold contamination, rancidity, gas or other deterioration, and a small amount of precipitate easily dispersed on shaking allowed. Such as Xiao'er Zhike Syrup: This product is a red-brown translucent viscous liquid; sweet taste.

（5）合剂　应为澄清的液体，在贮存期间不得有发霉、酸败、异物、变色、产生气体或其他变质现象，允许有少量摇之易散的沉淀。

(5) Mixture　It should be clear liquid. During the storage period, there must be no mold contamination, rancidity, foreign matters, color changing, gas or other deterioration, and a small amount of precipitate easily dispersed on shaking allowed.

（6）散剂　应干燥、疏松、混合均匀，色泽一致，无潮解和结块等现象。如六一散：本品为浅黄白色的粉末；具甘草甜味，手捻有润滑感。

(6) Powder　It should be dry, loose, mixed well, consistent color, no deliquescent and agglomeration. Such as Liuyi San: This product is a pale yellow-white powder; it has a sweet taste of licorice and has a lubricious feel when twisted by hand.

（7）颗粒剂　应干燥，颗粒均匀，色泽一致，无吸潮、结块、潮解等。如一清颗粒：本品为黄色的颗粒；味微甜、苦。

(7) Granules　It should be dry, uniform in partical size and color, no moisture absorption, agglomeration, deliquescence, etc. Such as Yiqing Granules: This product is yellow granules; slightly sweet and bitter.

（8）贴膏剂　膏料应涂布均匀，膏面应光洁，色泽一致，无脱膏、失黏现象；背衬面应平整、洁净、无漏膏现象。涂布中若使用有机溶剂的，必要时应检查残留溶剂。如红药贴膏：本品为淡红色片状橡胶膏；气芳香。

(8) Cataplasms　The plasters of cataplasms should be spread uniformly. while the surface should be smooth and clean, uniform in color, not unglued and not viscous. Backing liner should be smooth and clean, no leaking plaster. When organic solvents are used in spreading, residual solvents should be examined if necessary. Such as Hongyao Plaster: this product is a light red flake rubber paste; gas aroma.

### 三、物理常数的测定
### 3.1.3　Determination of Physical Constants

物理常数是鉴定中药质量的重要指标，其测定结果不仅对中药有鉴别意义，还可以反映中药的纯度。在药品质量标准中物理常数，包括溶解度、相对密度、馏程、熔点、凝点、比旋度、折光率和 pH 等。如松节油相对密度应为 0.850~0.870；馏程为 154~165℃馏出的数量不得少于90.0%（ml/ml）；折光率应为 1.466~1.477。牡荆油胶丸取含量测定项下的挥发油，依法测定折光率应为 1.485~1.500。

The physical constants are important index for identifying the quality of traditional Chinese medicine, and its measurement results not only have identification significance for traditional Chinese medicine, but also reflect its purity. Physical constants in pharmaceutical quality standards include solubility, relative density, distillation range, melting point, freezing point, specific rotation, refractive index and pH value. Such as the relative density of Turpentine Oil should be 0.850-0.870; Distillation range is 154-165℃, and the amount of distillation should not be less than 90.0% (ml /ml); the refractive index should be 1.466-1.477. The refractive index of volatile oil should be determined use the volatile oil in determination item of Mujingyou gum pills, should be 1.485-1.500.

## 第二节　显微鉴别
## 3.2　Microscopic Identification

PPT

　　显微鉴别是利用显微镜对药材或饮片切片、粉末、解离组织或表面制片及含饮片粉末的制剂中饮片的组织、细胞或内含物等特征进行鉴别的一种方法，以鉴别中药的真伪。适用于中药性状鉴别不易识别或者性状相似及粉末入药的中药制剂，尤其适合粉末入药的中药制剂中化学成分不清楚或尚无化学鉴别方法的药味。显微鉴别操作简便，耗费少，专属性强。

Microscopical identification is a method with the application of the microscope to identify the characters of tissues, cells or cell contents in sections, powders, disintegrated tissues or surface slides of decoction pieces of crude drugs and dosage forms including powders of prepared slices of crude drugs. It is used in identification the authenticity of traditional Chinese medicine. Microscopic identification is suitable for traditional Chinese medicine with similar appearance or difficult to identify authenticity using trait identification and Chinese medicinal preparations containing decoction pieces power, especially suitable for Chinese medicinal preparations containing decoction pieces power with unclear chemical composition or without chemical identification methods. Microscopic identification has the advantages of easy operation, and low cost, strong specificity.

### 一、特点
### 3.2.1　Characteristics

　　中药制剂的显微鉴别与单味药材相比要复杂得多。这是由于中药制剂一般多由两味以上中药饮片制备而成，可能存在几种药味具有相似的显微特征；或者由于制备方法的影响，一些在药材中易检出的显微特征在制剂中会消失或难以检出。因此，在对复方制剂进行显微鉴别时，应首先了解制剂处方及制法，明确相关原料的药用部位及其显微特征。然后，选取该复方制剂中各药味明显易查，且专属性强的特征进行鉴别。如六味地黄丸中的牡丹皮的显微鉴别选择草酸钙簇晶作为鉴别依据，而归勺地黄丸中的牡丹皮的显微鉴别则采用了淡红色至微紫色的长方形木栓细胞作为鉴别特征。即在不同的中药制剂中，对同一药味的鉴别选取了不同的显微特征。又如大黄药材粉末的显微鉴别特征是导管和草酸钙结晶，而在牛黄解毒丸中，因制剂加工时导管被破坏，因而只选择草酸钙簇晶作为鉴别依据。

Microscopic identification of traditional Chinese medicine preparations is much more complicated than that of single Chinese medicines. This is because traditional Chinese medicine preparations are usually prepared from two or more Chinese herbal pieces. There may be several kinds of medicine with similar microscopic characteristics; or due to the influence of the preparation method, some microscopic characteristics that are easily detectable in medicinal materials disappear or be difficult to detect in the preparation. Therefore, in the microscopic identification of compound preparations, the prescription and preparation method should be understood first, and the medicinal parts of the relevant raw materials and their microscopic characteristics should be clarified. Then, selecting Chinese medicine materials with obvious the microscopic characteristics and strong specificity to identify. For example, the microscopic identification of Moutan Cortex in Liuwei Dihuang Pills, calcium oxalate cluster crystals as the basis for identification, and the microscopic identification of Moutan Cortex in Guishao Dihuang Pills, rectangular pale-red to purplish cork cells as the identifying feature. That is, in different Chinese medicine preparations, different microscopic characteristics are selected for the identification of the same single Chinese medicines. Another example, microscopic identification feature of Rhei Radix et Rhizoma is the catheter and calcium oxalate crystals. In Niuhuang Jiedu Pill, because the catheter is destroyed during the preparation process, only calcium oxalate cluster crystals are used as the basis for identification.

## 二、制片方法
## 3.2.2　Microscopical Slides Preparation Methods

### （一）中药材、饮片
### 1. Chinese Medicinal Materials and Decoction Pieces

中药材的显微制片方法繁多，可分为切片法和非切片法。切片法是指利用切片刀徒手或借助特定的机械设备将材料切成一定厚度的薄片，适合对微细结构进行观察，且对比明显。对于根、茎、叶、皮等药材，可直接制作横切片观察；果实、种子类药材需制作横切片和纵切片观察；而木类药材需观察三维切片（横切、径向纵切，切向纵切）。非切片法则是利用物理或化学的方法将材料组织分离成单个细胞或薄片，或将整个材料进行整体封藏。该方法可以确保药材组织器官的原有状态及其完整性，主要包括整体封藏法、粉末制片法、表面制片法、磨片法等。

There are many methods for microsopical slides of Chinese medicinal materials. They can be divided into slice method and non-slice method. The slicing method refers to the use of a slicing knife to cut the material into thin slices with hand or with the specific mechanical equipment. It is suitable for observing fine structures, and the contrast is obvious. For root, stem, leaf, bark and other medicinal materials, you can directly make transverse sections observation; fruit and seed medicinal materials need to be made transverse sections and longitudinal slice observation; while wood-type medicinal materials need to be observed in three-dimensional slices (transverse, diametral longitudinal, tangential longitudinal). Non-slicing method is the use of physical or chemical methods to separate material tissue into individual cells or slices, or to seal the entire material as a whole. This method can protect the original state and integrity of medicinal materials, tissues and organs, and mainly includes the whole sealing method, slide of powder method, slide of surface method, and slide of ground method.

中药饮片的制片方法与中药材的制片方法相同，但炮制后的中药饮片，由于已进行了净选和切制处理，比如分离不同的药用部位，或除去非药用部位，故植物药的部分组织已不完整。如根类药材地骨皮，属根皮入药，炮制时需去除木质心，故镜检中不应有木质部位组织细胞存在。另外，经特殊炮制工艺加工而成的饮片，经长时间的蒸制后，又常经"整形"处理，故切片后的组织结构、细胞特征及其排列已非正常，如熟地黄应与生饮片作相应的对照鉴别。

The microscopical slides preparation method of Chinese medicine decoction pieces is the same as that of Chinese medicinal materials, but the processed Chinese medicine decoction pieces have been cleaned and cut, such as separating different medicinal parts or removing non-medicinal parts, so the plant some tissues of the drug are incomplete. For example, Lycii Cortex belongs to the root bark. The woody core must be removed during processing. Therefore, there should be no tissue cells of the xylem during microscopy. In addition, the decoction pieces processed through a special processing technology are often subjected to "shaping" treatment after long-time steaming, so the tissue structure, cell characteristics and arrangement of cells are abnormal, such as Radix Rehmanniae Preparata. It should be identified with the corresponding raw pieces.

（二）中药制剂

## 2. Chinese Medicine Preparations

中药制剂的制片方法与中药材（饮片）的制片方法不尽相同。散剂和胶囊剂可直接取适量粉末（内容物为颗粒状，应研细）装片或适当透化后装片；片剂取 2~3 片，水丸、糊丸、水蜜丸、锭剂等取数丸或 1~2 锭（包衣者除去包衣）分别置于乳钵中磨成粉末，取适量装片；蜜丸可先加水搅拌洗涤，离心后取沉淀物装片。

The method of slides of preparation of traditional Chinese medicine preparations is not the same as the Chinese medicinal materials and decoction pieces. Powders and capsules can be directly taken from an appropriate amount of powder (the contents are granular and should be finely ground) or proper permeabilization; tablets are taken from 2-3 tablets, watered pills, pasted pills water, honeyed pills, troches, etc., put a few pills or 1-2 troches (coater removes the coating) into a mortar and grind them into powder, then take an appropriate amount of powder; honeyed pills add water, stir, and centrifuge, take precipitate to make microscopical slides.

若观察细胞内含物，应选用不同试剂装片。例如，观察淀粉粒用水或甘油醋酸试液，糊粉粒用甘油；水溶性内含物用乙醇或水合氯醛试液。

If the contents of cells are to be observed, different reagents should be used for slides. For example, observe starch granules with water or glycerol-acetic acid TS, aleurone granules with glycerol; water-soluble contents with ethanol or chloral hydrate TS.

## 三、应用实例
## 3.2.3 Application Examples

例 3-1 龙胆泻肝丸的显微鉴别

Example 3-1 Longdan Xiegan Pills

【处方】龙胆 120g 柴胡 120g 黄芩 60g 栀子（炒）60g 泽泻 120g 木通 60g 盐车前子 60g 酒当归 60g 地黄 120g 炙甘草 60g

**Ingredients** Gentianae Radix et Rhizoma 120g; Bupleuri Radix 120g; Scutellariae Radix 60g; Gardeniae Fructus (stir-baked) 60g; Alismatis Rhizoma 120g; Akebiae Caulis 60g; Plantaginis Semen (stir-baked with salt) 60g; Angelicae Sinensis Radix (stir-baked with wine) 60g; Rehmanniae Radix 120g; Glycyrrhizae Radix et Rhizoma Curm Melle 60g.

【制法】以上十味，粉碎成细粉，过筛，混匀，用水泛丸，干燥，即得。

**Procedure** Pulverize the above ten ingredients to fine powder, sift and mix well. Make pills with water and dry.

【鉴别】取本品，置显微镜下观察：纤维素周围薄壁细胞含草酸钙方晶，形成晶纤维（炙甘草）。韧皮纤维淡黄色，梭形，壁厚，孔沟细（黄芩）。种皮石细胞淡黄色或淡棕，多破碎，完整者长多角形、长方形或形状不规则，壁厚，有大的圆形纹孔，胞腔棕红色（栀子）。薄壁细胞类圆形，有椭圆形纹孔，集成纹孔群；内皮层细胞垂周壁波状弯曲，较厚，木化，有稀疏细孔沟（泽泻）。种皮内表皮细胞表面观类长方形，壁微波状，以数个细胞为一组，略作镶嵌状排列（盐车前子）。薄壁组织淡灰棕色至黑棕色，细胞多皱缩，内含棕色核状物（地黄）。油管含淡黄色或黄棕色条状分泌物，直径 8~25μm（柴胡）。

**Identification**   Microscopical: Fibre bundles surrounded by parenchymatous cells containing prisms of calcium oxalate, forming crystal fibres (Glycyrrhizae Radix et Rhizoma Preaparaca Cum Melle). Fibres pale yellow, fusiform, with thickened walls and fine pit-canals (Scutellariae Radix). Stone cells of testa yellow or brownish, mostly broken, the whole ones elongated polygonal, rectangular or irregular, with thicked walls and large rounded pits, lumina brownish-red (Gardeniae Fructus). Parenchymatous cells subrounded, with elliptical pits gathered into pit groups the anticlinical walls of the endodermis cell sinuous, thickened, lingnified, with slender pit-canals (Alismatis Rhizoma). Hypodermal cells of testa narrow and long in surface view, walls slightly sinuous, several cells arranged in a group and somewhat parqueted (Plantaginis Semen, stir-baked with salt). Parenchyma greyish-brown to blackish-brown, cells mostly shrunken, and each containing a nucleus-like mass (Rehmanniae Radix). Vittae containing yellow or brownish-yellow strip secretion, 8-25μm in diameter (Bupleuri Radix).

### 四、显微化学鉴别法
### 3.2.4   Microscopic and Chemical Identification Methods

显微化学鉴别法是利用显微镜，观察试剂与中药的目标成分产生沉淀、结晶、颜色等特殊变化的反应，或通过检查中药的细胞壁或细胞内含物的化学物质的性质，达到鉴别真伪的目的，包括显微化学反应和显微组织化学定位。

The microscopic and chemical identification method refers to observing precipitation, crystals, color or special changes produced the reagent and target components of traditional Chinese medicine, or to check the nature of chemical substances in the cell wall or cell contents of traditional Chinese medicine by microscope to identify the authenticity of traditional Chinese medicine, Including microscopic and chemical reaction and microscopic histochemical localization.

（一）显微化学反应

### 1.  Microscopic and  Chemical  Reaction

显微化学反应是将中药粉末、切片、升华物或浸出液少量，置于载玻片上，滴加适宜的化学试剂使产生沉淀、结晶或特殊的颜色，在显微镜下观察化学反应结果，以此鉴别中药真伪。此法简便、快速，需用的样品和试剂量少。当中药供试样品数量较少且某些化学反应灵敏度高时，可采用显微化学鉴别法。

The microscopic and chemical reaction refers to putting a small amount of Chinese medicine powder, slices, sublimates or extracts on a glass slide, and add appropriate chemical reagents to cause precipitation, crystals or special colors. Observe the results of the chemical reaction under a microscope to identify the authenticity of Chinese medicine. This method is simple, fast, and requires a small amount of samples and reagents. When the number of Chinese medicines to be tested is small and the sensitivity of some chemical reactions is high, microscopic and chemical reaction can be used.

例 3-2   天麻的显微化学鉴别

Example 3-2   Identification of Gastrodiae Rhizoma

【鉴别】将粉末用醋酸甘油水装片，置显微镜下观察，可见含糊化多糖类物的薄壁细胞无色，有的细胞可见长卵形、长椭圆形或类圆形颗粒；滴加碘试液，显棕色或淡棕紫色。

**Identification**   When powder mounted in glycerin-acetic acid TS, parenchymatous cells containing gelatinized polysaccharides colorless, and some cells containing long-ovoid, long-ellipsoid or subrounded granules, showing a brown or brownish-purple color on adding iodine solution.

（二）显微组织化学定位

## 2. Microscopic Histochemical Localization

显微组织化学定位是指在中药有效成分明确的情况下，选择对有效成分具有特殊反应的化学试剂，使产生结晶或特殊颜色，用显微镜确定有效成分的存在部位。也可用于细胞壁和细胞内含物的性质鉴别。

The microscopic histochemical localization refers to the selection of chemical reagents that have a special reaction to the active ingredient when the active ingredient of the Chinese medicine is clear, so that crystals or special colors are produced, and the existence of the active ingredient is determined in different parts of Chinese medicine with a microscope. It can also be used to identify the properties of cell walls and cell contents.

## 第三节　理化鉴别

## 3.3　Physicochemical Identification

PPT

理化鉴别是根据中药中所含某些化学成分或成分群的理化特征，利用化学反应法、光谱法、色谱法等分析方法和技术检测中药中的某些成分，判断其真伪。常用的方法有：化学反应鉴别法、光谱鉴别法、色谱鉴别法、指纹图谱及特征图谱鉴别技术等。

The physicochemical identification refers to detecting certain ingredients in traditional Chinese medicine to identify of the authenticity of TCM based on the property of chemical components in traditional Chinese medicine by chemical reaction, spectral method, chromatographic method and so on. The commonly used methods are identification method based on reaction, spectral identification, chromatographic identification, fingerprint or characteristic chromatogram technology.

中药化学成分复杂，特别是中药复方制剂，在对处方中的每味药逐一鉴别有困难时，应进行处方分析，首选君药（主药）、臣药（辅药）、毒剧药及贵重药等，并根据待测定成分的结构性质及共存干扰物情况，建立专属性强、灵敏度高的鉴别方法。其他药味的选择应根据该药味的研究情况而定。

The chemical composition of traditional Chinese medicine is complicated, especially the traditional Chinese medicine compound preparation. When it is difficult to identify each medicine in the prescription one by one, prescription analysis should be performed, firstly, monarch drug (main medicine), minister medicine (auxiliary medicine), poisonous medicine and precious medicine, etc. are preferred, based on the structural properties of the components to be determined and the situation of coexisting interferences, an identification method with strong specificity, high sensitivity is established. The choice of other medicine should be based on itself research.

一、化学反应鉴别法

## 3.3.1　Chemical Reaction Identification Methods

中药中含有各类不同结构特征的化学成分，可与某些特定试剂发生化学反应，产生颜色变化、生成沉淀等现象，以此判断该药味或者某成分（群）的存在与否，鉴别其真伪。如：生物碱与碘化铋钾等生物碱沉淀试剂的反应；羟基蒽醌类与碱液的反应；黄酮类与盐酸–镁粉的反应；香豆素等内酯类化合物与异羟肟酸铁的反应；鞣质的明胶沉淀反应；氨基酸与茚三酮的反应；糖类的苯酚–硫酸反应等。

Traditional Chinese medicine contains various types of chemical components with different structural characteristics, which can react with certain specific reagents to produce color changes, precipitation, etc., they are used to determine the existence of the specific drug or a certain component (group), identify the authenticity of traditional Chinese medicine. Such as: the reaction of alkaloids with alkaloid precipitation reagents such as bismuth potassium iodide; the reaction of hydroxyanthraquinones with lye; the reaction of flavones with hydrochloric acid-magnesium powder; the reaction of lactones with hydroxamic acid iron; reaction of amino acid and ninhydrin; reaction of phenol-sulfuric acid and sugars, etc.

由于中药中化学成分复杂，干扰成分多，而中药的化学反应鉴别法多数基于官能团的反应，因此，专属性不强。为了提高其专属性：①慎用专属性不强的化学反应；②分析前对样品进行必要的纯化；③供试品溶液的颜色较深时可采用空白试验，进行对比；④采用阳性对照和阴性对照，提高反应结果判断的准确性。

Due to the complex the chemical compositions and the numerous interference components in Chinese medicine, the many chemical reaction identification methods in traditional Chinese medicine analysis are based on the reaction of functional groups, so the specificity is not strong. In order to improve the reliability and specificity of chemical reaction identification in TCM analysis, ① use weakly specific chemical reactions with caution; ② purify the sample before analysis if necessary; ③ use a blank test for comparison when the color of the sample solution is dark; ④ use positive controls negative control, improve the accuracy of judgment of reaction results.

例 3-3　麻黄的鉴别

Example 3-3　Identification of Ephedrae Herba

【鉴别】取本品粉末 0.2g，加水 5ml 与稀盐酸 1~2 滴，煮沸 2~3 分钟，滤过。滤液置分液漏斗中，加氨试液数滴使呈碱性，再加三氯甲烷 5ml，振摇提取。分取三氯甲烷液，置两支试管中，一管加氨制氯化铜试液与二硫化碳各 5 滴，振摇，静置，三氯甲烷层显深黄色；另一管为空白，以三氯甲烷 5 滴代替二硫化碳 5 滴，振摇后三氯甲烷层无色或显微黄色。（鉴别麻黄中以麻黄碱为主的生物碱类成分）

**Identification**　To 0.2g of the powder, add 5ml of water and 1-2 drops of dilute hydrochloric acid, boil for 2-3 minutes and filter. Place the filtrate in the separation funnel, and a few drops of ammonia solution be added to make it alkaline. Then add 5ml of trichloromethane and shake to extract the filtrate. Trichloromethane liquid is separated and placed in two tubes, one tube is added with ammoniated cupric chloride TS and carbon disulfide, 5 drops of each. After shaking and standing, the trichloromethane layer will be dark yellow. The other tube is blank, with 5 drops of trichloromethane instead of 5 drops of carbon disulfide. After shaking, the trichloromethane layer is colorless or slightly yellow. (Identify the alkaloids in Ephedrae Herba such as ephedrine.)

## 二、微量升华法
## 3.3.2　Microsublimation Methods

微量升华法是利用中药中所含成分的升华性对其进行鉴别的方法。此法简单、快速，需用的

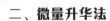

样品和试剂量少；当中药中存在具有升华性质的化学成分时，可采用微量升华法。通常将制备的升华物在显微镜下观察晶型，在可见光下观察颜色，在紫外灯下观察荧光，或加入合适的试液或试剂与其发生显色反应或荧光反应等。

The microsublimation method is a method of identifying the traditional Chinese medicine based on sublimation properties of the ingredients contained in traditional Chinese medicine. This method is simple, fast, and requires a small amount of samples and reagents. When there are chemical components with sublimation properties in traditional Chinese medicine, microsublimation method can be used. Usually, the prepared sublimate is observed under the microscope for the crystal form, the color is observed under visible light, the fluorescence is observed under ultraviolet light, or a suitable test solution or reagent is added to cause a color reaction or fluorescence reaction to occur.

例 3-4　安息香的鉴别

Example 3-4　Identification of Benzoinum

【鉴别】取本品约 0.25g，置干燥试管中，缓缓加热，即发生刺激性香气，并产生多数棱柱状结晶的升华物。（鉴别芳香酸类成分）

**Identification**　Take about 0.25g, place it in a dry test tube, and slowly heat it, which will produce irritant aromatic odor and most prismatic crystalline sublimates. (Identification of aromatic acids)

### 三、光谱鉴别法
### 3.3.3　Spectral Identification Methods

中药的光谱鉴别是利用中药中所含成分的光谱特性，判断中药真伪的分析方法。光谱鉴别法操作简单、样品用量少、检测速度快、信息量大，一定程度上可以得到反映中药整体特征的信息。但是由于中药化学成分的复杂性，所得光谱的专属性和特征性不强，因此经典光谱鉴别在中药鉴别中的应用受到限制。随着光谱技术与化学计量学等学科的交叉融合，使光谱法在中药分析中的有效作用得到了一定的发展和突破。目前用于中药鉴别的光谱法主要有荧光法（FS）、紫外 – 可见光谱法（UV-Vis）、红外光谱法（IR）、X- 射线衍射法（XRD）等。

Spectral identification of traditional Chinese medicine is a method of identifying based on spectral characteristics of the ingredients contained in traditional Chinese medicine, to identify the authenticity of traditional Chinese medicine. With simple operation, less sample consumption, fast detection speed and large amount of information, spectral method can obtain the informations reflecting the overall characteristics of TCM to a certain extent. However, due to the complexity of the chemical compositions of TCM, the specificity and characteristics of the obtained spectra are not strong. Therefore, the classical spectral method has not been widely used in identification of TCM. With the cross fusion of spectroscopy and chemometrics, the effective role of spectroscopy in the analysis of TCM has been developed and made a certain breakthrough. In recent years, the main spectral methods used for the identification of TCM include fluorescence (FS) method, Ultraviolet-visible spectrometry (UV-Vis) method, infrared spectroscopy (IR) method, X-ray diffraction (XRD) method, etc.

（一）荧光法

### 1. Fluorescence (FS) Methods

中药中的某些化学成分或其衍生物，在可见、紫外光照射下能产生荧光，其荧光颜色可以作为中药鉴别的依据。荧光法具有灵敏度高、选择性好、样品用量少、方法快捷等优点。但干扰因素多，应用具有一定的局限性。

Some chemical components or their derivatives of TCM can produce fluorescence under visible and ultraviolet light, and the fluorescence color can be used as the basis for identification. Fluorescence method has the advantages of high sensitivity, good selectivity, less sample consumption, fast detection speed, etc. But fluorescence is affected many interference factors, has not been widely used in identification of TCM certain limitation.

荧光法主要有两种，一是直接荧光法，适于自身能产生荧光的成分；另一种是间接荧光法，有些化合物自身不具有荧光，但经衍生化处理后（如经酸、碱或其他化学方法处理），能产生荧光。

Two kinds of fluorescence methods can be used. One is direct fluorescence method, which is suitable for components that can produce fluorescence by themselves. The other is indirect fluorescence, that mean some compounds do not have fluorescence on their own, but can produce fluorescence after derivatization, such as acidize, alkalify or other chemical treatment.

鉴别时，通常将中药的供试品溶液滴在滤纸或白瓷板上，置紫外灯下（365nm 或 254nm）观察，甚至有些在日光下也可观察到，如秦皮的水浸出液在日光下可见碧蓝色荧光。少数中药材也可直接取饮片、断面或粉末进行荧光鉴别。如黄连饮片显金黄色荧光；川牛膝饮片显淡蓝色荧光；怀牛膝饮片显黄白色荧光；麦冬薄切片显浅蓝色荧光；牛蒡子显蓝白色荧光；大黄粉末显深棕色荧光；浙贝母粉末显亮淡绿色荧光等。甚至还可利用显微镜观察荧光，判断化学成分存在的部位，如黄连饮片木质部的金黄色荧光尤为显著，说明木质部中小檗碱含量较高。

Usually, test solution of TCM is placed on filter paper or white porcelain plate, and observed the color of under ultraviolet lamp (365nm or 254nm). Some of them can even be observed in sunlight. For example, the water leach liquor of Fraxini cortex appear blue fluorescent in sunlight. A few Chinese medicine can also be taken fluorescence identification directly with pieces, section or powder. Such as Coptidis Rhizoma slices shows golden yellow fluorescence; Achyranthis bidentatae Radix slices shows yellow and white fluorescence; Cyathulae Radix slices shows light blue fluorescence; Ophiopogonis Radix in thin slice shows light blue fluorescence; Arctii Fructus shows blue-white fluorescence; Rhubarb powder shows dark brown fluorescence; Fritillariae thunbergii bulbus powder shows bright light green fluorescence. The fluorescence can even be observed under a microscope to determine where the chemical components exist, such as the xylem of Coptidis Rhizoma slices, where the golden yellow fluorescence is particularly significant, indicating that the content of berberine in the xylem is relatively high.

例 3-5　地枫皮的鉴别

Example 3-5　Identification of Illicii Cortex

【鉴别】取本品粗粉 2g，加三氯甲烷 5ml，振摇，浸渍 30 分钟，滤过。取滤液点于滤纸上，干后置紫外光灯（254nm）下观察，显猩红色至淡猩红色荧光。

**Identification**　Take 2g of the powder, add 5ml of trichloromethane, shake, steeping for 30 minutes, filter. Spot the filtrate to filter paper, and observe scarlet to slight scarlet fluorescence under the uv lamp (254nm) after drying.

（二）紫外－可见光谱法

## 2. Ultraviolet-Visible Spectrometry (UV-Vis) Methods

中药中常含具有共轭双键或芳香环等不饱和结构的化合物，在紫外－可见光区有选择性吸收，产生特征吸收光谱，可用于鉴别。紫外－可见光谱法具有操作简单、快速等优点，但光谱的特征性不强，常会遇到紫外光谱相似而成分不同的现象，如红景天苷与酪醇的紫外吸收光谱就非常相似，难以区别，尤其中药中成分复杂，干扰物质多，得到的谱图信息为诸多成分叠加而成，专属性和特征性较差。因此，需要一种合适且稳定的样品溶液制备方法，以有效地提高所获得光谱图的特性和特异性。除非另有说明，否则用于制备样品溶液的同一批溶剂应用作测定中的空白对照。

Compounds with unsaturated structures such as conjugated double bonds or aromatic rings often contained in TCM, which have selectively absorbed in UV-Vis region and generate characteristic absorption spectra can be used for identification. UV-Vis spectrometry has the advantages of simple operation and rapid, but the characteristic of spectrum are not strong and often faced the phenomenon of different ingredients with similar spectrograms. Such as the ultraviolet absorption spectrum of salidroside is very similar with tyrosol, and difficult to distinguish. Especially the spectra information of TCM geted are the superposition of spectrometry of many components because the complicated composition and interfering substance, so with poor characteristic and specificity. Therefore, a suitable and stable preparation method of sample solution is necessary to effectively improve the characteristic and specificity of the obtained spectrogram. Unless otherwise specified, the same batch of solvent used to prepare the sample solution shall be used as blank control in the determination. Common methods are as follows.

1. 规定吸收波长法　样品经规定方法处理后测定其吸收光谱，在规定波长处应有最大吸收。《中国药典》规定以最大吸收波长（$\lambda_{max}$）作为鉴别参数，样品应在规定波长 ±2nm 内有最大吸收。

(1) Specified absorption wavelength method　The absorption spectrum shall be measured after the sample being processed by the prescribed method, and the maximum absorption shall be at the specified wavelength. The *Chinese Pharmacopoeia* stipulates that the maximum absorption wavelength ($\lambda_{max}$) shall be used as the identification parameter. The maximum absorption of the sample shall be within ±2nm of the specified wavelength.

2. 对照品比较法　经规定方法处理并测定后，比较供试品与对照品或对照药材吸收光谱的一致性。

(2) Comparison of reference substance　To compare the consistency of absorption spectra between the samples and the reference substance or the reference herb after treatment and determination by prescribed methods.

3. 规定吸收波长和吸收度法　经规定方法处理并测定后，在所得吸收光谱中，样品在若干规定波长下应有相应的吸收峰及吸收强度值。

(3) Specified absorption wavelength and absorbance method　After treatment and determination by the specified method, the sample shall have corresponding absorption peaks and absorption intensity values at certain specified wavelengths in the obtained spectrogram.

4. 规定吸收波长和吸收度比值法　以规定波长下样品的吸收度比值是否达到规定范围做分析。此法也可同时采用对照品或对照药材作参照。

(4) Specified absorption wavelength and absorbance ratio method　Analyzing by the ratio of absorbance of samples whether reaches the specified range at specified wavelength. This method can also use reference substance or reference herb at the same time.

5. 多溶剂光谱法（紫外 – 可见光谱谱线组法）　对同一样品测定多种不同溶剂提取液的紫外光谱，通过综合比较其吸收差异，寻找吸收特征，可获得有参考价值的鉴别信息。

(5) Several different kinds of solvents spectrum (group method of ultraviolet spectrum) method　Determine the ultraviolet spectra of several different kinds of solvents extracts of the same sample. And through comprehensive comparison of their absorption differences to search for absorption

characteristics, can obtain valuable identification information.

例 3-6　阿魏的鉴别

Example 3-6　Identification of Ferulae Resina

【鉴别】取本品粉末 0.2g，置 25ml 量瓶中，加无水乙醇适量，超声处理 10 分钟，加无水乙醇稀释至刻度，摇匀，滤过，取滤液 0.2ml，置 50ml 量瓶中，加无水乙醇至刻度，摇匀。照紫外 – 可见分光光度法（《中国药典》通则 0401）测定。在 323nm 的波长处应有最大吸收。

**Identification**　Take 0.2g of the powder, put into a 25ml volumetric flask, add appropriate amount of anhydrous ethanol, ultrasonicate for 10 minutes, dilute with anhydrous ethanol to volume, shake well, filter, take 0.2ml of filtrate, put into a 50ml volumetric flask, add anhydrous ethanol to volume, shake well. Determination by UV-visible spectrophotometry (*Chinese Pharmacopoeia*, general chapters 0401). There should be maximum absorption at the wavelength of 323nm.

（三）红外光谱法

### 3. Infrared spectroscopy (IR)

红外光谱的特征性很强，特别是在"指纹区"。对于单体化合物来说，若样品与相同制样和测试条件下得到的对照品的光谱完全相同，或与某物质的标准图谱完全相同，便可以肯定是同一化合物。常用的标准图谱集有萨特勒红外标准图谱集、DMS 穿孔卡片、"API" 红外光谱数据。

The characteristics of IR are very strong, especially in the "fingerprint region". For a monomer compound, if the sample spectrogram is identical to the reference spectrogram under the same preparation and test conditions, or identical to the standard spectrogram of a substance, it is definitely the same compound. The commonly used standard spectrograms are the sadtler standard infrared spectroscopy atlas, DMS card with hole, and "API" infrared spectral data.

中药成分复杂，其红外光谱是各组分各基团吸收峰的叠加（分子间发生作用除外），吸收峰相互干扰，往往难以区分。此外，品种、产地、加工等的差异都会导致多组分体系的变化，从而导致所得红外光谱发生变化。但是只要中药中各成分相对稳定，样品处理方法一致，其红外光谱也会相对稳定，具有一定的特征性，借助于 IR 标准库或者计算机软件，可用于中药的真伪鉴别。红外光谱法具有特征性强、操作简便、快速、灵敏、样品用量少、不破坏样品等特点，广泛的用于贝母和六味地黄丸等中药的鉴别。

TCM contain complex components, so IR of them are the superposition of absorption peaks of various components and groups (except intermolecular interaction), and the absorption peaks interfere with each other, so often difficult to distinguish. In addition, the variety, origin, processing and other differences will lead to the change of absorption peak in IR spectrum. However, as long as the components of samples are relatively stable and the treatment methods are consistent, the IR spectrum will also be relatively stable, which has certain characteristics, can be used to identify the authenticity of traditional Chinese medicine with the help of IR standard database or computer software. IR is simple, fast, sensitive, less sample consumption and does not destroy the sample, widely used in the identification of traditional Chinese medicines such as Fritillaria and Liuwei Dihuang Pill.

近红外光谱技术可从未经处理的中药样本中直接获取鉴别信息，最大限度的保留样品的整体信息特点，即使是同种药材不同产地间的微小差异也可以体现出来。近年来，应用化学计量学方法，将反映样品结构或性质特点的近红外光谱信息，与标准方法测得的信息建立校正模型，达到快速预测样品组成或性质的分析方法得到认可，特别是大量样品的快速鉴别和水分测定。与中红外光谱相比，近红外光谱具有不破坏样品、重现性好、可在线分析等特点，该法除可以得到化合物组成和结构信息外，还可以得到如密度、粒子尺寸、大分子聚合度等一系列信息。对于中药的真伪鉴别、产地判断、有效成分定量分析均非常有效，可用于中药生产的在线检测，提高生产过程的可控性和产品的均一性。

Near infrared spectroscopy (NIR) technology can directly obtain the identification information from the untreated samples of TCM, so as to retain the overall information characteristics of the samples to the maximum extent, even the slight differences between different regions of the same medicinal materials can be reflected. In recent years, with the application of stoichiometric methods, the NIR information reflecting the structure or property characteristics of samples and the information measured by standard methods are banded together to establish a correction model, so as to achieve predicting the composition or property of samples rapidly, especially the rapid identification and moisture measurement of a large number of samples. Compared with the mid-infrared spectrum (MIR), the NIR has the characteristics of non-destructive sample, better reproducibility and on-line analysis, etc. Besides the information of compound composition and structure, the method can also obtain a series of information such as density, particle size and macromolecule polymerization degree. It is very effective for the authenticity identification, origin place judgment and quantitative analysis of effective components of TCM. NIR can be used for the online detection of TCM production to improve the controllability of production process and uniformity of products.

（四）X- 射线衍射法

## 4. X-ray diffraction (XRD) Methods

当某物质（晶体或非晶体）被 X 射线照射，产生不同程度的衍射现象时，会形成由该物质的组成、晶型、分子内成键方式、分子构型与构象等决定的特有衍射图谱。X 射线衍射法获得的图谱信息量大，指纹性强，样品用量少，且不破坏样品，特征信息能作为鉴别复杂体系的可靠依据。其中 X 射线衍射傅立叶指纹图谱，既能反映混合物质的整体结构特征，又能表现其局部变化，可根据衍射图谱的几何拓扑图形及特征标记峰值实现对混合物质的鉴别。

When substance (crystal or non-crystal) is irradiated by X-ray and produce different degrees of diffraction phenomenon, form special diffraction spectrum determined based on the composition, crystal form, intramolecular bonding mode, molecular configuration and conformation of the substance. XRD can obtain a large amount of information, with strong fingerprint, less sample consumption and do not damage the sample. The characteristic information of XRD can be used as a reliable basis for the identification of complex systems. Among them, X-ray diffraction Fourier fingerprint can reflect the overall structural characteristics of the mixture, and show its local changes, which can be used to identify mixed substances according to the geometric topological graph of the diffraction spectrum and the characteristic mark peak.

中药材由于所含组成、成分不同，被 X 射线照射，产生不同程度的衍射现象，产生特有的衍射图谱，可用于中药材的鉴别。中药制剂虽然成分复杂，所得衍射图是各成分衍射效应的叠加，但只要处方统一、生产工艺规范、原料药材合格的同一中药制剂，仍可获得特征相同的衍射图谱，与对照药材同法处理还可明确衍射峰的归属。不同的中药制剂因所含组成、成分不同，而产生特有的衍射图谱，以此实现对中药制剂的鉴别。

Chinese medicinal materials are irradiated by x-rays due to their different composition and ingredients, which produce different degrees of diffraction phenomena and unique diffraction patterns, which can be used to identify Chinese medicinal materials. Although the composition of traditional Chinese medicine preparations is complex, the obtained diffraction pattern is the superposition of the diffraction effects of each component. However, as long as the prescription is uniform, the production process is standardized, and Chinese medicinal materials is qualified, the same traditional Chinese medicine preparation can be obtain the same diffraction patterned. Treated in the same way as reference medicinal materials, the assignment of diffraction peaks can be clarified. Different traditional Chinese medicine preparations have unique diffraction patterns due to their different compositions and ingredients, so as to identify traditional Chinese medicine preparations.

### 四、色谱鉴别法
### 3.3.4　Chromatography Identification Methods

#### （一）纸色谱法
#### 1. Paper Chromatography Methods

纸色谱法是以滤纸为载体的分配色谱，适用于极性物质的分离。滤纸上所含水分或其他物质为固定相，用与水互不相溶的有机溶剂为流动相。用于中药的鉴别时，需要有对照物质（如对照品或对照药材）做参照，以斑点的位置与颜色作为判断鉴别结果的依据。鉴别时，供试品色谱中所显主斑点的位置、颜色（或荧光）应与对照物质在相应位置的斑点相同。纸色谱法操作简便、价格低廉，但其分离效果和重现性较差。除用于氨基酸等少数成分的分析外，纸色谱法已很少应用。

Paper chromatography (PC) is a partition chromatography, is suitable for separation of polar substances. filter paper is the carrier, the stationary phase is water or other substance in the filter paper, and the mobile phase is organic solvent that is not soluble with water. When PC is used to identify Chinses medicine, a reference substance (such as reference substance or reference Chinese medicinal materials) is required. The location and color of the spots are the basis of identification. When identifying, the test sample should have the same color (or fluorescent) spots as the reference substance in the corresponding position. PC is simple and inexpensive, but its separation effect and reproducibility are poor. Except for the analysis of a few components such as amino acids, PC has been rarely used.

#### （二）薄层色谱法
#### 2. Thin Layer Chromatography Methods

薄层色谱法是中药鉴别中最常用的方法。根据中药中所含待检成分的性质，采用适当的方法制备供试品溶液，选择适当的吸附剂和展开剂，与对照物（对照品、对照药材、对照提取物）点样在同一个板上，经展开、显色后，获得斑点清晰、$R_f$ 值稳定的色谱图。通过比较样品色谱应与对照物色谱在相应位置上，是否显相同颜色的斑点或主斑点来鉴别中药的真伪。

Thin layer chromatography (TLC) is the most commonly used method for the identification of TCM. Based on the nature of the components contained in TCM, using appropriate methods to prepare the sample solution, select the appropriate adsorbent and mobile phase. And the samples should be pointed with the reference (reference substance, reference herbs, reference extract) on the same plate. After developing and coloring, get chromatogram with clear spots and stable Rf. The sample chromatogram should show the same color spots in the corresponding position with the reference substance chromatogram.

TLC 既可用于定性鉴别，又可用于含量测定。其设备简单，样品用量少，方法专属性强、成本低、分析速度快，可选用的固定相种类较多（如硅胶、氧化铝、聚酰胺等），各种流动相及显色剂使用灵活，可同时分析比较多个样品，结果直观，灵活性强，是中药鉴别的首选方法。为了提高色谱的分离度和重现性，更好的达到分析效果和准确鉴别的目的，薄层色谱鉴别需要进行规范化操作。

TLC can be used for qualitative identification and content determination. Simple equipment, low sample consumption, strong method specificity, low cost, fast analysis speed, and the more types of stationary phase can be select (such as silica, alumina, polyamide, etc.). All kinds of mobile phase and visualization reagent are applicable. TLC can compare multiple samples at the same time, the results intuitive, with strong flexibility. TLC is the preferred method of TCM identification. In order to improve the separation and reproducibility, better to achieve the purpose of analysis and accurate identification, TLC identification requires standardization.

1. 操作方法

**(1) Operation Method**

（1）供试品溶液的制备　中药成分复杂，待测成分受其他未知"杂质"干扰，常常分离度差，甚至难以辨认。为了得到清晰的色谱结果，可采用一定的制备过程，使待检成分得到纯化富集。根据待检目标成分及干扰物质的性质，选用适宜的溶剂及方法进行提取纯化，并进行适当的浓缩富集。且最终用于点样的溶剂，黏度不宜太大，沸点不宜太高（如正丁醇）或太低（如乙醚），最常选用的是甲醇或乙醇。当然一般只要待检测的成分斑点分离度好、清晰可见即可，因此如果简单的制备就可以得到好的色谱结果，便无须繁杂的纯化过程。

① *Preparation of the Sample Solution*　The components of TCM are complicated and the components to be tested are disturbed by other unknown impurities, so the separation degree is often poor and even difficult to identify. In order to obtain clear chromatographic results, a certain preparation process can be used to purify and concentrate the components to be detected. The suitable solvent and method should be selected for extraction and purification according to the properties of tested composition and the interfering substances, and carry out appropriate concentration. And the final solvent for spotting, viscosity is unfavorable too high, boiling point is unfavorable too high (n-butanol) or too low (ethyl ether). The most often choose is methanol or ethanol. Of course, as long as the component to be detected has a good separation degree and can be clearly seen, so if simple preparation can get good chromatographic results, with no need for complicated purification process.

（2）对照物与对照方式的选择　薄层色谱法鉴别中药时，一般采用阳性对照、阴性对照和阴阳对照的方式。阳性对照采用的对照物有对照品、对照药材或对照提取物。阴性对照是为了验证薄层色谱法鉴别的专属性。在中药复方制剂的鉴别中必须采用阴阳对照方式。

② *Selection of Reference Substance and Reference Method*　in the identification of TCM by TLC, the methods of positive control, negative control and positive-negative control are generally adopted. The positive control uses the reference substance mainly are reference substance, reference herb or the reference extract. Negative control is used to verify the specificity of TLC identification. The positive-negative control method must be used in the identification of TCM compound preparations.

对照品对照：在薄层色谱法中确定的待检测成分，一般是中药中的某一有效成分或特征成分，以该成分的对照品作对照。样品应在相应位置上与对照品有相同颜色（荧光）的斑点。

Control based on reference substance, the component to be determined by TLC is usually an active component or characteristic component in TCM. The sample shall have spots of the same color (fluorescence) as the reference substance in the corresponding position.

阳性对照：将中药制剂中待检的某味药的对照药材按照与供试品溶液制备方法相同的方法，制备阳性对照溶液，并与样品溶液点样在同一薄层色谱板上，展开，显色，检视。样品应在相应位置上与对照药材有相同颜色（荧光）的主斑点。

Positive control, the reference herb is prepared in the same way as the preparation method of the sample solution, and expanded, colored and inspected on the same TLC plate as the sample. The sample should have the same color (fluorescent) main spots as the reference herb in the corresponding position.

对照品与对照药材同时对照：一般情况下选用对照品可满足薄层鉴别的需要，而有些情形需结合对照药材才能确定制剂的真实性。如：黄连和黄柏等多种植物均含有小檗碱，仅以小檗碱为对照不具有鉴别黄连的专属性，尤其在既含黄连又含黄柏的中药复方制剂中，无法确认投料的是黄连，还是黄柏甚至其他植物，此时可采用对照品与对照药材同时对照的方式，除对应鉴别小檗碱斑点的存在外，还应与黄连对照药材中除小檗碱以外的，与黄柏相区别的其他主斑点相比对，以提供鉴别黄连药材存在与否的专属性依据。

Control method based on reference substance and reference herb, In general, the reference substance can meet the needs of TLC identification, while in some cases, the authenticity of the preparation can be determined by combining with the reference herb. Such as Coptidis Rhizoma and Phellodendri Chinensis Cortex and so on the many kinds of plants are containing berberine. Berberine as the only reference substance can not make specificity identification of Coptidis Rhizoma, especially of compound preparation including Coptidis Rhizoma and Phellodendri Chinensis Cortex. It is unable to confirm the Coptidis Rhizoma or Phellodendri Chinensis Cortex even other plants be used in preparation. At this time, reference substance and reference herb can be used at the same time. Besides identifying the existence of berberine spots, also should be compared with other main spots of reference herb of Coptidis Rhizoma, in order to provide the identification of Coptidis Rhizoma existence specificity.

阴性对照：对于单味中药材、饮片或粉末，阴性对照其实就是供试品溶液的空白溶剂。对于中药复方制剂，阴性对照溶液的制备就尤为重要。在鉴别一个中药复方制剂中某味中药的存在时，除了制备供试品溶液和相应的阳性对照物溶液以外，还需要制备阴性对照溶液。即从中药制剂的处方中除去要鉴别的药味，其余各味药按该复方制剂的制法，制备阴性制剂，再将阴性制剂以与供试品溶液相同的制备方法，制备其阴性对照溶液。

Negative control, for single herb, medicinal slices or powder, negative control is the blank solvent of the sample solution in fact. For TCM compound preparation, the preparation of negative control solution is particularly important. In order to identify the existence of a kind of herb in a compound preparation, a negative control solution lacking this kind of herb should be prepared in addition to the preparation of the sample solution and the positive control solution. That is, according to the preparation process of the compound preparation, the negative preparation composed of other herbs but without this kind of herb was prepared, and then the negative control solution was prepared in the same preparation method as the sample solution.

阴阳对照：将供试品溶液、阳性对照溶液、阴性对照溶液点于同一薄层色谱板上，展开、显色、检视。供试品在相应位置上应与阳性对照物有相同颜色的斑点，为鉴别某味中药的存在与否提供依据；而阴性对照在相应位置应无干扰，以确定该鉴别方法的专属性。采用阴阳对照方式时，最好选择几种不同的色谱条件分别展开，进行验证，因为对一些结构性质相近的化合物，只用一种色谱条件，有时可能不能完全分离，甚至不同化合物出现斑点重合的现象，而导致误判。

Positive-negative control, Test solution, positive control solution, negative control solution should be pointed on the same TLC plate, developed, colored and inspected. The samples should have spots of the same color with the positive control in the corresponding position to provide a basis for the identification of the existence of a kind of herb. And the negative control should have no interference in the corresponding position to determine the specificity of the method. When using the positive-negative control method, it is best to choose several different chromatographic conditions to separate for verification. Because some compounds with similar structure and properties may not be completely separated sometimes only by one chromatographic condition, and even different compounds appear the same spot coincidently, leading to misjudgment.

（3）吸附剂的选择与薄层板的制备　吸附剂的性能对各种化合物的吸附力有很大影响，酸性吸附剂（如硅胶和酸性氧化铝）一般适用于分离含酸性基团的化合物，如黄酮、有机酸等；而碱性氧化铝适于分离生物碱等碱性化合物，但对碱敏感的化合物如含酯基的化合物不宜用碱性氧化铝，而以中性氧化铝较适宜。吸附剂的活度或含水量对分离也有影响，制备好的薄层板使用前一般需在105~110℃活化30分钟，使含水量降低。特别是氧化铝作为吸附剂时要选择适当的活度，才能有效地达到分离的目的。硅胶 G 长期贮放可使黏合力降低，且不同厂家或批次的商品硅胶质量不可能完全相同，常常会影响分析结果的重现性，在重复试验时应注意。

③ *The Selection of the Adsorbent and Preparation of Thin Layer Plate*　The performance of adsorbent has a great influence on the various compounds of adsorption, acid adsorbent (silica gel and acidic alumina) generally is suitable for the separation of compounds containing acidic groups, such as flavonoids, organic acids, etc. And alkaline alumina is suitable for separating alkaloids and other alkaline compounds. But alkali sensitive compounds such as compounds containing ester groups should not be used by alkaline alumina, and neutral alumina is more appropriate. The activity or water content of the adsorbent also has an effect on the separation. The prepared thin layer plate should be heated at 105-110℃ for 30min to reduce the water content before using. In particular, alumina as adsorbent should choose the appropriate activity, in order to effectively achieve the purpose of separation. Long-term storage of silica gel G can reduce the adhesive force. And the quality of silica gel from different manufacturers or batches of products cannot be completely the same, which often affects the reproducibility of analysis, so attention should be paid to the repeated tests.

薄层板有市售薄层板和自制薄层板，市售薄层板有普通薄层板和高效薄层板，如硅胶 H 薄层板、硅胶 G 薄层板、硅胶 $GF_{254}$ 薄层板、聚酰胺薄层板、铝基片薄层板等。高效薄层板的粒径一般为 5~7μm，分离效能更高、效果更好；聚酰胺薄层板不需要活化；铝基片薄层板可根据需要剪裁，但需注意不得使薄层板底边的硅胶层破损。

Thin layer plate has the tow kinds of market and self-made. The market thin layer plate has ordinary thin layer plate and high efficiency thin layer plate, such as silica gel thin layer plate, silica gel $GF_{254}$ thin layer plate, polyamide thin layer plate, aluminum substrate thin layer plate,etc. The particle size of high efficiency thin layer plate is generally 5-7μm, with the higher separation efficiency. Polyamide thin layer plate do not require activation. Aluminum substrate TLC plate can be cut according to the need, but should care not make the bottom edge damaged.

（4）点样　采用专用毛细管手动点样或采用半自动、自动点样仪点样。点样形状一般为圆点状或窄细的条带状。点样时需注意控制调整好点样点与点之间的距离、点与薄层板边缘之间的距离、点或条带的直径与宽度，以免在展开过程中产生由于扩散导致的相邻样品间斑点的相互干扰。可采用在同一个位置重复多次点样的方式积累点样量，但需注意点在同一圆心上，以免出现复斑；点样时切勿损坏薄层表面。

④ *Spot sample*　Use special capillary manual spot sample or semi-automatic and automatic spot sample meter. The shape is generally round or narrow strip. The attention should be paid to the control and adjustment of the distance between the sample point and point, between the point and edge of the plate, and the diameter and width of the point or strip. So as to avoid the mutual interference of the spots between adjacent samples caused by diffusion during the developing process. It is possible to accumulate samples by repeating many times in the same position. But need to pay attention to the point should in the same center of the circle, so as not to appear double spot, and do not damage the thin surface of plate.

（5）展开　选择合适的展开剂是分离成败的关键因素，展开剂的选择和优化主要考虑溶剂的极性和选择性，原则上应根据化合物性质，选用便于主斑点被展开分离的展开剂。此外，分离碱性物质（如生物碱）时，展开剂中可加入少量碱性试剂，分离酸性物质（如蒽醌、黄酮、有机酸等）时，展开剂中可加入少量酸性试剂，以减少斑点的拖尾与扩散。应使用两种或两种以上的溶剂系统，使被测成分展开后都能被检出，且与对照物表现一致。对于难分离的物质，必要时，可进行二次展开或双向展开进行分离。

⑤ *Developing*　The selection of appropriate developing solvent is a key factor of separation, and solvent polarity and selectivity should be mainly considered. In principle, should base on compound property to choose the developing solvent easy to separate master spots. In addition, when separating alkaline substances (such as alkaloids), a small number of alkaline reagents can be added in developing solvent; when separating acidic substances (such as anthraquinone, flavonoids, organic acids, etc.), a small number of acidic reagents can be added in developing solvent, in order to reduce the drag and diffusion of spots. Two or more solvent systems should be used so that the components under test can be detected and behave in accordance with the reference. For materials that are difficult to separate, secondary developing or bidirectional developing can be carried out when necessary.

展开之前，层析缸内溶剂蒸气的饱和平衡是必要的，可减少边缘效应。展开时，薄层板浸入展开剂的深度以距原点 5mm 为宜，要保证在整个展开过程中，层析缸放置在平整、避光、室温的环境中，保持密闭状态，且有足够量的展开剂。一般上行展开 8~15cm，高效薄层板也可上行展开至 5~8cm，取出薄层板后，及时标记溶剂前沿，晾干展开剂，待检视。

Before developing, the balance of solvent vapor in the chromatographic cylinder is necessary to reduce the edge effect. During the development, the depth of the TLC plate immersed in the developing solvent is 5mm away from the origin appropriately. To ensure that during the whole development process, the chromatographic cylinder should be placed in a flat, avoid light, room temperature environment, keep closed, and have sufficient amount of developing solvent. Generally, the developing distance is about 8-15cm upward, and the high-efficiency TLC plate can also be developing upward to 5-8cm. Take out plate and mark the solvent front timely after developing, and dry for inspection.

（6）显色与检视　有颜色的物质可直接在可见光下检视；有荧光的物质可在紫外光灯（365nm 或 254nm）下检视；无色或无荧光的物质可通过喷雾、浸渍、蒸汽熏蒸等方法以显色剂显色后再检视；对于在紫外光下有吸收的物质，还可用含有荧光剂的薄层板（如硅胶 $GF_{254}$），在紫外光灯下检视薄层板上荧光淬灭形成的斑点。

⑥ *Coloring and viewing*　Substances with colors can be viewed directly in visible light. Substances with fluorescence can be examined under UV lamps (365nm or 254nm). Colorless or non-fluorescent substances can be sprayed, impregnated, steam fumigation and other methods with coloring reagent and then viewing. For substances with absorption under UV light, adsorbent containing fluorescent agent (e.g. $GF_{254}$) can also be used. Spots formed by fluorescence quenching on the plate and can be examined under uv lamp.

（7）色谱结果记录与保存　鉴别用的薄层色谱结果，多采用数码相机等设备尽快拍摄或扫描成彩色电子照片保存，也可同时在薄层色谱扫描仪上记录扫描结果。

⑦ *Recording and preservation of chromatographic results* The use of digital cameras and other equipment as soon as possible to take or scan TLC chromatographic results into color electronic photos for preservation, and also can use the TLC scanner to record the scanning results.

### 2. 影响薄层色谱分析的主要因素

### (2) The Main Factors Affecting Thin Layer Chromatography

影响薄层色谱的因素很多，如供试液的净度、吸附剂的性能和薄层板的质量、点样、展开剂的组成及饱和情况、相对湿度和温度等。

There are many factors that affect thin-layer chromatography, such as the purity of the test solution, the performance of the adsorbent and the quality of the thin-layer plate, spotting, the composition and saturation of the developing agent, relative humidity and temperature.

薄层色谱的重现性与操作环境的相对湿度和温度密切相关。有些中药成分的薄层色谱行为极易受环境湿度和温度影响，相对湿度有时可用饱和盐溶液控制，如 $KNO_3$ 饱和溶液（25℃相对湿度 92.5%）、NaCl 饱和溶液（15.5~60℃ 相对湿度 75%±1%）、$NaNO_3$ 饱和溶液（25~40℃相对湿度 64%~61.5%）等。相对湿度对苍术薄层色谱的影响见图 3-1。温度对人参薄层色谱的影响见图 3-2。2020 年版《中国药典》（一部）收载的复方皂矾丸中西洋参的 TIC 鉴别要求在温度 10~25℃、相对湿度小于 60% 的条件下展开。

The reproducibility of TLC is closely related to the relative humidity and temperature of the operating environment. The TLC behavior of some traditional Chinese medicine ingredients is extremely susceptible to environmental humidity and temperature. Relative humidity can sometimes be controlled by saturated salt solutions, such as $KNO_3$ saturated solution (25℃,relative humidity 92.5%), NaCl saturated solution (15.5-60℃, relative humidity 75%±1%), $NaNO_3$ saturated solution (at 25-40℃, relative humidity 64%-61.5%), etc. The effect of relative humidity on Rhizoma Atractylodis TLC is shown in Fig. 3-1. The effect of temperature on thin layer chromatography of ginseng is shown in Fig. 3-2. The TIC identification of Panacis Quinquefolii Radix in Fufang Zaofan pills contained in the 2020 edition *Chinese Pharmacopoeia* (Volume Ⅰ) of is required to be carried out at a temperature of 10-25℃ and a relative humidity of less than 60%.

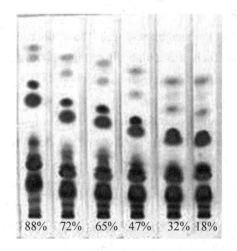

88% 72% 65% 47% 32% 18%

图 3-1 不同相对湿度下苍术的 TLC 图

Fig. 3-1 TLC diagram of Rhizoma Atractylodis under different relative humidity

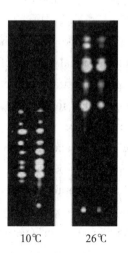

10℃ 26℃

图 3-2 不同温度下人参的 TLC 图

Fig. 3-2 TLC diagram of Ginseng Radix et Rhizoma under different temperature

薄层色谱－生物自显影技术是一种将薄层色谱分离和生物活性测定相结合的方法，集分离、鉴定、活性检测于一体。该方法不需要特殊设备，具有操作简单、耗费低、灵敏度好、专属性强等优点，可同时快速测定数个样品。如 1,1- 二苯基 -2- 苦肼基自由基（DPPH）是一种稳定的以氮为中心的自由基，若被测物能清除 DPPH，则提示被测物具有降低羟自由基、烷自由基或过氧自由基等的作用，及打断脂质过氧化链反应的作用，还可得到其有效浓度。DPPH 本身显紫色，具有清除 DPPH 自由基能力的物质能使其还原成黄色的二苯基苦肼。该技术对于中药的质量评价控制和活性成分筛选均有很好的应用价值。

TLC-Bioautography is a method combining TLC separation and bioactivity determination, which integrates separation, identification and activity detection. This method requires no special equipment, has the advantages of simple operation, low cost, sensitivity and high specificity, and can quickly determine several samples at the same time. For example, 1,1-diphenyl-2-pierylhydrazyl (DPPH) is a kind of stable nitrogen-centered free radical. If the tested substance can eliminate DPPH, it indicates that the tested substance has the function of reducing hydroxyl free radical, alkyl free radical or peroxide free radical, and the function of interrupting lipid peroxidation chain reaction, also the effective concentration can also be obtained. DPPH itself is purple, and the substances with the ability to remove DPPH radicals can revert it to the yellow diphenylpicrylhydrazine. This technique has a good application value for the quality evaluation and control of TCM and the screening of active substances.

例 3-7　大黄药材中五种成分的薄层色谱鉴别

Example 3-7　TLC identification of rhein, rheum emodin, chrysophanol, emodin methyl ether and aloe emodin in Rhei Radix Et Rhizoma

【鉴别】取本品粉末 0.1g，加甲醇 20ml，浸泡 1 小时，滤过，取滤液 5ml，蒸干，残渣加水 10ml 使溶解，再加盐酸 1ml，加热回流 30 分钟，立即冷却，用乙醚分 2 次振摇提取，每次 20ml，合并乙醚液，蒸干，残渣加三氯甲烷 1ml 使溶解，作为供试品溶液。另取大黄对照药材 0.1g，同法制成对照药材溶液。再取大黄酸、大黄素、大黄酚、大黄素甲醚、芦荟大黄素对照品各适量，加甲醇制成混合对照品溶液。照薄层色谱法（《中国药典》通则 0502）试验，吸取上述三种溶液各 4μl，分别点于同一以羧甲基纤维素钠为黏合剂的硅胶 H 薄层板上，以石油醚（30~60℃）- 甲酸乙酯 – 甲酸（15：5：1）的上层溶液为展开剂，展开，取出，晾干，置紫外光灯（365nm）下检视。供试品色谱中，在与对照品及对照药材色谱相应的位置上，显相同的五个橙黄色荧光主斑点，置氨蒸气中熏后，斑点变为红色（图 3-3）。

**Identification**　Take 0.1g of the powder, add 20ml of kmethanol, soak for 1 hour, filter, the filtrate 5ml, dry, dissolve residual in 10ml of water, add 1ml of hydrochloric acid, heating reflux 30 minutes, cool immediately. Shak to extract with ether for 2 times, every time 20ml, merge ether liquid, dry, dissolve residual in 1ml of chloroform as the test solution. Take 0.1g of the reference herb, with the same method to produce the reference herb solution. Take few rhein, rheum emodin, chrysophanol, emodin methyl ether and aloe emodin, added methyl alcohol to make a mixed reference substance solution. According to the general principles of thin layer chromatography (TLC) (*Chinese Pharmacopoeia*, general chapters 0502), take each of the above three solution 4μl separately to the same silica gel H thin layer plate which with sodium carboxymethyl cellulose as adhesive, with petroleum ether (30-60℃)-ethyl format-formic acid (15：5：1) upper layer solution for developing solvent. After developing dry in air, examine under a UV lamp (365 nm). In the sample chromatography, the same five orange yellow fluorescent spots should be found in the corresponding positions of the reference substances and the reference herb chromatography (Fig.3-3). After fumigating in ammonia vapor, the spots turn red. As shown in Fig.3-3.

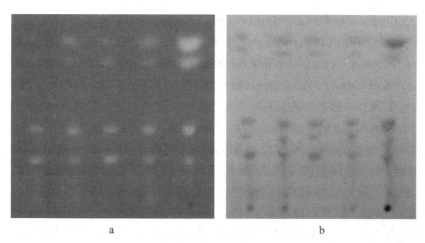

图 3-3　大黄药材中大黄素、大黄素、大黄酚、大黄素甲醚、芦荟大黄素的薄层色谱鉴别

Fig. 3-3　TLC identification of rhein, rheum emodin, chrysophanol, emodin methyl ether and aloe emodin in Rhei Radix Et Rhizoma

a. 紫外光下［under UV-light (365nm)］; b. 可见光下 (under visible light)

## （三）气相色谱法
## 3. Gas Chromatography (GC) Methods

气相色谱法适于分析具有挥发性且热稳定的成分或衍生化后能够被气化的成分，如麝香酮、薄荷醇、冰片、龙脑、麻黄碱等。气相色谱法以对照物的保留时间为参照，鉴定已知物，分离效率好、灵敏度高、快速、准确，可同时完成定性鉴别与定量分析。

Gas chromatography (GC) is suitable for the analysis of volatile and thermally stable components, or components that can be vaporized by derivation. Such as muscone, menthol, borneol, ephedrine. GC can identify the known substance with the retention time of the reference material as a basis. GC can complete qualitative identification and quantitative analysis at the same time with good separation efficiency, high sensitivity, fastdetection speed and good accuracy.

GC 用于中药鉴定时，特别要考虑样品前处理及供试溶液的制备方法对检测结果准确性的影响，尽量避免在此过程中待测成分的损失，以便实验结果更为稳定可靠。此外，为了避免几种结构性质相似的组分可能会在同一根色谱柱上有相同的保留时间，方法建立的过程中应采用双柱或多柱进行验证，若在每根色谱柱上已知物和未知物的保留值都一致，可认为是同一化合物。

It is particularly necessary to take into account the influence of sample pretreatment and preparation method of sample on the accuracy of test results when GC is used for the identification of TCM. Try to avoid the loss of components to be tested in this process, so as to make the experimental results more stable and reliable. In addition, in order to avoid the possibility that several components with similar structural properties may have the same retention time on the same chromatographic column. The method should be verified by using two or several chromatographic columns during the establishment of the method. If the retention time of known substance and unknown substance are the same on each chromatographic column, they can be considered the same compound.

一般气相色谱法在中药中很少只用于定性鉴别，多是在含量测定的同时达到鉴别的目的，或以指纹图谱、特征图谱的形式对中药这个复杂样品进行分析。如《中国药典》中满山红油的气相色谱特征图谱、薄荷素油的气相色谱指纹图谱等。

GC is rarely used for the qualitative identification of a certain component in TCM, but to achieve the purpose of identification at the same time of content determination. And also can analyze the complex sample of TCM in the form of fingerprint and characteristic chromatogram. Such as GC characteristic chromatogram of Dahurian rhododenron leaf oil (Manshanhong You) and fingerprint of Peppermint oil (Behesu You) recored in *Chinese Pharmacopoeia*.

例 3-8　安宫牛黄丸中麝香酮的鉴别

Example 3-8　Identification of muscone in Angong Niuhuang Pills

【鉴别】取本品 3g，剪碎，照挥发油测定法（《中国药典》通则 2204）试验，加环己烷 0.5ml，缓缓加热至沸，并保持微沸约 2.5 小时，放置 30 分钟后，取环己烷液作为供试品溶液。另取麝香酮对照品，加环己烷制成每 1ml 含 2.5mg 的溶液，作为对照品溶液。照气相色谱法（《中国药典》通则 0521）试验，以苯基（50%）甲基硅酮（OV-17）为固定相，涂布浓度为 9%，柱长为 2m，柱温为 210℃。分别吸取对照品溶液和供试品溶液适量，注入气相色谱仪。供试品色谱中应呈现与对照品色谱峰保留时间相同的色谱峰。

**Identification**　Cut 3g of the pills into small pieces, according to *Chinese Pharmacopoeia*, general chapters 2204 to test, add 0.5ml of cyclohexane, heat gently to boil and keep boiling for 2.5 hours. Allow to stand for half an hour, use the cyclohexane solution as the test solution. Dissolve musc-one CRS in cyclohexane to produce a solution containing 2.5mg per ml as the reference solution. according to *Chinese Pharmacopoeia*, general chapters 0521 to test, using a 2m long column packed with 9% phenylmethyl polysiloxane (OV-17) as the stationary phase, and maintain the column temperature at 210℃. Inject a quantity of each of the test solution and the reference solution respectively into the column. The peak in the chromatogram obtained with the test solution corresponds in retention time to the peak in the chromatogram obtained with the reference solution.

（四）高效液相色谱法

## 4. High Performance Liquid Chromatography Methods

高效液相色谱法具有快速、灵敏、准确的特点，不受样品挥发性和热稳定性的影响，色谱柱和流动相选择性广，因此，应用比 GC 广泛。和气相色谱法一样，高效液相色谱法也是采用保留时间定性，即在相同的色谱条件下，通过比较供试品色谱中是否存在与对照物色谱峰保留时间一致的色谱峰，判断被检成分（药味）的存在与否。

High performance liquid chromatography (HPLC) has the characteristics of rapid, sensitive and accurate. Unaffected by sample volatility and thermal stability, wide selective of chromatographic column and mobile phase, so wider application than GC. The same as GC, high performance liquid chromatography identify the authenticity of Chinese medicine based on retention time. That is, under the same chromatographic conditions, by comparing whether there is a chromatographic peak in the chromatogram of the test substance that is consistent with the retention time of the chromatographic peak of the reference substance, judge the presence or absence of the test ingredient (single medicine).

例 3-9　牛黄上清丸中黄芩苷、栀子苷、连翘酯苷 A、芍药苷的鉴别

Example 3-9　Identification of baicalin, geniposide, forsythiaside A and paeoniflorin in Niuhuang Shangqing pills

【鉴别】色谱条件及系统适用性试验　以十八烷基硅烷键合硅胶为填充剂；以乙腈为流动相 A，以 0.05% 磷酸为流动相 B，按下表中的规定进行梯度洗脱；检测波长为 240nm。理论板数按黄芩苷峰计算应不低于 3000。

**Identification**　*Chromatographic system and system suitability*　Use octadecylsilane bonded silica gel as the stationary phase, acetonitrile as the mobile phase A, and 0.05% solution of phosphoric acid as the mobile phase B, elute in gradient as the following. As detector a spectrophotometer set at 240nm. The number of theoretical plates for the column is not less than 3000, calculated with the reference to the peak of baicalin.

| 时间（Time, min） | 流动相 A（Mobile Phase A, %） | 流动相 B（Mobile Phase B, %） |
|---|---|---|
| 0~18 | 10 → 23 | 90 → 77 |
| 18~30 | 23 → 27 | 77 → 73 |
| 30~35 | 27 → 35 | 73 → 65 |
| 35~40 | 35 | 65 |
| 40~45 | 35 → 50 | 65 → 50 |
| 45~50 | 50 → 10 | 50 → 90 |

供试品溶液的制备 取小蜜丸或重量差异项下的大蜜丸，剪碎，混匀；或取水丸适量，研细。取约 1g，精密称定，置具塞锥形瓶中，精密加入 70% 甲醇 50ml，称定重量，超声处理（功率 500W，频率 40kHz）30 分钟，再加热回流 1 小时，放冷，再称定重量，用 70% 甲醇补足减失的重量，摇匀，滤过，取续滤液，即得。

*Test solution* Cut small honeyed pills or big honeyed pills obtained under the test of weight variation into pieces, mix well, or pulverize quantities of watered pills to fine powder. Weigh accurately 1g into a stoppered conical flask, add accurately 50ml of 70% methanol, weigh, ultrasonicate (power 500W, frequency 40kHz) for 30 minutes and heat under reflux for 1 hour, cool and weigh again, replenish the loss of weight with 70% methanol, and mix well, filter and use the successive filtrate as the test solution.

对照品溶液的制备 取黄芩苷对照品、栀子苷对照品、连翘酯苷 A 对照品、芍药苷对照品，加甲醇分别制成每 1ml 含黄芩苷 60μg、栀子苷 20μg、连翘酯苷 A 10μg、芍药苷 10μg 的溶液，作为对照品溶液。

*Reference solution* Dissolve separately baicalin CRS, geniposide CRS, forsythiaside A CRS and paeoniflorin CRS in methanol to produce solutions containing 60μg of baicalin per ml, 20μg of geniposide per ml, 10μg of forsythiaside A per each ml, and 10μg of paeoniflorin per ml as the reference solution.

测定法 分别吸取供试品溶液和对照品溶液各 10μl，注入液相色谱仪，测定。供试品色谱图中，应呈现与对照品色谱峰保留时间相对应的色谱峰。

*Procedure* Inject 10μl of each of the test solution and the above reference solutions into the column. The retention time of the peaks obtained with the test solution and reference solution is concordant with each other.

### 五、色谱－质谱联用鉴别法
### 3.3.5 Chromatography-Mass Spectrometry Identification Methods

高效液相色谱法和气相色谱法只能以对照物的保留时间为参照，鉴定已知化合物，对未知化合物的鉴别必须与质谱或红外光谱等其他仪器联用。如液相色谱－质谱（LC-MS）、气相色谱－质谱（GC-MS）、气相色谱－傅立叶变换红外光谱（GC-FTIR）等是鉴别未知化合物的有效工具。色谱法的高效快速分离，结合质谱对未知物高灵敏度、高选择性的定性分析，可获取复杂混合物的整体轮廓信息和其中各单一成分的结构信息，是定性定量分析含有许多未知成分的中药复杂体系的有效方法。如《中国药典》中的阿胶、龟角胶、鹿角胶等的鉴别均已采用 LC-MS 分析。

HPLC and GC only can identify known compounds with the retention time of reference material. And the identification of unknown compounds must be combined with other instruments such as mass spectrometer or infrared spectrometer. Such as LC-MS, GC-MS and GC-FTIR are effective tools for identifying unknown compounds. The efficient and rapid separation of chromatography, combined with the high sensitivity and selectivity of mass spectrometry for the qualitative analysis of unknown substances, can obtain the overall contour information of the complex mixture and the structure information of each single component. Chromatography-mass spectrometry is an effective method for the qualitative and quantitative analysis of the complex system of TCM containing many unknown components. For example, the identification of Asini corii Colla, Testudinis carapacis Et Plastri Colla, Cervi Cornus Colla in *Chinese Pharmacopoeia* has been analyzed LC-MS.

# 岗 位 对 接
# Post Docking

本章为中药、中药制药和中药资源专业学生必须掌握的内容，为成为合格的中药质量评价与控制人员奠定坚实的基础。

This task is the content that students of traditional Chinese medicine major must master and lays a solid foundation for becoming qualified personnel of quality evaluation and control of traditional Chinese medicine.

本章内容对应岗位包括中药药师、中药购销员、中药调剂员、中药材种植员、中药材生产管理员的相关工种。

The corresponding positions of this task include TCM pharmacist, TCM buyer and seller, TCM dispensing staff, TCM material planting staff and TCM production manager.

上述从事中药服务、中药购销和中药材生产种植相关所有岗位的从业人员均需要掌握中药鉴别的意义、任务、方法及内容；掌握理化鉴别中各方法的基本原理和实验技能等，学会应用本任务开展中药学服务工作。

The above practitioners engaged in TCM service, TCM purchase and sale, and TCM production and planting need to master the significance, task, method and content of TCM identification. Master the basic principles and experimental skills of physical and chemical identification methods, and learn to apply this task to carry out traditional Chinese medicine service.

# 重 点 小 结
## Summary of Key Points

中药的鉴别是中药质量检验工作的首要任务，主要包括性状鉴别、显微鉴别、理化鉴别等。性状鉴别是鉴别中药形状、形态、色泽、气和味等外观性状，主要用于中药材和中药饮片的真伪鉴别；显微鉴别是利用显微镜观察动植物药材、饮片或含饮片粉末的制剂的内部组织结构，细胞形状、大小、排列状况，细胞壁和细胞内含物等特征，主要用于外观相似或者破碎但显微特征不同的中药材和饮片以及含药材粉末的中药制剂；而理化鉴别是根据中药所含化学成分的理化性质、色谱、光谱特征进行真伪的鉴别，常用的方法有化学法、光谱法、色谱法等，是中药常用的鉴别方法，特别是色谱法中的 TLC 法。

The identification is the primary task of the quality inspection of traditional Chinese medicine. The identification of TCM mainly includes character identification, microscopic identification, physicochemical identification and other methods. Trait identification is identification of the appearance, shape, color, qi and taste of Chinese medicine, mainly used for authenticity identification of Chinese medicinal materials and decoction pieces. Microscopic identification is the use of a microscope to observe the internal tissue structure, cell shape, size, arrangement, cell wall and cell contents of animal and plant medicinal materials, medicinal slices or preparations containing medicinal slices powder, mainly used for Chinese medicinal materials and decoction pieces with similar appearance or broken but different microscopic characteristics, and Chinese medicinal preparations containing medicinal powder. The physical and chemical identification is based on the physical and chemical properties, chromatographic and spectral characteristics of the chemical components contained in traditional Chinese medicine, to identify the authenticity of Chinese medicine, commonly used methods include chemical method, spectroscopy, chromatography, etc., which are the common identification methods of traditional Chinese medicine, especially the TLC method in chromatography.

# 目 标 检 测

题库

**一、选择题**

（一）单项选择题

1. 对中药制剂分析时的显微鉴别最适用于
   A. 用药材提取物制成制剂的鉴别
   B. 用水煎法制成制剂的鉴别
   C. 用制取挥发油方法制成制剂的鉴别
   D. 用蒸馏法制成制剂的鉴别

2. 在中药的理化鉴别中，最常用的方法为
   A. UV 法　　　　　　B. Vis 法　　　　　　C. TLC 法　　　　　　D. HPLC 法

3. 在中药的薄层定性鉴别中，最常用的吸附剂是
   A. 硅胶 G　　　　　　B. 微晶纤维素　　　　　　C. 硅藻土　　　　　　D. 氧化铝

4. 气相色谱法最适宜分析测定中药中哪些成分
   A. 大分子苷类成分　　　　　　　　　　B. 不挥发性的成分

    C. 热不稳定性成分                             D. 挥发性的成分

5. 应用 HPLC 或 GC 法进行中药的定性鉴别中，主要依据是

    A. 吸收度             B. 保留时间            C. 色谱峰面积          D. 色谱峰峰高

6. 影响薄层色谱分析主要因素之一为

    A. 供试品数量         B. 对照品数量         C. 原药材来源         D. 相对湿度

7. 在薄层色谱鉴别中，硅胶薄层板需在什么条件下活化

    A. 410℃烘 30 分钟                    B. 310℃烘 30 分钟

    C. 210℃烘 30 分钟                    D. 110℃烘 30 分钟

8. 在中药分析的化学反应法鉴别中，应尽量采用

    A. 专属性强，简单易行的方法            B. 专属性不强，简单易行的方法

    C. 专属性强，较复杂的方法              D. 专属性不强，较复杂的方法

9. 采用薄层色谱进行中药复方制剂鉴别时，阴性对照的目的是考察

    A. 灵敏度             B. 专属性             C. 准确性         D. 重现性

10. 在薄层色谱鉴别中，如制剂中同时含有黄连、黄柏原药材，宜采用

    A. 阳性对照                          B. 阴性对照

    C. 化学对照品对照                  D. 对照药材和化学对照品同时对照

11. 显微鉴别可作为以下哪一项的定性鉴别

    A. 含有饮片粉末的丸剂                   B. 酒剂

    C. 注射剂                            D. 口服液

12. 中药制剂的性状是指去除包装后，成品的形状、形态、颜色、气味等，其描述的顺序是

    A. 形状、颜色、气、味              B. 颜色、形状、气、味

    C. 形状、颜色、味、气              D. 颜色、形状、味、气

（二）多项选择题

1. 中药的鉴别包括

    A. 性状鉴别                  B. 显微鉴别            C. 理化鉴别

    D. 杂质检查                  E. 生物鉴别

2. 以下属于中药的理化鉴别的有

    A. 化学反应法              B. 微量升华法           C. 光谱法

    D. 色谱法                 E. 砷盐检查法

3. 可用于中药鉴别的色谱方法有

    A. 纸色谱法              B. 薄层色谱法           C. 聚酰胺薄层色谱法

    D. 高效液相色谱法         E. 气相色谱法

4. 影响薄层色谱分析的主要因素有

    A. 样品预处理及供试液制备           B. 薄层色谱的点样技术

    C. 吸附剂的活性与相对湿度的影响     D. 温度的影响

    E. 展开剂的选择

5. 气相色谱法鉴别，适宜的制剂样品为含有何种成分的制剂

    A. 挥发油                   B. 挥发性成分

    C. 无机元素                D. 可被分解气化的成分

    E. 本身不挥发但可制成挥发性衍生物的成分

**二、思考题**

根据下述中药复方制剂的组成与制法，试设计在对该制剂进行定性鉴别时都可采用哪些方法。

名称：养胃舒胶囊

组成：人参、麦冬、五味子、黄芪、丹参、川芎、山楂

制法：人参粉碎成细粉备用。五味子、丹参用 85% 乙醇回流提取 2 次，合并提取液，减压浓缩至相对密度 1.12~1.15，得浸膏。其余四味加水煎煮两次，合并煎液，浓缩至约 500ml，加入等量 85% 乙醇，搅拌、静置、过夜，过滤，滤液浓缩至相对密度 1.30~1.36。将两种浸膏合并后，加入人参细粉和适量淀粉，混合均匀，制粒、干燥，装胶囊，即得。

# 第四章 中药的检查

# Chapter 4 Physic-Chemical Examination of Chinese Medicine

 学习目标 | Learning Goal

**知识要求：**

1．**掌握** 中药杂质的概念与杂质限量的计算方法，重金属、砷盐、水分、干燥失重、灰分等的检查原理、方法和注意事项。

2．**熟悉** 炽灼残渣、二氧化硫残留量、甲醇量、内源性有害物质、农药残留量的检查原理、方法以及制剂通则的检查项目。

3．**了解** 残留溶剂、黄曲霉毒素和酸败度测定方法

**能力要求：**

学会应用中药的一般杂质检查、特殊杂质检查和制剂通则检查等方法解决中药的杂质检查。

**Knowledge Requirements**

**1. Master** The concept of Chinese medicine impurities and the calculation method of the limit of impurities, the inspection principles, methods and precautions of heavy metals, arsenic, water, loss on drying, ash, etc.

**2. Familiar** Inspection principles and methods of ignition residue, sulfur dioxide residue, methanol, endogenous harmful substances, pesticide residues, and general requirements of preparations.

**3. Understand** Method for determination of residual solvents, aflatoxin and rancidity.

**Ability Requirements**

Learn to apply the methods of general impurities inspection, special impurities inspection and general requirements of preparations of traditional Chinese medicine to solve the impurity inspection of traditional Chinese medicine.

PPT

## 第一节 概述

## 4.1 Overview

### 一、中药检查的主要内容
### 4.1.1 Main Contents of Chinese Medicine Examination

药材和饮片的检查是指对药材和饮片的纯净程度、可溶性物质、有害或有毒物质进行限量检查，包括水分、灰分、杂质、毒性成分、重金属及有害元素、二氧化硫残留、农药残留、黄曲霉毒素等；除另有规定外，饮片水分通常不得过13%；药屑杂质通常不得过3%，药材及饮片（矿物类除外）的二氧化硫残留量不得过150mg/kg；药材及饮片（植物类）禁用农药（《中国药典》通则0212）不得过定量限。

"Test"of crude drugs and decoction pieces refers to purity and soluble substances tests, as well as limit test of harmful or poisonous substances, including water, ash, foreign matters, heavy metals, harmful elements, sulfur dioxide residues, pesticides residues, aflatoxins, and so on. Unless otherwise specified, the water of the decoction pieces should not exceed 13%; the impurities of medicinal crumbs should not exceed 3%, and the sulfur dioxide residues of medicinal materials and decoction pieces (except minerals) should not exceed 150mg/kg. The Content of prohibited pesticides (*Chinese Pharmacopoeia* general chapters 0212) of medicinal materials and decoction pieces (plants) Should not more than the limit.

重金属及有害元素一致性限量指导值：药材及饮片（植物类）中铅不得过5mg/kg，镉不得过1mg/kg，砷不得过2mg/kg，汞不得过0.2mg/kg，铜不得过20mg/kg。

Guidance value for consistency limit of heavy metals and harmful elements, lead must not exceed 5mg/kg, cadmium must not exceed 1mg/kg, arsenic must not exceed 2mg/kg, mercury must not exceed 0.2mg/kg, and copper must not exceed 20mg/kg in medicinal materials and decoction pieces (plants).

中药提取物和植物油脂检查应根据原料药材中可能存在的有毒成分、生产过程中可能造成的污染情况、剂型要求、贮藏条件等建立检查项目。如相对密度、pH值、水分、灰分、总固体、干燥失重、碘值、酸败度、炽灼残渣、酸值、皂化值、重金属与有害元素、农药残留、有机溶剂残留、大孔树脂残留物等。作为注射剂原料的提取物除上述检查项外，还应按照相应注射剂品种项下规定选择检查项目，如色度、总固体、蛋白质、鞣质、树脂、草酸盐、钾离子、有害元素（铅、镉、汞、砷、铜）、溶剂残留等。

"Test"of Chinese herbal extracts and vegetable oils based on the possible poisonous ingredients in raw materials, the possible pollution in the production process, the dosage form requirements, storage conditions, and so on, to establish inspection items .Such as relative density, pH value, water, ash, total solid, loss on dryness, iodine value, rancidity, residue on ignition, acid value, saponification value, heavy metals and harmful elements, pesticides residues, organic solvent residues, macroporous resin residues and so on. In addition to the above inspection items, the extracts used as raw materials for injections should also be selected according to the provisions of the corresponding injection product categories, such as color, total solids, protein, tannin, resin, oxalate, potassium ion, harmful elements (lead, cadmium, mercury, arsenic, copper), solvent residues, etc.

中药制剂除按制剂通则进行检查外，还应针对各品种规定相应检查项目，如水分、炽灼残渣、重金属及有害元素、农药残留量、有毒有害物质、有机溶剂残留量、树脂降解产物检查等。

"Test" of traditional Chinese medicine preparation, in addition to the general requirements of preparation, the examination items should also be specified for each kind of preparation, such as the determination of water, residue on ignition, heavy metals and harmful elements, pesticides residues, poisonous and harmful substances, residual solvents, resin degradation products, and so on.

### 二、中药杂质的分类及来源
### 4.1.2　Types and Sources of Impurities in Chinese Medicine

杂质是药品的关键质量属性，可影响产品的安全性和有效性。药品质量标准中的杂质系指在按照经国家药品监督管理部门依法审查批准的工艺和原辅料生产的药品中，由其生产工艺或原料带入的杂质，或在贮存过程中产生的杂质，不包括变更生产工艺或变更原辅料而产生的新杂质，也不包括掺入或污染的外来物质。

Impurities are key quality attributes of pharmaceuticals and can affect the safety and effectiveness of the product. Impurities in drug quality standards refer to impurities brought in by the production process or raw materials of pharmaceuticals produced according to the process and raw and auxiliary materials that have been reviewed and approved by the national drug regulatory authority according to law, or impurities generated during storage. No including new impurities produced by changing the production process or the original auxiliary materials, it also does not include foreign substances that are adulltered or contaminated.

《中国药典》将药材和饮片中混存的杂质定义成下列各类物质，一是来源与规定相同，但其性状或药用部位与规定不符的物质，如决明子、白扁豆中的果皮，党参中的芦头等；二是来源与规定不同的物质；三是无机杂质，如砂石、泥块等。

*Chinese Pharmacopoeia* defines the impurities mixed in medicinal materials and decoction pieces as the following types of substances. One is the substance whose source is the same as the regulations, but whose properties or medicinal parts are inconsistent with the regulations, such as the peel of Cassiae semen, Lablab semen album, and root stock of Codonopsis radix and so on; the second is a substance with a different source from the regulations; the third is inorganic impurities, such as gravel and mud.

#### （一）中药杂质的分类
#### 1. Types of Impurities in Chinese Medicine

药品的杂质可分为：有机杂质、无机杂质、残留溶剂。有机杂质可在药品的生产或贮存中引入，也可由药物与辅料或包装结构的相互作用产生，这些杂质可能是已鉴定或者未鉴定的、挥发性的或非挥发性的，包括起始物、副产物、中间体、降解产物、试剂、配位体和催化剂；化学结构与活性成分类似或具渊源关系，通常称为有关物质。无机杂质可能来源于生产过程，如反应试剂、配位体、催化剂、元素杂质、无机盐和其他物质（例如：过滤介质，活性炭等），一般是已知和确定的。药品中的残留溶剂系指原料药或辅料的生产中，以及制剂制备过程中使用的，但在工艺操作过程中未能完全去除的有机溶剂，一般具有已知的毒性。

Drug impurities can be divided into organic impurities, inorganic impurities, and residual solvents. Organic impurities can be introduced during the production or storage of pharmaceuticals, or can be generated by the interaction of drugs with excipients or packaging structures. These impurities may be identified or unidentified, volatile or non-volatile, including starting materials, by-products, intermediates, degradation products, reagents, ligands and catalysts; the chemical structure is similar or related to the active ingredients, and is often referred to as related substances. Inorganic impurities may originate from production processes, such as reaction reagents, ligands, catalysts, elemental impurities, inorganic salts and other substances (such as filter media, activated carbon, etc.), which are generally known and determined. Residual solvents in pharmaceuticals refer to organic solvents used in the production of bulk drugs or excipients and in the preparation of preparations, but which cannot be completely removed during the process operation, and generally have known toxicity.

（二）中药杂质的来源

## 2. Sources of Impurities in Chinese Medicine

1. 生产过程中引入　中药材生长在自然界，其生长过程中由于产地水源、土壤、空气等生长环境的污染及农药和化肥滥用而引入杂质。在中药材和饮片的收购和生产过程中由于采收、炮制、加工和所接触到的设备、用具、管道等，不可避免的引入泥沙、水分、重金属、无机盐、非药用部位等杂质。中药提取物和制剂的生产过程中使用的各种溶剂、试剂等可能会残留在产品中而产生杂质。

**(1) Introduced in the production process**　Chinese medicinal materials are grown in nature. During the growth process, impurities are introduced due to pollution of the growing environment such as the source of water, soil, and air, and abuse of pesticides and fertilizers. During the acquisition and production of Chinese medicinal materials and decoction pieces, due to the harvest season, processing and equipment, utensils, pipes, etc. that are in contact, it is inevitable to introduce sediment, moisture, heavy metals, inorganic salts, non-medicinal parts, etc impurities. Various solvents and reagents used in the production of traditional Chinese medicine extracts and preparations may remain in the product and produce impurities.

2. 储藏过程中引入　中药在贮藏过程中受外界条件的影响，引起其理化特性发生变化而产生杂质。中药在包装、贮存、运输过程中，在外界条件（日光、空气、温度、湿度等）影响或微生物作用下，其内部成分发生聚合、分解、氧化还原、水解等变化，使药品中产生杂质；由于处理不当，可能发生霉变、酸败、虫蛀等而引入杂质；为了防虫、保鲜或漂白，使用超量的硫黄熏蒸导致 $SO_2$ 残留等。

**(2) Introduced during storage**　Traditional Chinese medicine is affected by external conditions during storage, causing its physical and chemical properties to change. During the packaging, storage, and transportation of Chinese medicine, under the influence of external conditions (sunlight, air, temperature, humidity, etc.) or under the action of microorganisms, the internal components of the Chinese medicine undergo polymerization, decomposition, oxidation-reduction, hydrolysis, and other changes, produce impurities in the medicine; Due to improper treatment, impurities such as mildew, rancidity, worms, etc. may be introduced; in order to prevent insects, freshness or bleaching, excessive sulfur fumigation is used to cause residual $SO_2$.

### 三、杂质的限量检查方法及有害残留物限量的制定

## 4.1.3　Inspection Method for Impurity Limit and Establishment of Harmful Residue Limits

（一）杂质的限量检查方法

## 1. Inspection Method for Impurity Limit

完全除尽药物中的杂质非常困难，且没有必要。因此，从中药安全性及有效性评价来看，中药中存在的杂质，在保证药物安全、有效、稳定、质量可控的前提下，只进行限量检查。中药中

所含杂质的最大允许量，称为杂质的限量。

It is very difficult and unnecessary to completely remove the impurities in the medicine. Therefore, considering the safety and effectiveness of Chinese medicine, the impurities in them only be executed limit test on the premise of ensuring the safety, efficacy, stability and controllable quality of the medicine. The maximum allowable amount of impurities in Chinese medicine is called the limit of impurities.

中药中杂质的直接检查方法有两种：①限量检查，是杂质检查常见的方法；②定量测定。限量检查不要求测定杂质的准确含量，只检查是否超过限量，多采用对照法，此外还可用灵敏度法。

There are two methods for checking impurities in traditional Chinese medicines: ①limit test, which is a common method for impurity tests. ②quantitative determination, limit inspection does not require the exact content of impurities to be determined. It only checks whether the limit is exceeded. The control method is often used. In addition, the sensitivity method can also be used.

1. 限量检查

**(1) limit test**

**对照法** 对照法系指取一定量被检杂质的标准溶液与一定量的供试品溶液，在相同条件下试验，比较反应结果，确定杂质是否超过限量规定。此时，供试品（$S$）中所含杂质的最大允许量可以通过杂质标准溶液的浓度（$C$）和体积（$V$）的乘积表示，故杂质限量（$L$）的计算公式为：

*Control method* The control method refers to taking a certain amount of the standard solution of the tested impurities and a certain amount of the test solution, and testing under the same conditions, comparing the reaction results to determine whether the impurities exceed the limit. At this time, the maximum allowable amount of impurities in the test product ($S$) can be expressed by the product of the concentration ($C$) and volume ($V$) of the impurity standard solution, so the formula for calculating the limit of impurities ($L$) is:

$$杂质的限量（L）= \frac{标准溶液体积（V）\times 标准溶液浓度（C）}{供试品量（S）} \tag{4-1}$$

中药中重金属及砷盐等检查均采用本方法。

This method is used for the limit test of heavy metals and arsenic in traditional Chinese medicine.

**灵敏度法** 灵敏度法系指在供试品溶液中加入某种试剂，在一定条件下反应，观察有无阳性结果出现，以判断杂质是否超过限量。

*Sensitivity method* The sensitivity method refers to adding a certain reagent to the test solution, reacting under certain conditions, observing whether there is a positive result, so as to judge whether the impurities exceeds the limit.

例 4-1 肉桂油中重金属的检查

Example 4-1 Limit Test of Heavy Metals in Cinnamon Oil

【检查】重金属 取本品 10ml，加水 10ml 与盐酸 1 滴，振摇后，通硫化氢气使饱和，水层与油层均不得变色。

**Inspection** *Heavy Metals* Take 10ml of this product, add 10ml of water and 1 drop of hydrochloric acid. After shaking, pass hydrogen sulfide to make it saturated, and the water layer and oil layer must not change color.

2. 定量测定 定量测定系指用规定的方法测定杂质的含量，与规定的限量比较，以判断杂质是否超限。

**(2) Quantitative assay** Quantitative measurement refers to the determination of the content of impurities by a prescribed method and comparison with a prescribed limit to determine whether the impurity exceeds the limit.

（二）有害残留物限量的制定

## 2. Establishment of Harmful Residue Limits

限量的制定需考虑如下因素：杂质及含一定限量杂质药品的毒理学和药效研究数据，原料药的来源，给药途径，每日剂量，给药人群，治疗周期等。

The formulation of the limit should take into account the following factors, toxicology and pharmacodynamic research data of impurities and drugs containing a certain amount of impurities, the source of the crud drug, the route of administration, the daily dose, the population administered, the treatment cycle, etc.

有害残留物限量制定以毒理学数据为基础，结合残留物的暴露情况和人类日常膳食摄入情况，进行分析评估的结果。有害残留物的毒性程度是限量控制考虑的首要因素。残留物的动物毒理学实验数据、中药使用剂量及频率，人类经膳食日常摄入量是推导有害残留物最大限量理论值计算公式的主要依据。通过以下公式计算得到的结果是基于毒理学评估的有害残留物最大限量的理论计算值，在残留物最大限量制定过程中，还应结合其他影响因素进行综合评价后，确定最终限量标准。

The establishment of harmful residue limits is based on toxicological data, combined with the exposure of residues and the daily dietary intake of human beings, and the results of analysis and evaluation are conducted. The degree of toxicity of harmful residues is prime factor for limiting control considerations. The animal toxicology experimental data of residues, the dosage and frequency of traditional Chinese medicine, and the daily intake of humans through diet are the main basis for deriving the theoretical formula for calculating the maximum limit of harmful residues. The result calculated by the following formula is a theoretical calculation value of the maximum limit of harmful residues based on toxicological evaluation. In the process of setting the maximum limit of residues, a comprehensive evaluation should be conducted in combination with other influencing factors to determine the final limit standard.

1. **农药残留量** 建立农药残留量限量标准时，可按下列公式计算其最大限量理论值。

**(1) Pesticide Residues** When establishing the limit standard of pesticide residues, the theoretical value of maximal limit of residues may be calculated by the following equation.

$$L = \frac{A \times W}{M \times 100} \times \frac{AT}{EF \times ED} \times \frac{1}{t} \tag{4-2}$$

式中，$L$ 为最大限量理论值（mg/kg）；$A$ 为每日允许摄入量（mg/kg）；$W$ 为人体平均体重（kg），一般按 63kg 计；$M$ 为中药材（饮片）每日人均可服用的最大剂量（kg）；$AT$ 为平均寿命天数，一般为 365 天 / 年 × 70 年；$EF$ 为中药材或饮片服用频率（天 / 年）；$ED$ 为一生服用中药的暴露年限；$t$ 为中药材及饮片经煎煮或提取后，农药的转移率（%）；100 为安全因子，表示每日由中药材及其制品中摄取的农药残留量不大于日总暴露量（包括食物和饮用水）的 1%。

$L$, The theoretical value of maximal limit (mg/kg)；$A$, Acceptable daily intake (mg/kg bw)；$W$, The human average body weight (kg), generally 63kg；$M$, The maximal dose of the Chinese medicinal materials and decoction pieces ices that can be taken daily per person (kg)；$AT$, The average lifespan, generally 365 days/year × 70 years；$EF$, Frequency of taking Chinese medicinal materials or decoction pieces (day/year)；$ED$, Years of exposure to taking Chinese medicine in Lifetime；$t$, Transfer rate of pesticides after decoction or extraction of Chinese medicinal materials (%)，The safety factor is set to 100, suggesting that pesticides taken daily from the Chinese material medica and its products is not more than 1% of total daily exposure dose including food and drinking water.

**2. 重金属及有害元素**　建立重金属及有害元素限量标准时，可按照下列公式计算其最大限量理论值。

**(2) Heavy Metals and Harmful Elements**　When estalishing the limit standard of heavy metals and harmful elements, the theoretical value of maximal limit of the residue may be calculated by the following equation.

$$L = \frac{A \times W}{M \times 10} \times \frac{AT}{EF \times ED} \times \frac{1}{t} \qquad (4\text{-}3)$$

式中，$L$ 为最大限量理论值（mg/kg）；$A$ 为每日允许摄入量（mg/kg）；$W$ 为人体平均体重（kg），一般按 63kg 计；$M$ 为中药材（饮片）每日人均可服用的最大剂量（kg）；$AT$ 为平均寿命天数，一般为 365 天/年 × 70 年；$EF$ 为中药材或饮片服用频率（天/年）；$ED$ 为一生服用中药的暴露年限；$t$ 为中药材及饮片经煎煮或提取后，重金属元素的转移率（%）；10 为安全因子，表示每日由中药材及其制品中摄取的重金属量不大于日总暴露量（包括食物和饮用水）的 10%。

$L$, The theoretical value of maximal limit (mg/kg); $A$, Acceptable daily intake (mg/kg bw); $W$, The human average body weight (kg), generally 63kg; $M$, The maximal dose of the Chinese medicinal materials and decoction pieces ices that can be taken daily per person (kg); $AT$, The average lifespan, generally 365 days/year × 70 years; $EF$, Frequency of taking Chinese medicinal materials or decoction pieces (day/year); $ED$, Years of exposure to taking Chinese medicine in Lifetime; $t$, Transfer rate of pesticides after decoction or extraction of Chinese medicinal materials (%), The safety factor is set to 10, suggesting the daily heavy metals taken from the Chinese material medica and its products is not more than 10% of total daily exposure dose including food and drinking water.

**3. 黄曲霉毒素**　由于黄曲霉毒素毒性强，目前国际上不建议设定黄曲霉毒素的安全耐受量和无毒作用剂量，也无最大限量理论值计算公式，限量越低越好。黄曲霉毒素限量标准的制定，应根据具体品种和具体污染状况，参考国外药典和各国、各国际组织相关限量标准等规定，尽可能地将其限量控制在最低范围内，以降低安全风险。通常要求规定黄曲霉毒素 $B_1$ 和黄曲霉毒素 $B_1$、黄曲霉毒素 $B_2$、黄曲霉毒素 $G_1$、黄曲霉毒素 $G_2$ 总和的限量标准。

**(3) Aflatoxins**　Due to strong toxicity of aflatoxins, it is now recommended not to establish its safety tolerance dose and non-toxic effect dose, therefore calculation formula of theoretical value of maximal limit is not available. The level of aflatoxins should be kept as low as possible. Depending on specific products and pollution degree, the establishment of the limit standard of aflatoxins should refer to corresponding limit standard in foreign pharmacopoeia or guidelines from related countries and international organizations and its limit should be kept as low as possible in order to reduce safety risk. It is generally required to determine the limit standard of both aflatoxin $B_1$ and the total amount of aflatoxin $B_1$, aflatoxin $B_2$, aflatoxin $G_1$ and aflatoxin $G_2$.

有害残留物的限量制定，除了应用上述计算公式得到最大理论值外，还应考虑其他影响因素，进行综合评价后，确定其标准限值。各国家和国际组织对于已经规定的农药、重金属等最大残留限量，也会根据影响因素进行调整。

During the establishment of limit of harmful residue, in addition to theoretical maximal limit calculated by the formula above, other affecting factors should be included. Determine the standard limit after comprehensive evaluation. National and international organizations will also revise the maximum residue limits for pesticides, heavy metals, and other regulations that have been set in accordance with influencing factors.

## 第二节　无机杂质检查
## 4.2　Analysis of Inorganic Impurities in Chinese Medicine

### 一、重金属检查
### 4.2.1　Limit Test for Heavy Metals

重金属系指在规定实验条件下能与硫代乙酰胺或硫化钠作用显色的金属杂质。这些金属杂质通常有 $Pb^{2+}$、$Hg^{2+}$、$Ag^+$、$Fe^{3+}$ 等金属离子，在生产过程中 $Pb^{2+}$ 最为常见，易在体内蓄积中毒，故重金属的检查以铅为代表物。《中国药典》收载了 3 种重金属的检查方法。

The term "heavy metals" refers to those metals that react with thioacetamide or sodium sulfide under the specified conditions to produce a colored compound. These metal impurities usually include metal ions such as $Pb^{2+}$, $Hg^{2+}$, $Ag^+$, $Fe^{3+}$, etc. $Pb^{2+}$ is the most common in the production process, and it is easy to accumulate poisoning in the body. Therefore, the limit test of heavy metals is the limit test lead. The *Chinese Pharmacopoeia* contains three methods for the limit test of heavy metals.

**标准铅溶液的配制**　称取硝酸铅 0.1599g，置 1000ml 量瓶中，加硝酸 5ml 与水 50ml 溶解后，用水稀释至刻度，摇匀，作为贮备液。精密量取贮备液 10ml，置 100ml 量瓶中，加水稀释至刻度，摇匀，即得（每 1ml 相当于 10μg 的 Pb）。该溶液仅供当日使用。

*Lead standard solution*　Dissolve 0.1599g of lead nitrate in 5ml of nitric acid and 50ml of water in 1000ml volumetric flask, dilute to volume with water, mix well as the stock solution. Transfer 10ml of the stock solution, accurately measured, to a 100ml volumetric flask, dilute with water to volume and mix well (each ml is equivalent to 10μg of lead). This solution should be prepared on the day of use.

制备与贮存用的玻璃容器均不得含铅。

All glassware used for the preparation and preservation of the lead standard solution should be free from lead.

### 第一法　硫代乙酰胺法
### Method 1　Thioacetamide Method

本法适用于供试品可不经有机破坏即可溶于水、稀酸和乙醇的重金属检查。

This method is applicable to the limit test of heavy metals in the Chinese medicine that can be dissolved in water, dilute acid and ethanol without organic destruction.

（1）原理　硫代乙酰胺在弱酸性（pH3~3.5）条件下发生水解产生的硫化氢，与重金属离子反应生成有色的硫化物。与一定量的铅标准液在相同条件下产生的颜色进行比较，判定供试品中重金属是否符合限量规定。

(1) *Principle*　Thioacetamide undergoes hydrolysis under weakly acidic conditions (pH 3-3.5) to generate hydrogen sulfide, which reacts with heavy metal ions to form colored sulfides. Compare it with the color produced by a certain amount of lead standard solution under the same conditions to determine whether the heavy metals in the test product exceed the limits.

$$CH_3CSNH_2 + H_2O \xrightarrow{pH3.5} CH_3CONH_2 + H_2S\uparrow$$

（2）检查方法　除有规定外，取 25ml 纳氏比色管三支，甲管中加标准铅溶液一定量与醋酸盐缓冲液（pH3.5）2ml 后，加水或各品种项下规定的溶剂稀释成 25ml，乙管中加入按各品种项下规定方法制成的供试液 25ml；丙管中加入与乙管相同重量的供试品，加配制供试品溶液的溶剂适量使溶解，再加与甲管相同量的标准铅溶液与醋酸盐缓冲液（pH3.5）2ml后，用溶剂稀释成25ml；若供试品溶液带颜色，可在甲管中滴加少量的稀焦糖溶液或其他无干扰的有色溶液，使之与乙管、丙管一致；再在甲、乙、丙三管中分别加硫代乙酰胺试液各2ml，摇匀，放置2分钟，同置白纸上，自上向下透视，当丙管中显出的颜色不浅于甲管时，乙管中显示的颜色与甲管比较，不得更深。如丙管中显出的颜色浅于甲管，应取样按第二法重新检查。

(2) *Procedure*　Unless otherwise specified, use three 25ml Nessler cylinders. To cylinder A add the specified volume of lead standard solution and 2ml of acetate BS (pH 3.5), dilute with water or other solvent as specified in the individual monographs to 25ml. To cylinder B add 25ml of the test product solution prepared according to the method specified under each item. To cylinder C and 25ml of another solution containing the same quantity of the substance being examined in the individual monographs, the same volume of lead standard solution as cylinder A, and 2ml of acetate BS (pH 3.5). If the original test solution is colored, it may be matched by the addition of a few drops of dilute caramel solution or other suitable solution to cylinder A. To each cylinder add 2ml of thioacetamide TS and mix well, allow to stand for 2 minutes, compare the color produced by viewing down the vertical axis of the three cylinders against a white background. The color produced in cylinder B is not more intense than that produced in cylinder A and the color produced in cylinder C is equal to or intense than that produced in cylinder A. If the color produced in cylinder C is lighter than that produced in cylinder A, use Method 2 instead of Method 1 for the substance being examined.

（3）注意事项　① 供试品如含高铁盐影响重金属检查时，可在甲、乙、丙三管中分别加入相同量的维生素C 0.5~1.0g，再照上述方法检查。② 配制供试品溶液时，如使用的盐酸超过1ml，氨试液超过2ml，或加入其他试剂进行处理者，除另有规定外，甲管溶液应取同样同量的试剂置瓷皿中蒸干后，加醋酸盐缓冲液（pH 3.5）2ml与水15ml，微热溶解后，移置纳氏比色管中，加标准铅溶液一定量，再用水或各品种项下规定的溶剂稀释成25ml。

(3) *Notes*　① If the substance being examined contains a ferric salt which interferes with the test, the same quantity of 0.5-1.0g of ascorbic acid should be added to each cylinder, then check as above method. ② Unless otherwise specified, evaporate the same quantity of the same reagents to dryness in a porcelain dish. Dissolve the residue in 2ml of acetate BS (pH 3.5) and 15ml of water. Transfer the solution to a Nessler cylinder, add the specified quantity of lead standard solution and water or other solvent as specified under individual monographs to 25ml. The solution is used as the reference solution for the test solution which is prepared by using more than 1ml of hydrochloric acid, 2ml of ammonia TS or by treating with other reagents.

第二法　炽灼后的硫代乙酰胺法

Method 2　Thioacetamide Method after Ignition

本法适用于不能用第一法直接进行重金属检查，而需将样品有机破坏后，金属离子游离方可进行重金属检查的中药及产品。

It is applicable to traditional Chinese medicines and preparations that can't be used for the heavy metal inspection directly by the first method, but after the samples are organically destroyed, the metal ions are released before the heavy metal inspection can be performed.

（1）原理　重金属离子与中药中的有机物质结合牢固，供试品需先炽灼破坏，使其游离，再加盐酸转化为易溶于水的金属氯化物，再照第一法检查。

(1) *Principle*　The heavy metal ions are firmly combined with the organic substances in the traditional Chinese medicine. The test product needs to be ignited to make metal ions free, and then add

hydrochloric acid to convert it into water-soluble metal chloride, and then check it according to the first method.

（2）检查方法 取各品种项下规定量的供试品，按炽灼残渣检查法（《中国药典》四部通则 0841）进行炽灼处理，然后取遗留的残渣；或直接取炽灼残渣项下遗留的残渣；如供试品为溶液，则取各品种项下规定量的溶液，蒸发至干，再按上述方法处理后取遗留的残渣；加硝酸 0.5ml，蒸干，至氧化氮蒸气除尽后（或取供试品一定量，缓缓炽灼至完全炭化，放冷，加硫酸 0.5~1ml，使恰湿润，用低温加热至硫酸除尽后，加硝酸 0.5ml，蒸干，至氧化氮蒸气除尽后，放冷，在 500~600℃ 炽灼使完全灰化），放冷，加盐酸 2ml，置水浴上蒸干后加水 15ml，滴加氨试液至对酚酞指示液显微粉红色，再加醋酸盐缓冲液（pH3.5）2ml，微热溶解后，移置纳氏比色管中，加水稀释成 25ml，作为乙管；另取配制供试品溶液的试剂，置瓷皿中蒸干后，加醋酸盐缓冲液（pH3.5）2ml 与水 15ml，微热溶解后，移置纳氏比色管中，加标准铅溶液一定量，再用水稀释成 25ml，作为甲管；再在甲、乙两管中分别加入硫代乙酰胺试液各 2ml，摇匀，放置 2 分钟，同置白纸上，自上向下透视，乙管中显出的颜色与甲管比较，不得更深。

(2) *Procedure* Take the specified amount of test products under each item, carry out ignition treatment according to the test for residue on ignition (*Chinese Pharmacopoeia*, general requirements 0841), and then take the remaining residue; or directly take the residue obtained in the test for residue on ignition. If the substance being examined is a liquid, evaporate a volume of the substance being examined as specified in the individual monographs to dryness, using the residue obtained in the test for residue on ignition, add 0.5ml of nitric acid, evaporate to dryness, heat until nitrous oxide fumes are no longer evolved (or alternatively, ignite a quantity of the substance being examined in a crucible until thoroughly charred, cool, moisten the residue with 0.5-1ml of sulfuric acid, ignite at a low temperature until sulfurous acid fumes are no longer evolved, add 0.5ml of nitric acid, evaporate to dryness, heat until nitrous oxide fumes are no longer evolved and ignite at 500-600℃ until the incineration is complete). Cool, add 2ml of hydrochloric acid, evaporate to dryness on a water bath, add 15ml of water, followed by ammonia TS dropwise until the solution is slight pink to phenolphthalein dissolution. Transfer the resulting solution to Nessler cylinder B, dilute with water to 25ml. Place the same quantity of the same reagents used for the preparation of test solution in a porcelain dish and evaporate to dryness, heat gently to dissolve in 2ml of acetate BS(pH3.5) and 15ml of water, transfer to the Nessler cylinder A and add the specified volume of lead standard solution, dilute with water to 25ml. To each cylinder add 2ml of thioacetamide TS and mix well, allow to stand for 2 minutes, compare the color produced by viewing down the vertical axis of the two cylinders against a white background. The color produced in cylinder B is not more intense than that produced in cylinder A.

### 第三法 硫化钠法

### Method 3 Sodium Sulfide Method

本法适用于易溶于碱而不溶于稀酸和稀乙醇或在稀酸中生成沉淀的药物中重金属检查。

This method is suitable for the inspection of heavy metals in medicines that are easily soluble in alkali but not in dilute acid and dilute ethanol or precipitate in dilute acid.

（1）原理 在碱性条件下，硫化钠与重金属离子作用生成不溶性硫化物，反应式如下：

(1) *Principle* Under alkaline conditions, sodium sulfide interacts with heavy metal ions to form insoluble sulfides.

$$Pb^{2+}+S^{2-}\rightarrow PbS\downarrow$$

（2）检查方法 取供试品适量，加氢氧化钠试液 5ml 与水 20ml 溶解后，置纳氏比色管中加硫化钠试液 5 滴，摇匀，与一定量的标准铅溶液同样处理后的颜色比较，不得更深。

(2) *Procedure* Dissolve a quantity of the substance being examined in 5ml of sodium hydroxide TS and 20ml of water. Transfer the solution to a Nessler cylinder, add 5 drops of sodium sulfide TS and mix well, the color produced is not more intense than that of a reference preparation containing the specified volume of lead standard solution and treated in the same manner.

（3）注意事项 硫化钠对玻璃有腐蚀作用，久置会产生絮状物，应临用时配制。

(3) *Notes* Sodium sulfide has a corrosive effect on glass, and it will produce flocculent after long-term storage. It should be prepared before use.

### 二、砷盐检查
### 4.2.2 Limit Test for Arsenic

砷盐检查系指用于药品中微量砷（以 As 计算）限量检查的方法。《中国药典》收载了两种砷盐检查方法，即古蔡氏法和二乙基硫代氨基甲酸银法（Ag-DDC 法）。

The limit test for arsenic refers to the method used for the limit test for trace arsenic (calculated as As) in medicines. *Chinese Pharmacopoeia* contains two methods, namely the Gutzeit method (Gutzeit) and silver diethylthiocarbamate method (Ag-DDC method).

**标准砷溶液的配制** 称取三氧化二砷 0.132g，置 1000ml 量瓶中，加 20% 氢氧化钠溶液 5ml 溶解后，用适量的稀硫酸中和，再加稀硫酸 10ml，用水稀释至刻度，摇匀，作为贮备液。临用前，精密量取贮备液 10ml，置 1000ml 量瓶中，加稀硫酸 10ml，用水稀释至刻度，摇匀，即得（每 1ml 相当于 1μg 的 As）。

*Arsenic standard solution* Dissolve 0.132g of arsenic trioxide in 5ml of 20% sodium hydroxide solution in a 1000ml volumetric flask, neutralize with dilute sulfuric acid and add 10ml in excess. Dilute with water to volume and mix well, as a stock solution. Transfer 10ml of the stock solution, accurately measured, to a 1000ml volumetric flask immediately before use, add 10ml of dilute sulfuric acid, dilute with water to volume and mix well (each ml is equivalent to 1μg of arsenic).

（一）古蔡氏法
### 1. Gutzeit's method

1. 原理 金属锌与盐酸反应作用产生新生态的氢，与供试品中微量砷盐反应，生成挥发性砷化氢气体，砷化氢再与溴化汞试纸作用生成黄色至棕色砷斑。与一定量的标准砷溶液在同一条件下所形成的砷斑进行比较，判定供试品中砷盐是否符合限量规定。

(1) *Principle* The reaction of zinc metal with hydrochloric acid produces new ecological hydrogen, which reacts with trace arsenic in the test product to produce volatile arsine gas. The arsine reacts with mercuric bromide test paper to produce yellow to brown arsenic spots. Compare the arsenic spots formed by a certain amount of standard arsenic solution with that formed by test sample under the same conditions to determine whether the arsenic meet the prescribed limit in the test sample.

$$AsO_3^{3-}+3Zn+9H^+\rightarrow AsH_3\uparrow+3Zn^{2+}+3H_2O$$
$$AsH_3+3HgBr_2\rightarrow 3HBr+As(HgBr)_3（黄色，yellow）$$
$$AsH_3+2As(HgBr)_3\rightarrow 3AsH(HgBr)_2（棕色，brown）$$
$$AsH_3+As(HgBr)_3\rightarrow 3HBr+As_2Hg_3（棕黑色，brown-black）$$

五价砷生成砷化氢的速度较三价砷慢，在实验条件下能被锌粒还原为砷化氢，但故在反应液中加入碘化钾及酸性氯化亚锡将五价砷还原为三价砷，有利于砷化氢的生成。碘化钾被氧化生成的碘又可被氯化亚锡还原为碘离子，维持反应过程中碘化钾还原剂的存在。溶液中的碘离子还能与反应中产生的锌离子形成配合物，使生成砷化氢的反应不断进行。

Pentavalent arsenic can formate can arsenic hydrogen, the rate of arsenic hydrogen formation is slower than trivalent arsenic, but can be deoxidated to arsenic hydrogen by zinc particles under experimental conditions, so potassium iodide and acidic stannous chloride are added to the reaction solution to deoxidate pentavalent arsenic to trivalent arsenic, which is conducive to the formation of arsine. The iodine generated by the oxidation of potassium iodide can be reduced to iodide ion by stannous chloride to maintain the presence of potassium iodide reducing agent during the reaction. The iodide ions in the solution can also form a complex with the zinc ions produced in the reaction, so that the reaction to generate arsenic hydride is continued.

氯化亚锡与碘化钾存在，可抑制锑化氢的生成，因锑化氢也能与溴化汞试纸作用生成锑斑，在试验条件下100g锑的存在不会干扰测定。氯化亚锡又可与锌作用，在锌粒表面形成锌锡齐，起去极化作用，使锌粒与盐酸作用缓和，从而使氢气均匀而连续地发生。

The presence of stannous chloride and potassium iodide can inhibit the formation of antimony hydrogen. Since antimony hydrogen can also react with mercury bromide test paper to form antimony spots, the presence of 100g antimony under the test conditions will not interfere with the measurement. Stannous chloride can also act with zinc to form zinc tin tin on the surface of the zinc particles, which acts as a depolarizer, so that the action of zinc particles and hydrochloric acid become moderating, so that hydrogen can occur uniformly and continuously.

**2. 测定方法**

**(2) Method**

**仪器装置**　见图 4-1（左）。A 为 100ml 标准磨口锥形瓶；B 为中空的标准磨口塞，上连导气管 C（外径 8.0mm，内径 6.0mm），全长约 180mm，D 为具孔的有机玻璃旋塞，其上部为圆形平面，中央有一圆孔，孔径与导气管 C 的内径一致，其下部孔径与导气管 C 的外径相适应，将导气管 C 的顶端套入旋塞下部孔内，并使管壁与旋塞的圆孔相吻合，黏合固定；E 为中央具有圆孔（孔径 6.0mm）的有机玻璃旋塞盖，与 D 紧密吻合。测试时，于导气管 C 中装入醋酸铅棉花 60mg（装管高度为 60~80mm），再于旋塞 D 的顶端平面上放一片溴化汞试纸（试纸大小以能覆盖孔径而不露出平面外为宜），盖上旋塞盖 E 并旋紧，即得。

*Apparatus* as Fig.4-1 (left). A is a 100ml conical flask with standard ground joint; B is a standard hollow ground glass stopper connected to glass conduit C (external diameter 8.0mm, internal diameter 6.0mm), the total length of B and C is about 180mm; D is a plastic screw, the upper part of which has an aperture 6.0mm in diameter and the lower part of which has an aperture 8.0mm in diameter; E is a plastic screw cap which has an aperture 6.0mm in diameter. A wad of lead of lead acetate cotton weighing about 60mg is packed into tube C to a depth of about 60-80mm. A disc of mercuric bromide paper is placed between the contacting surfaces of D and E.

**标准砷斑的制备**　精密量取标准砷溶液 2ml，置 A 瓶中，加盐酸 5ml 与水 21ml，再加碘化钾试液 5ml 与酸性氯化亚锡试液 5 滴，在室温放置 10 分钟后，加锌粒 2g，立即将照上法装妥的导气管 C 密塞于 A 瓶上，并将 A 瓶置 25~40℃水浴中反应 45 分钟，取出溴化汞试纸即得。

*Arsenic standard stain*　Place 2ml of standard arsenic solution, accurately measured, in flask A. Add 5ml of hydrochloric acid and 21ml of water. Then add 5ml of potassium iodide TS and 5 drops of acid

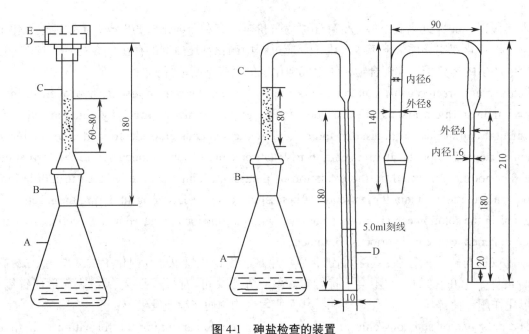

图 4-1　砷盐检查的装置

Fig.4-1　Apparatus of Gutzeit's method (left) and Ag-DDC method (right)

左：古蔡氏法检测砷装置；右：Ag-DDC 法检测砷装置

stannous chloride TS, allow to stand at room temperature for 10 minutes and add 2g of granulated zinc. Insert the stopper B and conduit C into the mouth of flask A and immerse the flask in a water bath at 25-40℃ for 45 minutes. Remove the mercuric bromide paper.

若供试品需经有机破坏后再行检砷，则应取标准砷溶液代替供试品，照该品种项下规定的方法同法处理后，依法制备标准砷斑。

Use arsenic standard solution instead of the substance being examined and treat it in the same manner described in the individual monographs. Then prepare the arsenic standard stain as described under Arsenic standard stain, if the substance being examined needs to be destroyed organically before carrying out the limit test for arsenic.

**检查法**　取按各品种项下规定方法制成的供试品溶液，置 A 瓶中，照标准砷斑的制备，自" 再加碘化钾试液 5ml" 起，依法操作。将生成的砷斑与标准砷斑比较，不得更深。

*Procedure*　Transfer the test solution prepared as described in the individual monographs to flask A and proceed as described under arsenic standard stain, beginning with the word "Then add 5ml of potassium iodide TS …". Any stain produced is not more intense than the standard stain.

（二）二乙基二硫代氨基甲酸银法

## 2. Silver Diethyldithiocarbamate Method

二乙基二硫代氨基甲酸银法，简称 Ag-DDC 法，也可用于微量砷盐的含量测定。

Silver diethyldithiocarbamate（Ag-DDC）method, an also be used for the determination of trace arsenic.

1. **原理**　金属锌与酸作用，产生新生态的氢，与供试品中的微量亚砷酸盐反应，生成具有挥发性的砷化氢，被二乙基二硫代氨基甲酸银溶液吸收，使 Ag-DDC 中的银还原成红色的胶态银。比较供试品与标准砷溶液在同一条件下生成红色胶态银颜色的深浅，判断供试品中砷盐是否符合限量规定。

**(1) Principle**　The reaction of zinc metal with hydrochloric acid produces new ecological hydrogen, which reacts with trace arsenic in the test product to produce volatile arsine gas. which is absorbed by silver diethyldithiocarbamate solution to make Ag in the DDC is reduced to red colloidal silver. Compare the shade of red colloidal silver produced by the test product and that of the standard arsenic solution under the same conditions to determine whether the arsenic in the test product meets the limit.

$$AsH_3 \ + \ 6 \quad \begin{matrix} C_2H_5 \\ \diagdown \\ \diagup \\ C_2H_5 \end{matrix} N-C \begin{matrix} \diagup S \\ \diagdown S \end{matrix} Ag \quad \rightleftharpoons \quad 6Ag \ + \ As \left[ \begin{matrix} C_2H_5 \\ \diagdown \\ \diagup \\ C_2H_5 \end{matrix} N-C \begin{matrix} \diagup S \\ \diagdown S \end{matrix} \right]_3 \ + \ 3 \begin{matrix} C_2H_5 \\ \diagdown \\ \diagup \\ C_2H_5 \end{matrix} N-C \begin{matrix} \diagup S \\ \diagdown SH \end{matrix}$$

二乙基二硫代氨基甲酸银　　　　　　　　　　　　　二乙基二硫代氨基甲酸
（Ag-DDC）　　　　　　　　　　　　　　　　　（HDDC）

### 2. 测定方法
### (2) Method

**仪器装置** 如图 4-1（右）。A 为 100ml 标准磨口锥形瓶；B 为中空的标准磨口塞，上连导气管 C（一端的外径为 8mm，内径为 6mm；另一端长为 180mm，外径为 4mm，内径为 1.6mm，尖端内径为 1mm）；D 为平底玻璃管（长为 180mm，内径为 10mm，于 5.0ml 处有刻度）。测试时，于导气管 C 中装入醋酸铅棉花 60mg（装管高度为约 80mm)，并于 D 管中精密加入 Ag-DDC 试液 5ml。

*Apparatus* as Fig. 4-1. (right). A is a 100ml conical flask with standard ground joint; B is a standard hollow ground glass stopper connected to conduit C (at one end, the external diameter is 8.0mm and the internal diameter is 6.0mm; the other end is in length of 180mm, in external diameter of 4mm and in internal diameter of 1.6mm, the internal diameter of sharp end is 1mm). D is a glass tube with flat bottom (length 180mm, internal diameter 10mm, and with a graduation at 5.0ml). A wad of lead acetate cotton weighing about 60mg is packed into conduit C to a depth of about 80mm, and measure accurately 5ml of silver diethyldithiocarbamate TS in tube D.

**标准砷对照液的制备** 精密量取标准砷溶液 2ml，置 A 瓶中，加盐酸 5ml 与水 21ml，再加碘化钾试液 5ml 与酸性氯化亚锡试液 5 滴，在室温放置 10 分钟后，加锌粒 2g，立即将导气管 C 与 A 瓶密塞，使生成的砷化氢气体导入 D 管中，并将 A 瓶置 25~40℃ 水浴中反应 45 分钟，取出 D 管，添加三氯甲烷至刻度，混匀，即得。

*Arsenic reference solution* Transfer 2ml of arsenic standard solution to flask A, accurately measured. Add 5ml of hydrochloric acid and 21ml of water. Then add 5ml of potassium iodide TS and 5 drops of acid stannous chloride TS, allow to stand at room temperature for 10 minutes and 2g of granulated zinc. Connect conduit C into flask A immediately, and allow the evolved arsine to enter tube D. Immerse the flask A in a water bath at 25-40℃ for 45 minutes. Remove tube D, add chloroform to the graduation, mix well.

若供试品需经有机破坏后再行检砷，则应取标准砷溶液代替供试品，照该品种项下规定的方法同法处理后，依法制备标准砷斑。

Use arsenic standard solution instead of the substance being examined and treat in the same manner in the individual monographs. Then prepare the arsenic reference solution as described above, if the substance being examined needs to be destroyed organically before carrying out the limit test for arsenic.

**检查法** 取照各药品项下规定方法制成的供试品溶液，置 A 瓶中，照标准砷对照液的制备，自 "再加碘化钾试液 5ml" 起，依法操作。将所得溶液与标准砷对照液同置白色背景上，从 D 管上方向下观察、比较，所得溶液的颜色不得比标准砷对照液更深。必要时，可将所得溶液转移至 1cm 吸收池中，照紫外 – 可见分光光度法（《中国药典》通则 0401）在 510nm 波长处以二乙基二硫代氨基甲酸银试液作空白，测定吸收度，与标准砷对照液按同法测得的吸收度比较，即得。

*Procedure*    Transfer the test solution prepared as described in the individual monographs to flask A and proceed as described under arsenic reference solution, beginning with the word "Then add 5ml of potassium iodide TS …". Compare the above two solutions against a white background. Any color produced by the test preparation is not more intense than that produced by the standard arsenic reference solution. If necessary, determine the absorbance at the wavelength of 510 nm, using silver diethyldithiocarbamate TS as the blank (*Chinese Pharmacopoeia*, general chapters 0401).

（三）注意事项

3.  Notes

（1）所用仪器和试液等照本法检查，均不应生成砷斑，或至多生成仅可辨认的斑痕。

(1)  Make sure that a blank test produces no arsenic stain or only a barely visible stain.

（2）制备标准砷斑或标准砷对照液，应与供试品检查同时进行。

(2)  The preparation of standard stain and test stain must be carried out simultaneously.

（3）本法所用锌粒应无砷，以能通过一号筛的细粒为宜，如使用的锌粒较大时，用量应酌情增加，反应时间亦应延长为 1 小时。

(3)  The granulated zinc should be arsenic free and the size is such that they will pass through a No.1 sieve. The quantity used should be increased and the reaction time should be extended up to 1 hour, if the granules are of larger size.

（4）醋酸铅棉花系取脱脂棉 1.0g，浸入醋酸铅试液与水的等容混合液 12ml 中，湿透后，挤压除去过多的溶液，并使之疏松，在 100℃ 以下干燥后，贮于玻璃塞瓶中备用。

(4)  Lead acetate cotton is prepared by immersing 1.0g of absorbent cotton in 12ml of a mixture of equal volumes of lead acetate TS and water. Drain off excess liquid and make the cotton fluffy, allow it to dry at a temperature below 100℃ and preserve in a well closed glass container.

### 三、铅、镉、砷、汞、铜测定法

### 4.2.3  Determination of Lead (Pb), Cadmium (Cd), Arsenic (As), Mercury (Hg) and Copper (Cu)

铅、镉、砷、汞、铜是目前公认的对人体有害的元素，《中国药典》采用原子吸收分光光度法、电感耦合等离子体质谱法检查上述 5 种元素。

Lead, cadmium, arsenic, mercury, and copper are currently recognized as harmful elements to the human body. The *Chinese Pharmacopoeia* uses atomic absorption spectrophotometry and inductively coupled plasma mass spectrometry to check the above five elements.

（一）原子吸收分光光度法

1.  Atomic absorption spectrophotometry

原子吸收分光光度计由光源、原子化器、单色器、背景校正系统、进样系统和检测系统等组成。其原理是将待测定元素原子化后，由待测元素灯发出的特征谱线通过样品经原子化产生的原子蒸气时，被蒸气中待测元素的基态原子所吸收，通过测定辐射光强度减弱的程度进行测定，依据标准曲线法求出样品中待测元素的含量。

The atomic absorption spectrophotometer is composed of a light source, an atomic generator, a monochromator, a background compensation system, a sampling system, and a detector system. The principle is that after the element to be measured is atomized, when the characteristic line emitted by the element to be measured passes through the atomic vapor generated by the atomization of the sample, it is absorbed by the ground state atoms of the element to be measured in the vapor, and the intensity of the radiated light is reduced by measuring the degree of determination is determined, and the content of the element to be measured in the sample is determined according to the standard curve method.

《中国药典》采用石墨炉法测定铅、镉的含量：将样品溶液干燥、灰化，以石墨作为发热体，经高温原子化使待测元素形成基态原子。采用氢化物法测定砷的含量：使用氢化物发生原子化器，将待测元素在酸性介质中还原成低沸点、易受热分解的氢化物，再由载气导入原子吸收池，在吸收池中加热分解形成基态原子。采用冷蒸气吸收法测定汞的含量：使用冷蒸气发生原子化器，将样品溶液中的汞离子还原成汞蒸气，再由载气导入石英原子吸收池，进行测定。采用火焰法测定铜的含量：使用火焰原子化器，将样品溶液雾化成气溶胶后，再与燃气（乙炔－空气）混合，进入燃烧灯头产生的火焰中，以干燥、蒸发、离解供试品，使待测元素形成基态原子。

*Chinese Pharmacopoeia* uses the graphite furnace method to determine the content of lead and cadmium: the sample solution is dried and free from carbon, using graphite as a heater, and the element to be measured form a ground state atom by high-temperature atomization; The arsenic content is determined by the hydride method: use a hydride generator to reduce the element to be tested into a low-boiling in acidic medium and easily pyrolyzed hydride. Then, hydride is swept by a stream of the carrier gas into the atomic absorption cell, pyrolyzed by heating to form the ground state atoms; Determination of mercury content by cold vapor absorption method: use a cold vapor atomizer to reduce the mercury ions in the sample solution to mercury vapor, and then the mercury vapor is swept by the carrier gas into a quartz atomic absorption cell for measurement; Use the flame method to determine copper content: using a flame atomizer, the sample solution is nebulize into an aerosol, then mixed with combustion gas (acetylene-air), enters the flame generated by the burner, and is dried, evaporated, and dissociated for the test article, so that the element to be measured forms a ground state atom .

（二）电感耦合等离子体质谱法

## 2. Inductively coupled plasma-mass spectrometry

样品由载气（氩气）引入雾化系统进行雾化后，以气溶胶形式进入等离子体中心区，在高温和惰性气体中被去溶剂化、气化解离和电离，转化成带正电荷的正离子，经离子采集系统进入质谱仪，质谱仪根据质荷比进行分离，根据元素质谱峰强度测定，依据标准曲线法求出样品中待测元素的含量。本法灵敏度高，专属性强，可同时对多种元素进行定性、定量分析，适用于各类药品从痕量到微量的元素分析，尤其是痕量有害元素的测定。

After the sample is introduced into the atomization system by the carrier gas (oxygen) for atomization, it enters the central area of the human plasma in the form of aerosol, is desolvated, vaporized, dissociated and ionized in high temperature and inert gas, and converted into positively charged the positive ions enter the mass spectrometer through the ion collection system. The mass spectrometer separates according to the mass-to-charge ratio. According to the peak intensity determination of the element mass spectrum, the content of the element to be measured in the sample is determined according to the standard curve method. The method has high sensitivity and strong specificity, and can perform qualitative and quantitative analysis of various elements at the same time. It is suitable for the analysis of trace elements to trace elements of various drugs, especially the determination of trace harmful elements.

例 4-1　山楂、金银花、丹参、甘草、三七、白芍、人参、西洋参等常用中药中重金属及有害元素的检查

Example 4-1　Test of heavy metals and harmful elements of crataegi fructus, lonicerae japonicae flos, radix et rhizoma salviae miltiorrhizae, nardostachyos radix et rhizome, notoginseng radix et rhizome, radix paeoniae alba, ginseng radix et rhizome, radix panacis quinquefolia and other Chinese medicines.

**重金属及有害元素**　照铅、镉、砷、汞、铜测定法（《中国药典》通则 2321 原子吸收分光光度法或电感耦合等离子体质谱法）测定，铅不得过 5mg/kg，镉不得过 1mg/kg，砷不得过 2mg/kg，汞不得过 0.2mg/kg，铜不得过 20mg/kg。

**Heavy metals and harmful elements**　Carry out the methods for determinations of lead, cadmium, arsenic, mercury and copper (*Chinese Pharmacopoeia*, general chapters 2321，absorption spectrophotometry, or inductively coupled plasma mass spectrometry), not more than 5 mg/kg of lead, 0.3 mg/kg of cadmium, 2 mg/kg of arsenic, 0.2 mg/kg of mercury and 20 mg/kg of copper.

### 四、汞、砷元素形态及价态测定法
### 4.2.4　Determination of Mercury, Arsenic Speciation and Valence States

由于元素存在的形态不同，其物理、化学性质与生物活性也不同，如不同形态的砷，其毒性大小也不同。《中国药典》采用高效液相色谱 – 电感耦合等离子体质谱法测定中药中汞、砷元素形态及价态（《中国药典》通则 2322 ）。

This method is provided for analysis of mercury or arsenic speciation and valence state in test samples using high performance liquid chromatography/ tandem inductively coupled plasma- mass spectrometry (HPLC/ICP MS) (*Chinese Pharmacopoeia*, general chapters 2322).

### 五、干燥失重测定法
### 4.2.5　Determination of Loss on Drying

干燥失重系指药品在规定的条件下，经干燥至恒重后所减失的重量。主要是检查药物中的水分、结晶水及其他挥发性的物质如乙醇等。由减失的重量和取样量计算供试品的干燥失重。药品中若含有较多的水分或其他挥发性物质，不仅使其成分的含量降低，而且会引起药物中某些成分水解或发霉变质。因此要进行干燥失重测定。

Loss on drying refers to the weight loss of a drug after drying to constant weight under prescribed conditions. Mainly check the water, crystal water and other volatile substances such as ethanol in the medicine. Calculate the loss on drying of the test sample from the weight loss and sampling quality. If the medicine contains more water or other volatile substances, not only will the content of its ingredients be reduced, but also some of the ingredients in the medicine will be hydrolyzed or mildewed. Therefore, the determination of loss on drying should be carried out.

（一）测定方法

## 1. Method

取供试品，混合均匀（如为较大的结晶，应先迅速捣碎使成 2mm 以下的小粒），取约 1g 或各品种项下规定的重量，置于与供试品相同条件下干燥至恒重的扁形称量瓶中，精密称定，除另有规定外，在 105℃ 干燥至恒重。由减失的重量和取样量计算供试品的干燥失重。

Mix the substance being examined thoroughly, If it is in the form of large crystals, reduce them to a size of about 2mm by quickly crushing. Place about 1g or the amount specified in the individual monographs of the substance being examined in a tared, shallow weighing bottle, previously dried to constant weight at 105℃, weigh accurately, unless otherwise specified, dried to constant weight at 105℃. Calculate the percentage content of loss on drying in the substance being examined according to the weight loss on drying and sample weight.

（二）注意事项

## 2. Notes

1. 供试品干燥时，应平铺在扁形称量瓶中，厚度不可超过 5mm，如为疏松物质，厚度不可超过 10mm。放入烘箱或干燥器进行干燥时，应将瓶盖取下，置称量瓶旁，或将瓶盖半开进行干燥；取出时，须将称量瓶盖好。置烘箱内干燥的供试品，应在干燥后取出置干燥器中放冷，然后称定重量。

(1) The substance being examined should be evenly distributed to form a layer of not more than 5mm in the thickness, or not more than 10mm in the case of bulky material. When the loaded bottle is placed in the drying chamber or desiccator, remove the stopper and put it beside the bottle, or leave it on the bottle in half open position. Upon the opening of the drying chamber or desiccator, the bottle should be closed promptly. If the substance is dried by heating, allow it to cool to room temperature in a desiccator before weighing.

2. 供试品如未达规定的干燥温度即融化时，应先将供试品在低于熔化温度 5~10℃ 的温度下干燥至大部分水分除去后，再按规定条件干燥。生物制品应先将供试品于较低的温度下干燥至大部分水分除去后，再按规定条件干燥。

(2) If the substance melts at a lower temperature than the specified drying temperature, unless otherwise specified, maintain the bottle with its content at about 5-10℃ below the melting point until most of the water is removed, and then dry it under the specified conditions. For biological products, dry it under the specified conditions after most of the water of the substance being examined was removed at a lower temperature.

3. 当用减压干燥器（通常为室温）或恒温减压干燥器（温度应按各品种项下的规定设置。生物制品除另有规定，温度为 60℃）时，除另有规定外，压力应在 2.67kPa（20mmHg）以下。干燥器中常用的干燥剂为五氧化二磷、无水氯化钙或硅胶；恒温减压干燥器中常用的干燥剂为五氧化二磷。干燥剂应及时更换，使其保持在有效状态。

(3) If a vacuum desiccator or constant temperature vacuum desiccator is to be used (Set the temperature as specified in the monograph. For biological products, set the temperature at 60℃ unless otherwise specified.) a pressure of 2.67 kPa (20mmHg) or less should be maintained unless otherwise directed. The desiccants used in a desiccator are usually phosphorus pentoxide, anhydrous calcium chloride or silica gel. Phosphorus pentoxide is often used in a constant temperature vacuum desiccator. The desiccants should be replaced in time.

## 六、水分测定法
## 4.2.6　Determination of Water

《中国药典》收载五种水分测定方法，分别为费休氏法、烘干法、减压干燥法、甲苯法和气相色谱法，其中后四种主要用于中药中水分的测定。

Methods for determining moisture in *Chinese Pharmacopoeia* include drying in oven method, drying under reduced pressure method, toluene distillation method and gas chromatography, of which the last four are mainly used for the determination of water in Chinese medicines.

### （一）烘干法
### 1.　Drying in Oven Method

本法适用于不含或少含挥发性成分的药品。

The method is used for the determination of water in drugs with little or no volatile constituents.

测定法：取供试品 2~5g，如果供试品的直径或长度超过 3mm，在称取前应快速制成直径或长度不超过 3mm 的颗粒或碎片。平铺于干燥至恒重的扁形称量瓶中，厚度不超过 5mm，疏松样品不超过 10mm，精密称定，打开瓶盖，在 100~105℃ 干燥 5 小时，将瓶盖盖好，移至干燥器中，放冷 30 分钟，精密称定重量，再在上述温度干燥 1 小时，放冷，称重，至连续两次称重的差异不超过 5mg 为止。根据减失的重量，计算供试品中含水量（％）。

*Procedure*　Place 2-5g of the substance being examined, accurately weighed, if the diameter or length of the test product exceeds 3mm, particles or fragments with a diameter or length not exceeding 3mm should be quickly made before weighing, in a flat weighing bottle previously dried to constant weight to form a smooth layer not exceeding 5mm in thickness, or not exceeding 10mm in thickness for substance of loose texture. Dry in an oven at 100-105℃ for 5 hours with the stopper of the bottle removed, upon opening the oven, close the bottle promptly and allow it to cool in a desiccator for 30 minutes. Weigh accurately and dry it again under similar condition for 1 hour, cool and weigh. Repeat the operation until the difference between two successive weighings is not more than 5mg. Calculate the percentage content of water in the substance being examined according to the weight loss on drying.

### （二）减压干燥法
### 2.　Drying under Reduced Pressure Method

本法适用于含有挥发性成分的贵重药品。中药测定用的供试品，一般先破碎并需通过二号筛。

The method is used for the determination of water in valuable drugs containing volatile constituents. The substance of Chinese Medicine for determination should be pulverized to pass through a No. 2 sieve.

测定法：先取直径 12cm 的培养皿，加入新鲜五氧化二磷干燥剂适量，使铺成 0.5~1cm 的厚度，放入直径 30cm 的减压干燥器中。取供试品 2~4g，混合均匀，分别取 0.5~1g，置已在供试品同样条件下干燥并称重的称量瓶中，精密称定，打开瓶盖，放入上述减压干燥器中，抽气减压至 2.67kPa（20mmHg）以下并持续抽气半小时，室温放置 24 小时。在减压干燥器出口连接无水氯化钙干燥管，打开活塞，待内外压一致，关闭活塞，打开干燥器，盖上瓶盖，取出称量瓶迅速精密称定重量，计算供试品中含水量（％）。

*Procedure*　Distribute 0.5-1 cm depth of phosphorous pentoxide into a Petri dish of 12 cm in diameter and put the dish in a vacuum desiccator of 30 cm in diameter. Mix thoroughly 2-4g of the substance being examined. Weigh accurately 0.5-1g in a weighing bottle, previously dried to constant weight under the conditions prescribed for the substance being examined, Place the loaded bottle in the vacuum desiccator, remove the stopper of the bottle and leave it also in the desiccator. Reduce the pressure of the desiccator by suction to 2.67 kPa (20mmHg) and last for 30 minutes. Allow to stand at room temperature for 24 hours, connect an anhydrous calcium chloride tube to the air inlet and open the desiccator plunger. Upon opening the desiccator, close the bottle promptly and weigh accurately. Calculate the percentage content of water in the substance being examined according to the weight loss on drying.

（三）甲苯法

### 3. Toluene Distillation Method

本法适用于含挥发性成分的药物。

The method is used for the determination of water in drugs containing volatile constituents.

**仪器装置**　如图 4-2 所示。A 为 500ml 的短颈圆底烧瓶；B 为水分测定管；C 为直形冷凝管，外管长 40cm。使用前，全部仪器应清洁，并置烘箱中烘干。

*Apparatus*　As Fig. 4-2. The apparatus consists of a 500ml round bottom flask (A), a graduated receiving tube (B) and a reflux condenser (C) approximately 40 cm in length. All parts of the apparatus should be cleaned and dried in an oven.

**测定法**　取供试品适量（相当于含水量 1~4ml）精密称定，置 A 瓶中，加甲苯约 200ml，必要时加入干燥、洁净的沸石（无釉小瓷片数片）或玻璃珠数粒，连接仪器，自冷凝管顶端加入甲苯至充满 B 管的狭细部分。将 A 瓶置电热套中或用其他适宜方法

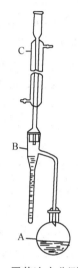

图 4-2　甲苯法水分测定装置
Fig.4-2　Apparatus for determination of water

缓缓加热，待甲苯开始沸腾时，调节温度，使每秒钟馏出 2 滴。待水分完全馏出，即测定管刻度部分的水量不再增加时，将冷凝管内部先用甲苯冲洗，再用饱蘸甲苯的长刷或其他适当方法，将管壁上附着的甲苯推下，继续蒸馏 5 分钟，放冷至室温，拆卸装置，如有水黏附在 B 管的管壁上，可用蘸甲苯的铜丝推下，放置，使水分与甲苯完全分离（可加亚甲蓝粉末少量，使水染成蓝色，以便分离观察）。检读水量，并计算成供试品中含水量（%）。

*Procedure*　Place a quantity of the substance being examined which is anticipated to yield about 1-4ml of water, accurately weighed, in the flask A. Add about 200ml of toluene and dry clean unglazed porcelain or a few glass beads if necessary. Assemble the apparatus and fill the receiving tube B with toluene through the condenser. Heat the flask gently, when toluene begins to boil, adjust the temperature and allow to distill at a rate of 2 drops per second, When the volume of water in the receiving tube does not increase anymore, rinse the inside of condenser with toluene and pushdown the toluene adhering to the wall with a brush or other suitable tools. Continue the distillation for 5 minutes, cool to room temperature and disconnect the apparatus. Push down any droplet of water adhering to the wall of the receiving tube with a copper wire wetted with toluene. Allow to stand until water is completely separated from toluene in the receiving tube (a small amount of methylene blue may be added to facilitate observation). Record the volume of water distilled and calculate the percentage content of water in the substance being examined.

**注意事项**　（1）测定用的甲苯须先加水少量充分振摇后放置，将水层分离弃去，经蒸馏后使用。

*NOTE* (1) The toluene to be used should be prepared as follows. Add a small quantity of water. Shake thoroughly and allow to stand for a while. Discard the water layer and distill the remainder.

(2) 中药测定用的供试品，一般先破碎成直径不超过 3mm 的颗粒或碎片；直径和长度在 3mm 以下的可不破碎。

(2) The substance of Chinese medicine for determination should be broken into granules or pieces with no more than 3mm in diameter. The substances which have less than 3mm in length and diameter, can be examined without further breaking.

### （四）气相色谱法
### 4. Gas Chromatography

该方法适用于各类型中药制剂中微量水分的精密称定。测定方法如下。

The method is used for the accurate determination of water in drugs containing. Methods as follows.

1. **色谱条件与系统适用性试验** 用直径为 0.18~0.25mm 的二乙烯苯－乙基乙烯苯型高分子多孔小球作为载体，柱温为 140~150℃，热导检测器检测。注入无水乙醇，照气相色谱法测定，应符合下列条件要求：①理论板数按水峰计算应大于 1000，理论板数按乙醇峰计算应大于 150。②水和乙醇两峰的分离度应大于 2。③用无水乙醇进样 5 次，水峰面积的相对标准偏差不得大于 3.0%。

(1) *Chromatographic system and system suitability* Carry out the method for gas chromatography, using porous polymer beads of divinylbenzene cross-linked ethylvinylbenzene with 0.18-0.25mm in diameter as the support, or capillary column with similar polarity. Maintain the column temperature at a range of 140-150℃, determine by conductivity detector. Inject anhydrous ethanol and carry out the method for gas chromatography, the performance of the instrument should comply with the following requirements. ① The number of theoretical plates for the column calculated with respect to the peak of water should be more than 1000, while the number of theoretical plates for the column calculated with respect to the peak of ethanol should be more than 150. ②The resolution between the peaks of water and ethanol is more than 2. ③Carry out 5 replicate injections of anhydrous ethanol, the RSD of the peak areas of water should not be more than 3.0%.

2. **对照溶液的制备** 取纯化水约 0.2g，精密称定，置 25ml 量瓶中，加无水乙醇至刻度，摇匀，即得。

(2) *Reference solution* Accurately weigh about 0.2g of purified water in a 25ml volumetric flask, dilute to volume with anhydrous ethanol and mix well.

3. **供试品溶液的制备** 取供试品适量（含水量约 0.2g），剪碎或研细，精密称定，置具塞锥形瓶中，精密加入无水乙醇 50ml，密塞，混匀，超声处理 20 分钟，放置 12 小时，再超声处理 20 分钟，密塞放置，待澄清后倾取上清液，即得。

(3) *Test solution* Place the pulverized test sample (containing about 0.2g water). accurately weighed, in a conical flask with stopper. Add anhydrous ethanol 50ml accurately and mix well. Ultrasonicate for 20 minutes, allow to stand for 12 hours, Ultrasonicate for another 20 minutes and allow to stand, After the solution becomes clarified, use the clear supernatant solution as the test solution,

4. **测定法** 取无水乙醇、对照溶液和供试品溶液各 1~5μl，注入气相色谱仪，测定，即得。

(4) *Procedure* Inject 1-5μl of anhydrous ethanol, reference solution and test solution respectively into the column. Determine and calculate the content of water.

5. **注意事项** 对照溶液与供试品溶液的配制须用新开启的同一瓶无水乙醇；用外标法计算供试品中的含水量，计算时应扣除无水乙醇中的含水量，方法如下：

(5) *Note* Use fresh opened anhydrous ethanol from the same bottle when preparing the reference solution and the test solution. Calculate the water content by the external standard method. The water contained in anhydrous ethanol should be deducted as follows:

对照溶液中实际加入的水的峰面积 = 对照溶液中总水峰面积 –K× 对照溶液中乙醇峰面积

供试品中水的峰面积 = 供试品溶液中总水峰面积 –K× 供试品溶液中乙醇峰面积

Peak area of water practically added into the reference solution = the total peak area of water in the reference solution – K× peak area of ethanol in the reference solution.

Peak area of water in test sample = the total peak area of water in test solution – K× peak area of ethanol in test solution.

$$K = \frac{无水乙醇中水峰面积\ (\text{peak area of water in anhydrous ethanol})}{无水乙醇中乙醇峰面积\ (\text{Peak area of ethanol in anhydrous ethanol})} \qquad (4\text{-}4)$$

## 七、灰分测定法
## 4.2.7　Determination of Ash

中药灰分包括总灰分和酸不溶性灰分。总灰分是指中药经加热炽灼灰化后遗留的非挥发性灰烬，包括生理灰分（药物本身所含的各种无机盐类，如草酸钙等）和外来的泥沙、砂石等。中药中的总灰分对于保证中药的品质和纯净有一定的意义。酸不溶性灰分是指总灰分加稀盐酸处理后得到的不溶性灰分，主要是不溶于盐酸的砂石、泥土等硅酸盐类化合物。凡易夹杂泥沙，且在生产、炮制等加工过程中不易除去的中药应规定总灰分；生理灰分高的中药（测定值大于10%，酸不溶性灰分测定值超过2%），除规定总灰分外还应规定酸不溶性灰分（如大黄）。

Chinese medicine ash includes total ash and acid-insoluble ash. The total ash refers to the non-volatile ash left after the traditional Chinese medicine is ignited until free from carbon by heating, including physiological ash (various inorganic salts contained in the medicine itself, such as calcium oxalate, etc.) and foreign sediment, sand and gravel. The total ash content in traditional Chinese medicine has certain significance for ensuring the quality and purity of traditional Chinese medicine. Acid-insoluble ash refers to the insoluble ash obtained after the treatment of total ash plus dilute hydrochloric acid, mainly silicate compounds such as sand, soil, etc. that are insoluble in hydrochloric acid. All traditional Chinese medicines that are easy to be mixed with sediment and are not easy to be removed during production, processing, etc. should be specified with total ash; Chinese medicines with high physiological ash content (measured value greater than 10%, acid-insoluble ash content measured value exceeds 2%), in addition to the specified total ash content, acid-insoluble ash (such as rhubarb) should be specified also.

（一）总灰分测定法
### 1. Total Ash

测定用的供试品需粉碎，使能通过二号筛，混合均匀后，取供试品 2~3g（如须测定酸不溶性灰分，可取供试品 3~5g），置炽灼至恒重的坩埚中，称定重量（准确至 0.01g），缓缓炽热，注意避免燃烧，至完全炭化时，逐渐升高温度至 500~600℃，使完全灰化并至恒重。根据残渣重量，计算供试品中总灰分的含量（%）。

Pulverize the sample to be examined through a No.2 sieve, and mix well. Weigh 2-3g (3-5g for the determination of acid- insoluble ash) of the powdered drug in a tared crucible accurate to 0.01g. Ignite the sample slowly till it is completely carbonized. To avoid burning, raise the temperature gradually to 500-600℃. Incinerate the sample until free from carbon and dry to constant weight. Calculate the percentage of ash with reference to the sample.

如供试品不易灰化，可将坩埚放冷，加热水或 10% 硝酸铵溶液 2ml，使残渣湿润，然后置水浴上蒸干，残渣照前法炽灼，至坩埚内容物完全灰化。

If a carbon-free ash cannot be obtained in this way, cool the crucible and moisten the charred mass with hot water or 2ml of 10% ammonium nitrate solution. Evaporate to dryness on a water bath, and incinerate the residue as described above until carbon-free ash is obtained.

### （二）酸不溶性灰分测定法
### 2. Acid-Insoluble Ash

取总灰分测定所得的灰分，在坩埚中小心加入稀盐酸约 10ml，用表面皿覆盖坩埚，置水浴上加热 10 分钟，表面皿用热水 5ml 冲洗，洗液并入坩埚中，用无灰滤纸滤过，坩埚内的残渣用水洗于滤纸上，并洗涤至洗液不显氯化物反应为止。滤渣连同滤纸移至同一坩埚中，干燥，炽灼至恒重。根据残渣重量，计算供试品中酸不溶性灰分的含量（%）。

To the crucible containing the residue from the determination of total ash, add 10ml of dilute hydrochloric acid with great care, cover with a watch glass, and heat on a water bath for 10 minutes. Wash the watch glass with 5ml of hot water and add the washings to the crucible, filter with an ashless filter paper, then transfer the residue to the filter paper with water, and wash till the filtrate yields no reactions of chlorides. Transfer the filter paper together with the residue to the original crucible, dry and ignite to constant weight. Calculate the percentage of acid- insoluble ash with reference to the sample.

### 八、炽灼残渣检查法
### 4.2.8  Determination of Residue on Ignition

有机药物经炽灼炭化，再加硫酸湿润，高温（700~800℃）炽灼至完全灰化，使有机物破坏分解变为挥发性物质逸出，或者使含有挥发性无机成分的中药受热挥发或分解，残留的非挥发性无机杂质的硫酸盐（多为金属的氧化物或无机盐类），称为炽灼残渣，也称硫酸灰分。其检查的目的是用于控制有机药物或挥发性无机药物中非挥发性的无机杂质。

Organic drugs are carbonized by ignition, moistened with sulfuric acid, and ignited at high temperature (700-800℃) to complete until free from carbon, which destroys and decomposes organic substances into volatile substances, or causes Chinese medicine containing volatile inorganic components to evaporate or heat decomposition, residual sulfate of non-volatile inorganic impurities (mostly metal oxides or inorganic salts), known as ignition residue, also known as sulfuric acid ash. The purpose of its inspection is to control non-volatile inorganic impurities in organic drugs or volatile inorganic drugs.

### （一）测定方法
### 1. Method

取供试品 1.0~2.0g 或各品种项下规定的重量，置已炽灼至恒重的坩埚中（如供试品分子结构中含有碱金属或氟元素，则应使用铂坩埚），精密称定，缓缓炽灼至完全炭化，放冷至室温；加硫酸 0.5~1ml 使湿润，低温加热至硫酸蒸气除尽后，在 700~800℃ 炽灼使完全灰化，移置干燥器内，放冷至室温，精密称定后，再在 700~800℃ 炽灼至恒重，即得。

Place 1.0-2.0g or the quantity specified in the individual monographs of the substance to be examined, accurately weighed, in a suitable crucible (If the substance to be examined contains alkali metals or fluorine element, the platinum crucible should be used). Previously ignited to constant weight. Heat gently until it is thoroughly charred, cool and moistens the residue with 0.5-1ml of sulfuric acid, unless otherwise directed. Heat gently until white fumes are no longer evolved and then ignite at 700-800℃ until the incineration is complete. Cool in a desiccator and weigh accurately, ignite again at 700-800℃ to constant weight.

如需将残渣留作重金属检查，则炽灼温度必须控制在 500~600℃。

If the residue is to be used in the limit test for heavy metals, the ignition temperature should be controlled at 500-600℃.

（二）注意事项

## 2.　Note

1. 取样量可根据炽灼残渣限量来决定，取样量过多，炭化及灰化时间长，取样量少，炽灼残渣量少，称量误差大。由于炽灼残渣限量一般在 0.1%~0.2%，所以取样量一般为 1~2g。

(1) The amount of sampling can be determined according to the limit of ignition residue. Too much sampling amount, long carbonization and ashing time, less sampling amount, less ignition residue, large weighing error. Since the limit of ignition residue is generally 0.1%-0.2%, the sampling volume is generally 1-2g.

2. 为了防止供试品在炭化时骤然膨胀而溢出，可将坩埚斜置，缓缓加热，直至完全灰化；在移至高温炉炽灼前，务必低温蒸发除尽硫酸蒸气，以免腐蚀炉膛，造成漏电事故。

(2) In order to prevent the test product from suddenly expanding and overflowing during carbonization, the crucible can be tilted and slowly heated until it is completely ashed; before moving to the high-temperature furnace to burn, be sure to evaporate sulfuric acid vapor at low temperature to avoid corrosion of the furnace , causing a leakage accident.

## 九、二氧化硫残留量测定法
## 4.2.9　Determination of Residue of Sulfur Dioxide

中药材在加工过程中用硫黄熏蒸具有漂白、增艳、防虫等作用，但硫黄熏蒸过程可能会造成二氧化硫的残留，影响人体健康。《中国药典》通则 2331 中采用酸碱滴定、气相色谱、离子色谱三种方法检查中药中二氧化硫的残留量。

Chinese medicinal materials fumigated use sulfur in the process has the effects of bleaching, brightening, insect control, etc., but the sulfur fumigation process may cause residual sulfur dioxide, affecting human health. *Chinese Pharmacopoeia* general chapters 2331 uses acid-base titration, gas chromatography, ion chromatography to check the residual of sulfur dioxide in Chinese medicine.

（一）原理

## 1.　Principle

**酸碱滴定法**　将中药材以蒸馏法进行处理，样品中的亚硫酸盐系列物质加酸处理转化为二氧化硫后，随氮气流带入到含有双氧水的吸收瓶中，双氧水将其氧化为硫酸根离子，采用酸碱滴定法测定，计算药材及饮片中的二氧化硫残留量。

*Acid-base Titration*   The method refers to that traditional Chinese medicines are treated via distillation. After the sulfite substances in the sample are converted to sulfur dioxide via acidification, they are carried together with nitrogen to an absorption bottle with hydrogen peroxide and oxidized through by hydrogen peroxide to sulfate ions. Determine and calculate the amount of sulfur dioxide residue in the medicine or decoction pieces via acid-base titration.

**气相色谱法**　将中药材以蒸馏法进行处理，样品中的亚硫酸盐系列物质加酸处理转化为二氧化硫后，通过顶空进样系统注入气相色谱仪，热导检测器检测二氧化硫的含量。

*Gas Chromatography*   The method refers to that traditional Chinese medicines are treated via distillation. After the sulfite substances in the sample are converted to sulfur dioxide via acidification, and then injected into the gas chromatograph through the headspace bottle gases of balanced, and thermal conductivity detector detects the sulfur dioxide content.

**离子色谱法**　将中药材以蒸馏法进行处理，样品中的亚硫酸盐系列物质加酸处理转化为二氧化硫，随水蒸气蒸馏，并被双氧水吸收，将其氧化为硫酸根离子后，通过离子色谱法测定，计算药材及饮片二氧化硫残留量。

*Ion Chromatography*   According to the method, traditional Chinese medicines are handled with steam distillation, so that sulfite series substances, in the sample which are converted to sulfur dioxide after acidification are absorbed by hydrogen peroxide and oxidized into sulfate ions; then such ions are measured and the amount of sulfur dioxide residue in the medicine or decoction pieces are calculated with ion chromatography.

（二）计算

## 2. Calculation

**酸碱滴定法**　照式（4-5）计算。

*Acid-base Titration*   Calculate according to the following formula:

供试品中二氧化硫残留量（Amount of sulfur dioxide residue in test sample, μg/g）=

$$\frac{(A-B) \times c \times 0.032 \times 10^6}{W} \tag{4-5}$$

式中，$A$ 为供试品消耗氢氧化钠滴定液的体积（ml）；$B$ 为空白消耗氢氧化钠滴定液的体积（ml）；$c$ 为氢氧化钠滴定液摩尔浓度（mol/L）；$W$ 为供试品的重量（g）；0.032 为每 1ml 氢氧化钠滴定液（1mo/L）相当的二氧化硫的质量（g）。

$A$ refers to the volume of titrant sodium hydroxide consumed by the test sample, ml; $B$ refers to the volume of titrant sodium hydroxide consumed by blank test, ml; $C$ refers to the mol concentration of titrant sodium hydroxide, mol/L; 0.032 refers to the mass of sulfur dioxide equivalent to 1ml of titrant sodium hydroxide (1mol/L), g; $W$ refers to the weight of test sample, g.

**气相色谱法**　按外标工作曲线法定量，计算样品中亚硫酸根含量，测得结果乘以 0.5079，即为二氧化硫含量。

*Gas Chromatography*   Quantify according to the external standard work curve method, calculate the sulfite content in sample and multiply the measured result with 0.5079 to obtain the sulfur dioxide content.

**离子色谱法**　采用外标工作曲线法，按照"$SO_2/SO_4^{2-}=0.6669$"计算样品中二氧化硫的含量。

*Ion Chromatography*   Calculate the content of sulfur dioxide residue in the sample according to "$SO_2/SO_4^{2-}=0.6669$".

# 第三节 有机杂质及残留溶剂检查

## 4.3 Analysis of Organic Impurities and Pesticide Residues in Chinese Medicine

PPT

### 一、农药残留量测定法
### 4.3.1 Determination of Pesticide Residues

农药残留是使用农药后残留于生物体和环境中微量的农药原型、有毒代谢物、降解物等杂质的总称。中药材有相当数量为人工栽培，为防治危害中药材生产的昆虫、真菌、霉菌及杂草，在生产过程中常需喷洒农药提高药材产量，不合理的使用农药以及环境污染均易产生农药残留。而农药对人体危害极大，故须控制中药材及其制剂中农药残留量。

Pesticide residues are the general term for trace pesticide prototypes, toxic metabolites, degradants and other impurities that remain in organisms and the environment after using pesticides. A considerable number of Chinese medicinal materials are cultivated artificially. In order to prevent insects, fungi, molds and weeds that harm the production of Chinese medicinal materials, pesticides are often sprayed in the production process to increase the yield of medicinal materials. Unreasonable use of pesticides and environmental pollution are prone to pesticide residues. Pesticides are extremely harmful to humans, so it is necessary to control pesticide residues in Chinese medicinal materials and their preparations.

（一）原理
### 1. Principle

农药品种繁多，迄今为止，常用的农药主要有：有机氯类、有机磷类、拟除虫菊酯、苯基羧酸类除草剂、氨基甲酸酯类、苯氧乙酸类等。有机氯类和有机磷类农药的毒性大，降解时间长，其他农药大多残留期较短，因此，在接触农药时间长短未知的情况下，应对中药进行有机氯类和有机磷类农药残留量的检查。《中国药典》采用气相色谱和质谱法测定药材、饮片及制剂中部分农药残留量。对于大多数热稳定性好、易挥发的农药采用 GC 法分离，可选择的检测器有：$^{63}$Ni 电子捕获检测器（ECD）、氮磷检测器（NPD）、火焰光度（FPD）和电子轰击源（EI）质谱；对于热不稳定的农药采用 HPLC 法分离，可选择电喷雾源（ESI）质谱。

This method is provided for the determination of pesticide residues in crude drugs, decoction pieces and preparations by gas chromatography and mass spectrometry. For most thermal stability, volatile pesticides are separated by GC method. The available detectors are, $^{63}$Ni-electron capture detector (ECD), nitrogen phosphorous detector (NPD) or flame photometric detector (FPD) and electron bombardment source (EI) mass spectrometry; for thermal Unstable pesticides are separated by HPLC, and electrospray source (ESI) mass spectrometry can be selected.

（二）方法
### 2. Method

《中国药典》收载的农药残留量测定方法有：第一法（有机氯类农药残留量测定法 – 色谱法）、第二法（有机磷类农药残留量测定法 – 色谱法）、第三法（拟除虫菊酯类农药残留量测定法 – 色谱法）和第四法（农药多残留量测定法 – 质谱法）。

The methods for determining the amount of pesticide residues in *Chinese Pharmacopoeia* included are: Method 1 (Determination of Organochloride Pesticide Residues by Chromatography), Method 2 (Determination of Organophosphorus Pesticide Residues by Chromatography), and Method 3 (Determination of Pyrethrin Pesticide Residues by Chromatography) and Method 4 (Determination of Multiple Pesticide Residues by Mass Spectrometry).

1. 气相色谱法

**(1) Gas Chromatography**

9 种有机氯类农药残留量测定法　用（14% – 氰丙基 – 苯基）甲基聚硅氧烷或（5% 苯基）甲基聚硅氧烷为固定液的弹性石英毛细管柱（30m×0.32mm×0.25μm），$^{63}$Ni-ECD 电子捕获检测器。进样口温度 230℃，检测器温度 300℃，不分流进样。程序升温：初始 100℃，每分钟 10℃ 升至 220℃，每分钟 8℃ 升至 250℃，保持 10 分钟。理论板数按 α-BHC 峰计算应不低于 $1×10^6$，两个相邻色谱峰的分离度应大于 1.5。

*Determination method of 9 kinds of organochlorine pesticide residues*　Column: a fused silica capillary column (30m×0.32mm) with a film(0.25μm) of 14% cyanopropyl phenyl-86% methyl polysiloxane or 5% phenyl-95% methyl polysiloxane; detector: $^{63}$Ni-electron capture detector (ECD); injection port temperature: 230℃; detector temperature: 300℃; injection mode: splitless; column temperature program: maintain the initial temperature at 100℃, increase the temperature at a rate of 10℃ per minute to 220℃, and then increase the temperature at a rate of 8℃ per minute to 250℃, hold for 10 minutes. The number of theoretical plates of the column is not less than $10^6$, calculated with reference to the peak of α-BHC. The resolution between two neighboring peaks is more than 1.5.

22 种有机氯类农药残留量测定法　分析柱：以 50% 苯基 –50% 二甲基聚硅氧烷为固定液的弹性石英毛细管柱（30m×0.32mm×0.25μm），验证柱：以 100% 二甲基聚硅氧烷为固定液的弹性石英毛细管柱（30m×0.32mm×0.25μm），$^{63}$Ni-ECD 电子捕获检测器。进样口温度 240℃，检测器温度 300℃，不分流进样，流速为恒压模式（初始流速为每分钟 1.3ml）。程序升温：初始 70℃，保持 1 分钟，每分钟 10℃ 升至 180℃，保持 5 分钟，再以每分钟 5℃ 升至 220℃，最后以每分钟 100℃ 升至 280℃，保持 8 分钟。理论板数按 α-BHC 计算应不低于 $1×10^6$，两个相邻色谱峰的分离度应大于 1.5。

*Determination of 22 organochlorine pesticide residues*　Column 1: a fused silica capillary column (30m×0.25mm) with a film(0.25μm) of 50% phenyl and 50% dimethyl polysiloxane; column 2: a fused silica capillary column (30m×0.25mm) with a film (0.25μm) of 100% dimethylsiloxane polymer; detector: $^{63}$Ni-electron capture detector (ECD); injection port temperature: 240℃; detector temperature: 300℃; injection mode: splitless; flow rate: constant pressure(initial flow rate is 1.3ml per min); column temperature program: maintain the initial temperature at 70℃ for 1 minute, increase the temperature at a rate of 10℃ per minute to 180℃, hold for 5 minutes, then increase the temperature at a rate of 5℃ per minute to 220℃, and then increase the temperature at a rate of 100℃ per minute to 280℃, hold for 8 minutes. The number of theoretical plates of the column is not less than $10^6$, calculated with reference to the peak of a-BHC. The resolution between two neighboring peaks is more than 1.5.

12 种有机磷农药残留量测定法　以 50% 苯基 –50% 二甲基聚硅氧烷或（5% 苯基）甲基聚硅氧烷为固定液的弹性石英毛细管柱（30m×0.32mm×0.25μm），氮磷检测器（NPD）或火焰光度检测器（FPD）。进样口温度 220℃，检测器温度 300℃，不分流进样。程序升温：初始 120℃，每分钟 10℃ 升至 200℃，每分钟 5℃ 升至 240℃，保持 2 分钟，每分钟 20℃ 升至 270℃，保持 0.5 分钟。理论板数按敌敌畏峰计算应不低于 6000，两个相邻色谱峰的分离度应大于 1.5。

*Determination of 12 organophosphorus pesticide residues*　Column: a fused silica capillary column

(30m×0.32mm) with a film (0.25μm) of 50% phenyl-50% dimethyl polysiloxane, or 5% phenyl-95% methyl polysiloxane; detector: nitrogen phosphorous detector (NPD) or flame photometric detector (FPD); injection port temperature: 220℃; detector temperature: 300℃; injection mode: splitless; column temperature program: maintain the initial temperature at 120℃, increase, the temperature at a rate of 10℃ per minute to 200℃, then increase the temperature at a rate of 5℃ per minute to 240℃, hold for 2 minutes, and then increase the temperature at a rate of 20℃ per minute to 270℃, hold for 0.5 minutes. The number of theoretical plates of the column is not less than 6000, calculated with reference to the peak of 2,2-dichlorovinyl dimethyl phosphate (DDVP). The resolution between two neighboring peaks is more than 1.5.

**3 种拟除虫菊酯类农药残留量测定法** 以（5% 苯基）甲基聚硅氧烷为固定液的弹性石英毛细管柱（30m×0.32mm×0.25μm），$^{63}$Ni-ECD 电子捕获检测器。进样口温度 270℃，检测器温度 330℃。不分流进样（或根据仪器设置最佳的分流比）。程序升温：初始 160℃，保持 1 分钟，每分钟 10℃ 升至 278℃，保持 0.5 分钟，每分钟 1℃ 升至 290℃，保持 5 分钟。理论板数按溴氰菊酯峰计算应不低于 $10^5$，两个相邻色谱峰的分离度应大于 1.5。

*Determination of 3 pyrethrin pesticide residues* Column: a fused silica capillary column (30m×0.32mm) with a film (0.25μm) of 5% phenyl and 95% methyl polysiloxane; detector: $^{63}$Ni-electron capture detector (ECD); injection port temperature: 270℃; detector temperature: 330℃; injection mode: splitless; column temperature program: maintain the initial temperature at 160℃ for 1 minute, increase the temperature at a rate of 10℃ per minute to 278℃, hold for 0.5 minute, and then increase the temperature at a rate of 1℃ per minute to 290℃, hold for 5 minutes. The number of theoretical plates of the column is not less than $10^5$, calculated with reference to the peak of deltamethrin. The resolution between two neighboring peaks is more than 1.5.

**2. 质谱法** 气相色谱 – 质谱联用法与液相色谱 – 质谱联用法对中药中农药残留的快速定性筛查，发现残留农药便于测量。采用气相色谱 – 串联质谱法和液相色谱 – 串联质谱法测定多种农药残量，结合各化合物的保留时间、监测离子对、碰撞电压 (CE) 可大幅提高定性和定量能力，可同时测定多种农药残留。为提高灵敏度，还可根据保留时间分段监测各农药。

**(2) Mass Spectrometry** Gas chromatography-mass spectrometry and liquid chromatography-mass spectrometry were used for rapid qualitative screening of pesticide residues in traditional Chinese medicine, and it was found that the residual pesticides were easy to measure. Using GC-MS and LC-MS to determine the residues of various pesticides, combined with the retention time of each compound, monitoring ion pair, and collision voltage (CE) can greatly improve the qualitative and quantitative of many pesticide residues. In order to improve the sensitivity, each pesticide can be monitored in stages according to the retention time.

用气相色谱 – 串联质谱法，对 91 种农药进行了定性测定；以氘代莠去津、氘代二嗪农和氘代倍硫磷为内标物，用内标标准曲线法对 88 种农药进行了定量分析。

91 kinds of pesticides were qualitatively determined by GC-MS; using deuterated atrazine, deuterated diazinon, and deuterated fenthion as internal standards, quantitative analysis of 88 pesticides were carried out by internal standard curve method.

受热易分解，挥发性差或极性较大的农药残留，可采用液相色谱 – 串联质谱法进行测定。用液相色谱 – 串联质谱法对 526 种农药进行了定性测定，以氘代莠去津、氘代二嗪农和氘代倍硫磷为内标物，用内标标准曲线法对 523 种农药进行了定量分析。

Pesticide residues that are easily decomposed by heat, poor in volatility or more polar, can be determined by LC-MS. The 526 pesticides were qualitatively determined by LC-MS, using deuterated atrazine, deuterated diazinon, and deuterated fenthion as internal standards, and quantitative analysis of 523 pesticides were carried out by the internal standard curve method.

### 二、黄曲霉毒素测定法
### 4.3.2　Determination of Aflatoxins

黄曲霉毒素是黄曲霉和寄生曲霉的代谢产物，具有极强的毒性和致癌性。因此，为保证用药安全，应该对中药及其制剂中黄曲霉毒素的含量进行控制。

Aflatoxins are metabolites of aspergillus flavus and aspergillus parasiticus, which has strong toxicity and carcinogenicity. Therefore, in order to ensure the safety of medication, the content of aflatoxins in Chinese medicine and its preparations should be controlled.

（一）原理
### 1.　Principle

黄曲霉毒素是一类结构相似的化合物，均为二呋喃香豆素的衍生物。在紫外线照射下，都能发出荧光，根据荧光颜色、比移值及结构等，分别命名为 $B_1$、$B_2$、$G_1$、$G_2$、$M_1$、$M_2$ 等。黄曲霉毒素耐热，280℃发生裂解，一般制药加工的温度很难将其破坏。黄曲霉毒素在水中溶解度低，易溶于油及三氯甲烷、丙酮和甲醇等有机溶剂，但不溶于乙醚、石油醚和己烷。

Aflatoxins are structurally similar compounds, all of which are derivatives of difuran coumarin. Under ultraviolet irradiation, they can emit fluorescence. According to the fluorescence color, specific shift value and structure, it is named $B_1$, $B_2$, $G_1$, $G_2$, $M_1$, $M_2$, etc. Aflatoxins are heat-resistant and crack at 280℃, which is difficult to destroy under the temperature of pharmaceutical manufacturing. Aflatoxins have low solubility in water, easily soluble in oil and some organic solvents such as chloroform, acetone and methanol, but insoluble in ether, petroleum ether and hexane.

（二）方法
### 2.　Method

《中国药典》采用高效液相色谱法和高效液相色谱 – 串联质谱法测定中药中的黄曲霉毒素（以黄曲霉毒素 $B_1$、黄曲霉毒素 $B_2$、黄曲霉毒素 $G_1$ 和黄曲霉毒素 $G_2$ 总量计）。

*Chinese Pharmacopoeia* uses high performance liquid chromatography and high performance liquid chromatography-tandem mass spectrometry to determine the aflatoxins in Chinese crude drugs and decoction pieces (calculated as the total amount of aflatoxin $B_1$, aflatoxin $B_2$, aflatoxin $G_1$ and aflatoxin $G_2$).

**高效液相色谱法**　以十八烷基硅烷键合硅胶为填充剂；以甲醇 – 乙腈 – 水（40：18：42）为流动相；采用柱后衍生法检测。①碘衍生法：衍生溶液为 0.05% 的碘溶液（取碘 0.5g，加入甲醇 100ml 使溶解，用水稀释至 1000ml 制成），衍生化泵流速每分钟 0.3ml，衍生化温度 70℃；②光化学衍生法：光化学衍生器（254nm）。以荧光检测器检测，激发波长 $\lambda$=360nm（或 365mm），发射波长 $\lambda$=450m，两个相邻色谱峰的分离度应大于 1.5。

*High performance liquid chromatography*　Use octadecylsilane bonded silica gel as the stationary phase and a mixture of methanol, acetonitrile and water (40：18：42) as the mobile phase. A post-column derivatization method is used as the detecting method. ① Derivatization with iodine: use a 0.05% of iodine solution (dissolve 0.5g of iodine with 100ml of methanol, and dilute with water to 1000ml) as derivatisation reagent, maintain the rate of derivatisation pump at 0.3ml per minute and the derivatisation temperature at 70℃. ②Derivatization with photochemical reactor (254nm). Detect with a fluorescence detector, and set the excitation wavelength at 360nm (or 365nm) and emission wavelength at 450nm. The resolution between the neighboring chromatographic peaks should be more than 1.5.

**高效液相色谱 – 质谱法**　以十八烷基硅烷键合硅胶为填充剂；以 10mmol/L 醋酸铵溶液为流动相 A，以甲醇为流动相 B（0~4.5min：65%→15%A；4.5~6min：15%→0A；6~6.5min：0~65%A；6.5~10min：65%A）梯度洗脱；柱温 25℃；流速每分钟 0.3ml 以三重四极杆串联质谱仪检测：电喷雾离子源（ESI），采集模式为正离子模式；各化合物监测离子对和碰撞电压（CE）见表 4-1。

*High performance liquid chromatography/tandem mass spectrometry*　Use octdcylslane bonded silica gel as the stationary phase. Use 10mmol/L ammomium acetate solution as mobile phase A, methanol as mobile phase B, at the rate of 0.3ml per minute the column temperature of 25℃. Elute with the following gradient elution program. Detector: triple-quadrupole mass spectrometer. Ion source: ESI. Acquisition mode: positive ion mode. Reference monitoring ion pair and collision energy (CE) are shown in the following Table 4-1.

| 时间 (Time, min) | 流动相 A (Mobile phase A, %) | 流动相 B (Mobile phase B, %) |
|---|---|---|
| 0-4.5 | 65→15 | 35-85 |
| 4.5-6 | 15→10 | 85→100 |
| 6-6.5 | 0→65 | 100→35 |
| 6.5-10 | 65 | 35 |

表 4-1　黄曲霉毒素 $B_1$、黄曲霉毒素 $B_2$、黄曲霉毒素 $G_1$、
黄曲霉毒素 $G_2$ 对照品的监测离子对、碰撞电压（CE）参考值

Table 4-1　Reference monitoring ion pair and collision energy (CE) of Aflatoxin $B_1$, $B_2$, $G_1$, $G_2$

| 编号（No.） | 名称（Name） | 母离子（Precursor ion） | 子离子（Product ion） | CE（V） |
|---|---|---|---|---|
| 1 | 黄曲霉毒素 $G_2$ (Aflatoxin $G_2$) | 331.1 | 313.1 | 33 |
| | | 331.1 | 245.1 | 40 |
| 2 | 黄曲霉毒素 $G_1$ (Aflatoxin $G_1$) | 329.1 | 243.1 | 35 |
| | | 329.1 | 311.1 | 30 |
| 3 | 黄曲霉毒素 $B_2$ (Aflatoxin $B_2$) | 315.1 | 259.1 | 35 |
| | | 315.1 | 287.1 | 40 |
| 4 | 黄曲霉毒素 $B_1$ (Aflatoxin $B_1$) | 313.1 | 141 | 50 |
| | | 313.1 | 285.1 | 40 |

**测定法**　采用外标工作曲线法计算黄曲霉毒素 $B_1$、黄曲霉毒素 $B_2$、黄曲霉毒素 $G_1$、黄曲霉毒素 $G_2$ 的量。

Quantitative analysis of Aflatoxins $B_1$, $B_2$, $G_1$, $G_2$ were carried out by the external standard working curve method.

### 三、甲醇量检查法
### 4.3.3　Determination of Methanol

（一）原理
### 1．Principle

甲醇可能会对人体的中枢系统、眼睛等产生毒性，由于乙醇中含有少量的甲醇，在含醇量比

较高酒剂或酊剂等制剂中需要进行甲醇量的测定。由于甲醇具有挥发性,《中国药典》采用气相色谱法测定甲醇的含量。

Methanol may be toxic to the human body's central system, eyes, etc. Because ethanol contains a small amount of methanol, the amount of methanol needs to be measured in preparations such as medicinal wines and tinctures, which have a relatively high alcohol content. Because methanol is volatile, *Chinese Pharmacopoeia* uses gas chromatography to determine the content of methanol.

（二）方法

## 2. Method

### 1. 毛细管柱法

### (1) Capillary Columns

**色谱条件与系统适用性试验**　采用（6%）氰丙基苯基 -（94%）二甲基聚硅氧烷为固定液的毛细管柱；起始温度为 40℃，维持 2 分钟，以每分钟 3℃ 的速率升温至 65℃，再以每分钟 25℃ 的速率升温至 200℃，维持 10 分钟；进样口温度 200℃；检测器（FID）温度 220℃；分流进样，分流比为 1：1；顶空进样平衡温度为 85℃，平衡时间为 20 分钟。理论板数按甲醇峰计算应不低于 10000，甲醇峰与其他色谱峰的分离度应大于 1.5。

*Chromatographic system and system suitability*　The gas chromatograph is equipped with a flame-ionization detector (FID), and a fused-silica capillary column bonded with a film of 6% cyanopropylphenyl siloxane 94% polydimethylsiloxane. Maintain the temperature of the column at 40℃ for 2 minutes, then raise the temperature at a rate of 3℃ per minute to 65℃, and then raise the temperature at a rate of 25℃ per minute to 200℃ and maintain it at 200℃ for 10 minutes. Maintain the temperature of the injection port at 200℃ and that of the detector at 220℃. The split ratio is 1：1. The head-space sampler parameters are set as follows: the equilibration temperature is 85℃ and the equilibration time is 20 minutes. The number of theoretical plates for the column is not less than 10000 calculated with reference to the peak of methanol, and the resolution of the peaks of methanol and other compounds is more than 1.5.

**测定法**　取供试液作为供试品溶液。精密量取甲醇 1ml，置 100ml 量瓶中，加水稀释至刻度，摇匀，精密量取 5ml，置 100ml 量瓶中，加水稀释至刻度，摇匀，作为对照品溶液。分别精密量取对照品溶液与供试品溶液各 3ml，置 10ml 顶空进样瓶中，密封，顶空进样。按外标法以峰面积计算，即得。

*Procedure*　Use the solution to be examined as the test solution. Measure accurately 1ml of methanol into a 100ml volumetric flask, dilute to volume with water and mix well. Measure accurately 5ml of this solution into a 100ml volumetric flask, dilute to volume with water and mix well as the reference solution. Transfer accurately 3ml of the reference solution and the test solution into separate 10ml head-space vials and seal the vials, respectively. Determine and calculate the content of methanol with respect to the peak area by the external standard method.

### 2. 填充柱法

### (2) Packed Columns

**色谱条件与系统适用性试验**　用直径为 0.18~0.25mm 的二乙烯苯 - 乙基乙烯苯型高分子多孔小球作为载体；柱温 125℃。理论板数按甲醇峰计算应不低于 1500；甲醇峰、乙醇峰与内标物质各相邻色谱峰之间的分离度应符合规定。

*Chromatographic system and system suitability*　Carry out the method for gas chromatography, using a column packed with porous polymer beads (0.18-0.25mm) of ethylvinyl-benzene cross-linked with divinylbenzene. The temperature of the column is maintained at 125℃. The number of theoretical plates for the column is not less than 1500 calculated with reference to the peak of methanol. The resolution of the peaks of methanol, ethanol, the internal standard and other compounds shall comply with the requirements.

**校正因子测定**　精密量取正丙醇 1ml，置 100ml 量瓶中，用水溶解并稀释至刻度，摇匀，作为内标溶液。另精密量取甲醇 1ml，置 100ml 量瓶中，用水稀释至刻度，摇匀，精密量取 10ml，置 100ml 量瓶中，精密加入内标溶液 10ml，用水稀释至刻度，摇匀，取 1μl 注入气相色谱仪，连续进样 3~5 次，测定峰面积，计算校正因子。

*Conection factor*　Measure accurately 1ml of n-propanol into a 100ml volumetric flask, dilute to volume with water and mix well, as the internal standard solution. Measure accurately 1ml of methanol into a 100ml volumetric flask, dilute to volume with water and mix well. Measure accurately 10ml of this solution and 10ml of the internal standard solution into a 100ml volumetric flask, dilute to volume with water and mix well, as the reference solution. Inject 1μl of the reference solution for 3-5 times successively and calculate the correction factor according to the peak area of each injection.

**测定法**　精密量取内标溶液 1ml，置 10ml 量瓶中，加供试液至刻度，摇匀，作为供试品溶液，取 1μl 注入气相色谱仪，测定，即得。

除另有规定外，供试液含甲醇量不得过 0.05%（ml/ml）。

*Procedure*　Measure accurately 1ml of the internal standard solution into a 10ml volumetric flask, dilute to volume with the solution to be examined and mix well, as the test solution. Inject 1μl of the test solution an calculate the content of methanol.

Unless otherwise specified, the content of methanol in the solution to be examined is not more than 0.05% (ml/ml).

（三）注意事项

### 3. Note

（1）如采用填充柱法时，内标物质峰相应的位置出现杂质峰，可改用外标法测定。

When using packed columns, if any peak corresponding to the location of the internal standard appears in the chromatogram, the assay method can be replaced by the external standard method.

（2）建议选择大口径、厚液膜色谱柱，规格为 30m×0.53mm×3.00μm。

It is recommended to use a column with wide internal diameter and thick film (30m×0.53mm×3.00μm).

**四、酸败度测定法**

### 4.3.4　Limit Tests of Rancidity

（一）原理

### 1. Principle

酸败是指油脂或含油脂的种子类药材和饮片，在贮藏过程中发生复杂的化学变化，生成游离脂肪酸、过氧化物和低分子醛类、酮类等产物，出现特异臭味，影响药材和饮片的感观和质量。通过测定酸值、羰基值和过氧化值，以检查药材和饮片中油脂的酸败度。

Rancidity means that the complex chemical reactions occur in fatty oils or seed medicinal herbs that contain fatty oils during the storage process, producing the decomposed components such as free fatty acids, peroxides, low molecular aldehydes and ketones, turning up distinctive smell and influencing the sense properties as well as the interior quality of the crude drugs and the processed pieces. This rancidity of crude drugs and the processed pieces are checked through the determination of acid value, carbonyl value and peroxide value.

（二）方法

## 2. Method

1. **油脂提取**　除另有规定外，取供试品 30~50g（根据供试品含油脂量而定），研碎成粗粉，置索氏提取器中，加正己烷 100~150ml（根据供试品取样量而定），置水浴上加热回流 2 小时，放冷，用 3 号垂熔玻璃漏斗滤过，滤液置水浴上减压回收溶剂至尽，所得残留物即为油脂。

**(1) Extraction of fatty oils**　Unless otherwise specified, pulverize 30-50g of the test sample (varying in according with the content of fatty oil) to coarse powder. Extract the coarse powder with 100-150ml of n-hexane in a Soxhlet type extractor under reflux for 2 hours. After allowing to cool, filter the mixture through a No.3 sintered-glass funnel. Recover the solvent to dryness in vacuum, and the fatty oil will be obtained.

2. **酸败度测定**

**(2) Determination of rancidity**

（1）**酸值测定**　酸值系指中和脂肪、脂肪油或其他类似物质 1g 中含有的游离脂肪酸所需氢氧化钾的重量（mg），但在测定时采用氢氧化钠滴定液（0.1mol/L）进行滴定。

*Determination of acid value*　Acid value refers to the weight (mg) of potassium hydroxide (0.1mol/L) required to neutralize the free fatty acids contained in 1g of fats, fatty oils or other similar substances.

（2）**羰基值测定**　羰基值系指每 1kg 油脂中含羰基化合物的毫摩尔数。

除另有规定外，取油脂 0.025~0.5g，精密称定，置 25ml 量瓶中，加甲苯适量溶解并稀释至刻度，摇匀。精密量取 5ml，置 25ml 具塞刻度试管中，加 4.3% 三氯醋酸的甲苯溶液 3ml 及 0.05% 2,4-二硝基苯肼的甲苯溶液 5ml，混匀，置 60℃ 水浴加热 30 分钟，取出冷却，沿管壁缓缓加入 4% 氢氧化钾的乙醇溶液 10ml，加乙醇至 25ml，密塞，剧烈振摇 1 分钟，放置 10 分钟，以相应试剂作空白，照紫外－可见分光光度法（《中国药典》通则 0401）在 453nm 波长处测定吸光度，按式（4-6）计算：

*Determination of carbonyl value*　The carbonyl value is the number that expresses in millimoles of carbonyl compounds in 1000g of fatty oils.

Unless otherwise specified, weigh accurately 0.025-0.5g of the fatty oil in a 25ml volumetric flask. Dissolve and dilute to the scale volume with toluene and mix well. Take accurately 5ml in a 25ml stoppered tube, add 3ml of a 4.3% solution of trichloroacetic acid in toluene and 5ml of a 0.05% solution of 2,4-dinitrophenylhydrazine in toluene, mix well and heat in a 60℃ water bath for 30 minutes. Stand for cool, add slowly 10ml of a 4% solution of potassium hydroxide in ethanol along the tube wall, then add ethanol to 25ml, stopper well, shake thoroughly for 1 minute and stand for 10 minutes. Carry out the method for ultraviolet-visible spectrophotometry (*Chinese Pharmacopoeia*, general chapters 0401), measure the absorbance at 453 nm, with the corresponding solvent solution as the blank. Calculate according to the following formula (4-6):

$$供试品的羰基值（\text{Carbonyl value}）= \frac{A \times 5}{854 \times W} \times 1000 \qquad （4\text{-}6）$$

式中，$A$ 为吸光度；$W$ 为油脂的重量，g；854 为各种羰基化合物的 2,4-二硝基苯肼衍生物的摩尔吸收系数平均值。

Where $A$=absorbance of the substance being examined; $W$=weight of the fatty oil (g); 854=

average value of the molar absorption coefficient of 2,4-dinitrophenylhydrazine derivatives of carbonyl compounds.

（3）过氧化值测定 过氧化值系指油脂中过氧化物与碘化钾作用，生成游离碘的百分数。

除另有规定外，取油脂 2~3g，精密称定，置 250ml 的干燥碘瓶中，加三氯甲烷 – 冰醋酸（1：1）混合溶液 30ml，使溶解。精密加新制碘化钾饱和溶液 1ml，密塞，轻轻振摇半分钟，在暗处放置 3 分钟，加水 100ml，用硫代硫酸钠滴定液（0.01mol/L）滴定至溶液呈浅黄色时，加淀粉指示液 1ml，继续滴定至蓝色消失；同时做空白试验，照式（4-7）计算：

*Determination of peroxide value* The peroxide value is the percentage of free iodine produced by the reaction of peroxide compounds in fatty oil with potassium iodide.

Unless otherwise specified, weigh accurately 2-3g of the fatty oil in a 250ml dried iodine flask. Add 30ml of a mixture of chloroform and glacial acetic acid (1:1) to dissolve the sample completely. Add accurately 1ml of a freshly prepared saturated solution of potassium iodide, stopper well, shake gently for 30 seconds, stand in a dark place for 3 minutes, and then add 100ml of water. Titrate with sodium thiosulfate VS (0.01mol/L) until the colour change to yellow, add 1ml of starch IS, and continue titrating until the blue colour disapper. Perform a blank determination. Calculate the peroxide value according to the following formula (4-7):

$$供试品的过氧化值（Peroxide\ value）= \frac{(A-B) \times 0.001269}{W} \times 100 \qquad （4-7）$$

式中，$A$ 为油脂消耗硫代硫酸钠滴定液的体积，ml；$B$ 为空白试验消耗硫代硫酸钠滴定液的体积，ml；$W$ 为油脂的重量，g；0.001269 为硫代硫酸钠滴定液（0.01mol/L）1ml 相当于碘的重量，g。

Where $A$=volume of sodium thiosulfate VS (ml); $B$= volume of sodium thiosulfate VS for blank determination (ml); $W$= weight of the fatty oil (g); 0.001269= weight (g) of iodine equivalent to 1ml of sodium thiosulfates VS (0.01 mol/L).

### 五、有关物质的检查
### 4.3.5 Test for Related Substances and Associated Substances

化学结构与活性成分类似或具渊源关系的有机杂质，通称为有关物质。中药中的有关物质包括：①在特定药物的采收、加工或贮存过程中引入或产生与该药物本身特性有关的物质。如附子中双酯型生物碱、大黄中的土大黄苷等。②由于药物的来源、生产工艺和剂型的不同及贮存过程中可能产生的分解产物，如薄荷脑中有关物质，注射用灯盏花素中有关物质等。上述有机杂质有些具有毒性，有些影响药物的纯度，因此，药品的检查应根据其特点引入有关物质和相关物质检查（表 4-2）。

Organic impurities whose chemical structure is similar to or related to active ingredients are commonly referred to as related substances. Related substances in Chinese medicine include: ① Impurities that related to the properties of the medicine were introduced or produced in the process of collection, processing or storage of the special medicine, such as diester alkaloids in aconite, rhaponiticin in rhubarb root and rhizome etc. ② Impurities were introduced or produced based on sources, production processes, dosage forms and storage processes. such as related substances of menthol, the related substances and associated substances in breviscapine for injection. Some of the above organic impurities are toxic, and some affect the purity of the drug. Therefore, the inspection of related substances and associated substances should be introduced according to their characteristics (Table 4-2).

表 4-2 部分有关物质种类、名称和检查方法

| 类别 | 名称 | 检查方法 | 中药 |
|------|------|----------|------|
| 双酯型乌头碱 | 乌头碱、次乌头碱、新乌头碱 | TLC、HPLC | 乌头类药材、附子理中丸、四逆汤等 |
| 吡咯里西啶类生物碱 | 阿多尼弗林碱 | HPLC-MS | 千里光、紫草等 |
| 莨菪烷类生物碱类 | 阿托品、莨菪碱、东莨菪碱 | HPLC、TLC | 洋金花、天仙子等 |
| 马钱子碱类 | 士的宁、马钱子碱 | HPLC、TLC | 马钱子、九分散等 |
| 马兜铃酸类 | 马兜铃酸、马兜铃酸 I | HPLC | 天仙藤、马兜铃、细辛等 |
| 银杏酸类 | 总银杏酸 | HPLC | 银杏叶提取物 |
| 其他 | 朱砂 (HgS) 中的可溶性汞盐；雄黄（$As_2S_2$）中的三氧化二砷；大黄中的土大黄苷 | | 朱砂、雄黄、大黄等 |

Table 4-2 Some related substance types, names and inspection methods

| Category | Name | Inspection Method | Chinese Medicine |
|----------|------|-------------------|------------------|
| Diester alkaloids | Aconitine, Hypaconitine, Mesaconitine | TLC、HPLC | Aconiti lateralis radix praeparaia, FuziLizhong pills, Sini Tang |
| Pyrrolizidine alkaloids | Adonifoline | HPLC-MS | Senecionis Scandentis hebra, Arnebiae Radix |
| Scopolamine alkaloids | Atropine, Hyoscyamine, Scopolamine | HPLC、TLC | flos daturae, Semen Hyoscyami |
| Brucines | Strychnine, Brucine | HPLC、TLC | Strychni semen, Jiufen powders |
| Aristolochic acids | Aristolochic acids、Aristolochic acids I | HPLC | Aristolochiae Herba, Aristolochiae Fructus, Asari Radix et Rhizoma |
| Ginkgolic acids | Total ginkgolic acid | HPLC | Ginkgo leaves extract |
| Other | Soluble mercury salts in Cinnabaris, $As_2O_3$ in Realgar, Rhaponiticin in Radix et Rhizoma Rhei | | Cinnabaris, Realgar, Radix et Rhizoma Rhei |

例 4-2 灯盏花素（供注射用）中有关物质和相关物质的检查

Example 4-2 The test for related substances and associated substances of breviscapine used to prepare injections.

**有关物质的检查** 取本品，加 1% 碳酸氢钠溶液溶解并稀释成每 1ml 含野黄芩苷 0.02mg 的溶液，除"树脂"外，照注射剂有关物质检查法（《中国药典》通则 2400）检查，应符合规定。

*Test for related substances* Dissolve the Breviscapine in 1% sodium bicarbonate solution to produce a solution containing scutellarin 0.02mg per ml. Except resin, carry out the test method (*Chinese Pharmacopoeia* general chapters 2400), which shall comply with the requirements.

**相关物质的检查** 取本品适量（相当于野黄芩苷 20mg），置 50ml 量瓶中，加甲醇适量，超声处理（功率 300W，频率 50kHz）45 分钟，放至室温，加甲醇稀释至刻度，摇匀，作为供试品

溶液；精密量取供试品溶液 1ml，置 100ml 量瓶中，加甲醇稀释至刻度，摇匀，作为对照溶液。照色谱条件 [ 以十八烷基硅烷键合硅胶为填充剂；以甲醇 -0.1% 磷酸溶液（40：60）为流动相；流速为每分钟 1.0ml；柱温为 40℃；检测波长为 335nm。理论板数按野黄芩苷峰计算应不低于 5000 ]，取对照溶液 5μl，注入液相色谱仪，调节检测灵敏度，使主成分色谱峰的峰高约为满量程的 10%。再精密量取供试品溶液与对照溶液各 5μl，分别注入液相色谱仪，记录色谱图至主成分峰保留时间的 2.5 倍。供试品溶液色谱图中各杂质峰峰面积的和不得大于对照溶液主峰峰面积的 2 倍。

*Test for associated substances*　Place the Breviscapine (equivalent to about 20mg of scutellarin) to a 50ml volumetric flask, add appropriate amount of methanol, ultrasonic treatment (power 300W, frequency 50kHz) for 45 minutes, put to room temperature, dilute to volume with methanol and mix well as the test solution. Pipet accurately 1ml of the test solution to a 100ml volumetric flask, dilute to volume with methanol and mix well as the reference solution. Under the Chromatographic conditions (Use octadecylsilane bonded silica gel as the stationary phase and a mixture of methanol and 0.1% phosphoric acid solution (40：60) as the mobile phase. The flow rate is 1.0ml per minute and the column temperature is 40℃. As detector a spectrophotometer set at 335nm. The number of theoretical plates of the column is not less than 5000, calculated with reference to the peak of scutellarin), inject 5μl of the reference solution into the column, adjust the detection sensitivity to the peak height of the main component chromatographic peak was 10% of the full range. Pipet accurately separately 5μl of the test solution and the reference solution into the column, record 2.5 times retention time from chromatogram to principal component peak. In test solution chromatogram, the sum of the peak areas of other components shall not be greater than 2 times of the main peak area of the reference solution.

### 六、残留溶剂测定法
### 4.3.6　Determination of Residual Solvents

药品中的残留溶剂系指在原料药或辅料的生产中，以及在制剂制备过程中使用的，但在工艺过程中未能完全去除的有机溶剂。除另有规定外，第一、第二、第三类溶剂的残留限度应符合《中国药典》（通则 0861）中的规定；对其他溶剂应根据生产工艺的特点，制定相应的限度，使其符合产品规范、药品生产质量管理规范（GMP）或其他基本的质量要求。照气相色谱法（《中国药典》通则 0521）测定。

Residual solvents in pharmaceutical products are defined as organic volatile chemicals that are used or produced in the manufacture of drug substances or excipients, or in the preparation of drug products, but not completely removed by practical manufacturing techniques. The general residual solvents in pharmaceutical products and the limits are listed in *Chinese Pharmacopoeia* general chapters. Unless otherwise specified, the residual content class 1, of class 2 and class 3 residual solvents should comply with the requirement in *Chinese Pharmacopoeia* general chapters 0861; for other solvents. According to the manufacture technology, relevant limits should be regulated in order to meet product specifications, good manufacturing practices (GMP) or other quality- based requirements. Carry out the method for gas chromatograph（*Chinese Pharmacopoeia* general chapters 0521）.

（一）限度检查
1. Limit test
除另有规定外，按各品种项下规定的供试品溶液浓度测定。以内标法测定时，供试品溶液所得被测溶剂峰面积与内标峰面积之比不得大于对照品溶液的相应比值。以外标法测定时，供试品溶液所得被测溶剂峰面积不得大于对照品溶液的相应峰面积。

Unless otherwise specified, determine the residual solvents in the test solution as specified in the monograph. When internal standard method is used, the ratio of the peak area of the residual solvent in the test solution to that of the internal standard is not more than the corresponding ratio in the reference solution. When the external standard method is used, the peak area of residual solvent being examined in the test solution is not more than the corresponding peak area in the reference solution.

（二）定量测定

## 2. Quantitative test

按内标法或外标法计算各残留溶剂的量。

The content of residual solvents can be calculated by internal standard method or external standard method.

PPT

## 第四节　其他检查

## 4.4　Other Test

### 一、制剂通则检查
### 4.4.1　General Requirements for Preparations Test

制剂通则检查是检查中药制剂是否达到制剂学方面的有关要求，是为了确保中药制剂的安全性、有效性和均一性而进行的检查项目。常见中药制剂的检查项目见《中国药典》四部制剂通则。

The general requirements for preparations test to check whether the Chinese medicine preparations meet the relevant requirements of preparation, and to ensure the safety, effectiveness and uniformity of Chinese medicine preparations. For the inspection items of common Chinese medicine preparations, please refer to the general requirements for preparations in volumes IV of the *Chinese Pharmacopoeia*.

### 二、非无菌产品微生物限度检查与标准
### 4.4.2　Non-Sterile Product Microbiological Limit Tests and Standards

微生物检查法是检查非规定灭菌制剂及其原料、辅料受微生物污染程度的方法。非无菌产品微生物限度检查包括微生物计数法（《中国药典》通则 1105）和控制菌检查法（《中国药典》通则 1106）等。非无菌药品的微生物限度标准是基于药品的给药途径和对患者健康潜在的危害以及药品的特殊性而制订的（表 4-3）。

Microbiological tests refer to check the degree of microbial contamination of non-specified sterilizing preparations and their raw materials and auxiliary materials. Microbiological limit tests of non-sterile pharmaceutical products containing microbial enumeration tests (*Chinese Pharmacopoeia*, general chapters 1105) and specified microorganisms tests (*Chinese Pharmacopoeia*, general chapters 1106). The microbial acceptance criteria of non-sterile preparations are drawn with full consideration of the administration routes, potential harm to the patients and the particularity of drugs (Table 4-3).

表 4-3　非无菌药品的微生物限度标准

| 给药途径 | | 需氧菌总数（cfu/g、cfu/ml 或 cfu/10cm²） | 霉菌和酵母菌总数（cfu/g、cfu/ml 或 cfu/10cm²） | 控制菌 |
|---|---|---|---|---|
| 非无菌化学药品制剂、生物制品制剂、不含药材原粉的中药制剂 | 口服给药[①]<br>　固体制剂<br>　液体制剂 | $10^3$<br>$10^2$ | $10^2$<br>$10^1$ | 不得检出大肠埃希菌（1g 或 1ml）；含脏器提取物的制剂还不得检出沙门菌（10g 或 10ml） |
| | 口腔黏膜给药制剂<br>齿龈给药制剂<br>鼻用制剂 | $10^2$ | $10^1$ | 不得检出大肠埃希菌、金黄色葡萄球菌、铜绿假单胞菌（1g、1ml 或 10cm²） |
| | 耳用制剂<br>皮肤给药制剂 | $10^2$ | $10^1$ | 不得检出金黄色葡萄球菌、铜绿假单胞菌（1g、1ml 或 10cm²） |
| | 呼吸道吸入给药制剂 | $10^2$ | $10^1$ | 不得检出大肠埃希菌、金黄色葡萄球菌、铜绿假单胞菌、耐胆盐革兰阴性菌（1g 或 1ml） |
| | 阴道、尿道给药制剂 | $10^2$ | $10^1$ | 不得检出金黄色葡萄球菌、铜绿假单胞菌、白色念珠菌（1g、1ml 或 10cm²）；中药制剂还不得检出梭菌（1g、1ml 或 10cm²） |
| | 直肠给药<br>　固体制剂<br>　液体制剂 | $10^3$<br>$10^2$ | $10^2$<br>$10^2$ | 不得检出金黄色葡萄球菌、铜绿假单胞菌（1g 或 1ml） |
| | 其他局部给药制剂 | $10^2$ | $10^2$ | 不得检出金黄色葡萄球菌、铜绿假单胞菌（1g、1ml 或 10cm²） |
| 非无菌含药材原粉的中药制剂 | 固体口服给药制剂<br>　不含豆豉、神曲等发酵原粉<br>　含豆豉、神曲等发酵原粉 | $10^4$（丸剂 $3×10^4$）<br>$10^5$ | $10^2$<br>$5×10^2$ | 不得检出大肠埃希菌（1g）；不得检出沙门菌（10g）；耐胆盐革兰阴性菌应小于 $10^2$cfu（1g） |
| | 液体口服给药制剂<br>　不含豆豉、神曲等发酵原粉<br>　含豆豉、神曲等发酵原粉 | $5×10^2$<br>$10^3$ | $10^2$<br>$10^2$ | 不得检出大肠埃希菌（1ml）；不得检出沙门菌（10ml）；耐胆盐革兰阴性菌应小于 $10^1$cfu（1ml） |
| | 固体局部给药制剂<br>　用于表皮或黏膜不完整<br>　用于表皮或黏膜完整 | $10^3$<br>$10^4$ | $10^2$<br>$10^2$ | 不得检出金黄色葡萄球菌、铜绿假单细菌（1g 或 10cm²）；阴道、尿道给药制剂还不得检出白色念珠菌、梭菌（1g 或 10cm²） |
| | 液体局部给药制剂<br>　用于表皮或黏膜不完整<br>　用于表皮或黏膜完整 | $10^2$<br>$10^2$ | $10^2$<br>$10^2$ | 不得检出金黄色葡萄球菌、铜绿假单细菌（1ml）；阴道、尿道给药制剂还不得检出白色念珠菌、梭菌（1ml） |
| 非无菌药用原料及辅料 | 药用原料及辅料 | $10^3$ | $10^2$ | * |
| 中药提取物及中药饮片 | 中药提取物 | $10^3$ | $10^2$ | * |
| | 研粉口服用<br>贵细饮片、直接口服及泡服饮片 | * | * | 不得检出沙门菌（10g）；耐胆盐革兰阴性菌应小于 $10^4$cfu（1g） |

注：①化学药品制剂和生物制品制剂若含有未经提取的动植物来源的成分及矿物质，还不得检出沙门菌（10g 或 10ml）。
②＊为未作统一规定。

109

**Table 4-3  Microbiological Acceptance Criteria for Nonsterile Preparations**

| | Administrate Route | Total Aerobic Microbial Count (cfu/g，cfu/ml or cfu/10cm$^2$) | Total Combined Yeast and Mold Counts (cfu/g，cfu/ml or cfu/10cm$^2$) | Specified Microorganisms |
|---|---|---|---|---|
| Nonsterile chemical preparation, biological products preparation and Chinese medicine preparations without crude power | Oral use[1] non-aqueous aqueous | $10^3$ $10^2$ | $10^2$ $10^1$ | Absence of *Escherichia coli* (1g or 1ml); Absence of *Salmonella* in preparations contain organ extracts (10g or 10ml) |
| | Oromcosal use Gingival use Nasal use | $10^2$ | $10^1$ | Absence of *Escherichia coli, Staphylococcus aureus, Pseudomonas aeruginosa* (1g, 1ml or 10cm$^2$) |
| | Auricular use Cutaneous use | $10^2$ | $10^1$ | Absence of *Staphylococcus aureus, Pseudomonas aeruginosa* (1g, 1ml or 10cm$^2$) |
| | Inhalation use | $10^2$ | $10^1$ | Absence of *Escherichia coli, Staphylococcus aureus, Pseudomonas aeruginosa*, Bile-tolerant Gram-negative bacteria (1g or 1ml) |
| | Vaginal use Urethra use | $10^2$ | $10^1$ | Absence of *Staphylococcus aureus, Pseudomonas aeruginosa, Candida albicans* (1g, 1ml or 10cm$^2$) Absence of *Clostridium* in Chinese medicine preparations (1g, 1ml or 10cm$^2$) |
| | Rectal use non-aqueous aqueous | $10^3$ $10^2$ | $10^2$ $10^2$ | Absence of *Staphylococcus aureus, Pseudomonas aeruginosa* (1g or 1ml) |
| | Other topical use | $10^2$ | $10^2$ | Absence of *Staphylococcus aureus, Pseudomonas aeruginosa* (1g, 1ml or 10cm$^2$) |

continued

| | Administrate Route | Total Aerobic Microbial Count (cfu/g, cfu/ml or cfu/10cm²) | Total Combined Yeast and Mold Counts (cfu/g, cfu/ml or cfu/10cm²) | Specified Microorganisms |
|---|---|---|---|---|
| Non-sterile Chinese medicine preparations with crude powder | Non-aqueous oral use Without fermented crude powder from bean, medicated leaven | $10^4$ (pill $3\times10^4$) | $10^2$ | Absence of *Escherichia coli* (1g) Absence of *Salmonella* (10g) Bile-tolerant Gram-negative bacteria are not more than $10^2$ (1g) |
| | With crude power above | $10^5$ | $5\times10^2$ | |
| | Aqueous oral use Without fermented crude powder from bean, medicated leaven | $5\times10^2$ | $10^2$ | Absence of *Escherichia coli* (1ml) Absence of *Salmonella* (10ml) Bile-tolerant Gram-negative bacteria are not more than $10^1$ (1ml) |
| | With crude power above | $10^3$ | $10^2$ | |
| | Non-aqueous topical use For wound epidermal or mucosal | $10^3$ | $10^2$ | Absence of *Staphylococcus aureus*, *Pseudomonas aeruginosa* (1g or 10cm²) Absence of *Candida albicans*, *Clostridium* in vagina/urethra preparations (1g or 10cm²) |
| | For intact epidermal or mucosal | $10^4$ | $10^2$ | |
| | Aqueous topical use For wound epidermal or mucosal | $10^2$ | $10^2$ | Absence of *Staphylococcus aureus*, *Pseudomonas aeruginosa* (1ml) Absence of *Candida albicans*, *Clostridium* in vagina/urethra preparation (1ml) |
| | For intact epidermal or mucosal | $10^2$ | $10^2$ | |
| Non-sterile raw material and excipients | Raw material and excipients | $10^3$ | $10^2$ | * |
| Chinese medicine extract and prepared pieces | Chinese medicine extract | $10^3$ | $10^2$ | * |
| | Prepared pieces for oral precious powder for oral directly, after soak | * | * | Absence of *Salmonella* (10g), Bile-tolerant Gram-negative bacteria are not more than $10^4$ cfu (1g) |

Note: ① *Salmonella* should be absent in 10g (10ml) if chemical/biological product preparation contain natural (botanical, animal ingredients or minerals) origin without extraction.

② * There is no unified requirement.

# 岗 位 对 接
# Post Docking

本章为中药学、中药制药和中药资源专业学生必须掌握的内容，为成为合格的中药学服务人员奠定坚实的基础。

This task is the content that students of traditional Chinese medicine major must master and lays a solid foundation for becoming qualified personnel of quality evaluation and control of traditional Chinese medicine.

本章内容对应岗位包括中药及相关领域的药品检验与管理的相关工种。

*The post docking corresponding to the content of this task include the related jobs of Chinese medicine and medicine test and management in related fields.*

上述从事中药学服务工作及药品质量监督相关所有岗位的从业人员均需要掌握有机杂质、无机杂质和残留溶剂的检查，能熟记制剂通则检查项目，学会应用本任务开展中药学服务工作。

The above practitioners engaged in TCM service, TCM purchase and sale, and TCM production and planting need to master the determination of inorganic impurities, organic impurities and Pesticide Residues in Chinese Medicine, memorize the general requirements for preparations, and learn to apply this task to carry out traditional Chinese medicine service.

# 重 点 小 结
# Summary of Key Points

中药的检查是中药分析的重要组成部分，通过中药的检查环节，可以确保药材的安全、有效。中药的检查主要涉及纯度、安全性和制剂通则三个方面检查。主要包括重金属、砷盐、有毒有害元素、水分、灰分、干燥失重、炽灼残渣等无机杂质的检查和农药残留量、黄曲霉素、残留溶剂等有机杂质以及残留溶剂的检查。制剂通则检查是检查中药制剂是否达到制剂学方面的有关要求，是为了确保中药制剂的安全性、有效性和均一性而进行的检查项目。

The test for Chinese medicine is an important measure to ensure the quality and human safety of medicine. The inspection of traditional Chinese medicine mainly involves three aspects of purity, safety and general requirements of preparation, It mainly includes the inspection of inorganic impurities such as heavy metals, arsenic salts, toxic and harmful elements, moisture, ash, loss on drying, Residue on ignition, and the inspection of organic impurities such as pesticide residues, aflatoxin and residual solvents. The general requirements of preparations check whether traditional Chinese medicine preparations meet the relevant requirements of pharmacology, and is an inspection item to ensure the safety, effectiveness and uniformity of traditional Chinese medicine preparations.

题库

# 目 标 检 测

（一）单项选择题

1. 中药制剂的杂质来源途径较多，不属于其杂质来源途径的是
   A. 原料不纯　　　　　　　　　B. 包装不当
   C. 服用错误　　　　　　　　　D. 产生虫蛀

2. 在酸性溶液中检查重金属常用何种试剂作显色剂
   A. 硫代乙酰胺　　　　　　　　B. 氯化钡
   C. 硫化钠　　　　　　　　　　D. 氯化铝

3. 硫代乙酰胺与重金属反应的最佳 pH 值是
   A. 2.5　　　　B. 2.0　　　　C. 3.0　　　　D. 3.5

4. 砷盐检查法中，制备砷斑所采用的滤纸是
   A. 氯化汞试纸　　　　　　　　B. 溴化汞试纸
   C. 氯化铅试纸　　　　　　　　D. 溴化铅试纸

5. 砷盐检查第一法（古蔡法）中，标准砷溶液（$1\mu gAs/ml$）的取用量为
   A. 0.5ml　　　B. 1.0ml　　　C. 1.5ml　　　D. 2.0ml

6. 砷盐限量检查中，醋酸铅棉花的作用是
   A. 将 $As^{5+}$ 还原为 $As^{3+}$　　　　B. 过滤空气
   C. 除 $H_2S$　　　　　　　　　　D. 抑制锑化氢的产生

7. 采用 Ag-DDC 法进行比色测定时，应采用的参比液为
   A. 甲醇　　　　　　　　　　　B. 三氯甲烷
   C. Ag-DDC 试液　　　　　　　D. 水

8. 炽灼残渣的组成主要是
   A. 有机物　　　　　　　　　　B. 硫酸盐
   C. 氯化物　　　　　　　　　　D. 硝酸盐

9. 采用甲苯法测定水分时，测定前甲苯需用水饱和，目的是
   A. 减少甲苯的挥发　　　　　　B. 增加甲苯在水中的溶解度
   C. 避免甲苯与微量水混合　　　D. 减少水的挥发

10. 进行炽灼残渣检查时，样品的炽灼温度为
    A. 400~500℃　　　　　　　　B. 500~600℃
    C. 600~700℃　　　　　　　　D. 700~800℃

11. 总灰分与酸不溶性灰分的组成差别在
    A. 钙盐　　　　　　　　　　　B. 硝酸盐
    C. 泥土　　　　　　　　　　　D. 沙石

（二）多项选择题

中药材中农药残留量的测定可采用的方法是
   A. 红外分光光度法　　　　　　B. 紫外分光光度法　　　　　　C. 气相色谱法
   D. 质谱法　　　　　　　　　　E. 电化学分析法

# 第五章　中药指纹图谱与特征图谱
# Chapter 5　Fingerprint and Characteristic Chromatogram of Chinese Medicine

 **学习目标｜Learning Goal**

**知识要求：**

1. **掌握**　中药指纹图谱。

2. **熟悉**　中药特征图谱。

**能力要求：**

学会应用色谱技术，特别是 HPLC 法解决中药化学指纹图谱和特征图谱的建立。

**Knowledge Requirements**

1. **Master**　Fingerprint of Chinese Medicine.

2. **Familiar**　Characteristic chromatogram of Chinese Medicine.

**Ability requirements**

Learn to apply chromatography, especially HPLC, to build fingerprint and characteristic chromatogram of Chinese medicine.

　　中药指纹图谱是指中药经适当处理后，采用一定的分析手段，得到的能够标示该中药特征的共有峰图谱。中药指纹图谱主要用于评价中药质量的真实性、稳定性和一致性，是一种综合、可量化的鉴别手段。其基本属性是"整体性"和"模糊性"。作为一种半定量的中药质量评价方法，指纹图谱分析强调准确的辨认，而不是精密的计算，比较图谱强调的是相似，而不是相同。

Traditional Chinese medicine (TCM) fingerprint refers to the map of common peaks that can mark the characteristics of TCM after proper treatment and analysis. TCM fingerprint is a comprehensive and quantifiable identification method, which is mainly used to evaluate the authenticity, stability and consistency of the quality of TCM, and wholeness and fuzziness are its basic attributes. As a semiquantitative method to evaluate the quality of TCM, fingerprint analysis emphasizes accurate identification rather than precise calculation, and comparison of fingerprint emphasizes similarity rather than sameness.

# 第一节 中药指纹图谱
# 5.1 Fingerprint of TCM

## 一、中药指纹图谱的分类
## 5.1.1 Classification of TCM Fingerprint

### （一）按应用对象分类
### 1. According to Application Objects

按应用对象分，中药指纹图谱可分为中药材（原料药材）指纹图谱、中药制剂原料药（包括饮片、配伍颗粒）指纹图谱、中间体（生产过程中间产物）指纹图谱和中药制剂指纹图谱。

According to the application objects, the fingerprint of traditional Chinese medicine can be divided into the fingerprint of traditional Chinese medicinal materials (raw materials), the fingerprint of raw materials of Chinese patent medicines (including Chinese herbal piece and compatibility granules), the fingerprint intermediate products and TCM preparations.

### （二）按研究方法分类
### 2. According to Research Methods

按研究方法分，中药指纹图谱又可分为中药化学指纹图谱和中药生物学指纹图谱。中药化学指纹图谱系指采用理化分析方法建立的用以表征中药化学成分特征的指纹图谱，包括色谱指纹图谱、光谱指纹图谱等。狭义的中药指纹图谱就是指中药化学（成分）指纹图谱。中药生物学指纹图谱系指采用生物技术手段建立的用以表征中药生物学特征的指纹图谱，包括中药的 DNA 指纹图谱、基因组学指纹图谱和蛋白组学指纹图谱等。

According to the research method, the fingerprint of TCM can be divided into chemical fingerprint and biological fingerprint. The spectrum of chemical fingerprinting of TCM refers to the fingerprint established by physical and chemical analysis to characterize the chemical components of TCM, including chromatographic fingerprint, spectral fingerprint, etc. In the narrow sense, the fingerprint of TCM refers to the chemical (composition) fingerprint. The biological fingerprint refers to the fingerprint established by biotechnology to represent the biological characteristics of TCM. Including DNA fingerprint, genomics fingerprint and proteomics fingerprint of TCM.

中药化学指纹图谱技术涉及色谱法（高效液相色谱法、气相色谱法、薄层色谱扫描法和高效毛细管电泳法等），光谱法（紫外光谱法、中红外光谱法、近红外光谱法），此外还有质谱法、核磁共振法和 X- 射线衍射法以及气相色谱 – 串联质谱和高效液相色谱 – 串联质谱等联用技术。其中使用最多的是色谱法，HPLC 因具有分离效能高、选择性高、检测灵敏度高、分析速度快、应用范围广等特点，已成为中药指纹图谱技术的首选方法。

Chemical fingerprint technology of TCM involves chromatography, such as high performance liquid chromatography (HPLC), gas chromatography (GC), thin layer chromatography (TLC) and high performance capillary electrophoresis (HPCE), spectroscopy, such as ultraviolet spectroscopy (UV), mid-infrared spectroscopy (IR) and near-infrared spectroscopy (NIR). In addition, mass spectrometry (MS), nuclear magnetic resonance (NMR) and X-ray diffraction (XRD), as well as GC-MS, HPLC-MS, HPLC-

MS-MS are used. Among them, the most commonly used method is chromatography, especially HPLC. Due to its high separation efficiency, high selectivity, high detection sensitivity, fast analysis speed and wide application range, so HPLC has become the preferred method for the fingerprinting of traditional Chinese medicine.

### 二、中药指纹图谱建立的原则
### 5.1.2　Principles of Establishment of TCM Fingerprint

建立中药指纹图谱，必须遵循系统性、专属性和稳定性的要求。

The establishment of TCM fingerprint must follow the requirements of systematic, specificity and stability。

（一）系统性

#### 1.　Systematic

系统性是指指纹图谱中所反映的化学成分群应包括该中药大部分药效物质，并与临床疗效相关联。对有效成分不清楚的中药，指纹图谱必须能反映大部分成分。可采用将样品按极性分级的方法，分别建立各极性萃取部位的指纹图谱，以尽可能多地反映其中所含化学物质。也可通过成分预试验方法，初步了解该中药所含主要化学成分的类型，然后有针对性地设计样品制备方法，再进行指纹图谱研究。

Systematic means that the chemical composition groups reflected in the fingerprint should include most of the medicinal substances of the TCM and be associated with the clinical efficacy. For TCM with unclear effective constituent, the fingerprint must be able to reflect most of the ingredients. The sample can be processed according to polarity, the fingerprint of each extraction is established to reflect the chemical substances contained in it as much as possible. It is also possible to get a preliminary understanding of the types of main chemical components contained in the TCM through the method of ingredient pre-test, and then design a specific sample preparation method, and then conduct fingerprint research.

（二）专属性

#### 2.　Specificity

中药指纹图谱必须能体现该中药的特征，即能用于区分中药的真伪与优劣，如区分不同来源的中药材，包括同属不同种，乃至同种不同产地、不同采收期的样品，以及不符合药用要求或变质的样品。

The fingerprint must be able to reflect the characteristics of the TCM and can use to distinguish the true or false in nature and good or bad in quality of TCM. Such as it can be used to distinguish Chinese medicinal materials of different origins, including samples of the same genus but different species, or even the same species with different origin and harvest period, as well as samples that do not meet medicinal requirements or have deteriorated.

中药制剂的指纹图谱除能鉴定处方中各药味的存在及其质量，有的还应能反映工艺过程的某些改变，以鉴别同一品种不同生产厂家的产品。只用一张指纹图谱不足以表现其全部特征的，常要采用几张指纹图谱来表现某种中药各个不同侧面的特征，从而构成其全貌。但对其中的每一张图谱均应符合专属性的要求。

In addition to identifying the presence and quality of each medicine in the prescription, the fingerprint of TCM preparations should also reflect changes in the technological process to identify products of the same variety produced by different manufacturers. One fingerprint is not enough to show all its characteristics, several fingerprint are often used to show the characteristics of different aspects of a certain Chinese medicine, so as to constitute the whole chromatogram. But each of spectrum should meet the requirements of specificity

（三）稳定性

### 3. Stability

稳定性是指同一样品在相同操作条件下，结果的重现性好。指纹图谱主要是用于表现、评价中药化学成分的整体，故要有较好的稳定性、通用性。因而要求包括样品制备、分析方法、实验过程及数据采集、处理、分析等全过程都要规范化操作，同时还应建立相应的评价方法，对其进行客观评价。

Stability refers to the reproducibility of the results of the same sample under the same operating conditions. Fingerprint is mainly used to express and evaluate the whole chemical composition of TCM, so it should have good stability and universality. Therefore, it is required that the whole process should be standardized, including sample preparation, analysis method, experiment process and data collection, processing and analysis, and corresponding evaluation methods should be established to make an objective evaluation.

### 三、中药指纹图谱的建立
### 5.1.3　Establishment of TCM Fingerprint

建立中药指纹图谱的基本程序包括：样品的收集、供试品溶液的制备、对照品（参照物）溶液的制备、方法建立、数据分析、样品评价和方法检验等。

The basic procedures of Chinese medicine fingerprint research include: sample collection, preparation of test solution, preparation of reference solution, method establishment, data analysis, sample evaluation and method test, etc.

（一）样品的收集

### 1. Collection of Samples

样品应具有真实性和代表性。研究指纹图谱用的样品应不少于10个批次，每批取样量应不少于3次检验量。中药材收集时要注意确定品种、药用部位、产地、采收期和炮制方法（或产地加工方法）等方面的因素，不能将同一样品人为分成若干份。在半成品和成品方面，样品收集时应重点选择工艺稳定、疗效确定、临床使用中很少出现不良反应的批次。

The collected samples should be authentic and representative. The sample for studying the study of fingerprint should be no less than 10 batches, and the sample quantity of each batch should be no less than 3 tests. When collecting Chinese medicinal materials, attention should be paid to the determination of varieties, medicinal parts, origin, harvesting period and processing method (or origin processing method). The same samples should not be artificially divided into several batches. In terms of semi-finished products and finished products, the focus of sample collection should be on selecting batches with stable process, confirmed curative effect and few adverse reactions in clinical use.

（二）供试品溶液的制备

### 2. Preparation of Test Solution

供试品溶夜制备的基本原则是整体性和专属性，必须既能保证充分反映出样品的特征性，又能保证待测样品所含特性的完整性。制备过程中应对不同的提取溶剂、提取方法、分离纯化方法等进行考察，力求最大限度地保留供试品中的化学成分，保证该中药中的主要化学成分或有效成分在指纹图谱中得以体现。

The basic principle of the preparation of the samples is integrity and specificity, which must not only fully reflect the characteristics of the samples, but also ensure the integrity of the characteristics of the samples to be tested. In the preparation process, different extraction agents, extraction methods, separation and purification methods should be investigated, so as to keep the chemical components in the samples to the maximum extent and ensure that the main chemical components or effective components in the TCM can be reflected in the fingerprint.

同一中药饮片在不同方剂中所起的作用不同，实际上是不同的药效成分群在不同方剂中所起的作用。所以理想的中药饮片指纹图谱应针对该饮片不同的药效成分群制备多种供试品溶液，获得多张指纹图谱。当作为原料饮片需考察与制剂指纹图谱的相关性时，其制备供试品溶液的溶剂宜尽可能与制剂提取溶剂一致。提取物或中间体的供试品溶液需根据所含成分的理化性质和检测方法的要求，参考制剂和相关产品的制备工艺，选择适宜的方法进行制备。在确保体现提取物或中间体中主要化学成分的同时，应可有效体现与制剂指纹图谱的相关性。各类制剂根据具体情况，制备供试品溶液。若制剂中不同类型化学成分性质差异较大，较难在一张图谱中体现，则可制备不同的供试品溶液，以获得针对不同类型成分的图谱。建立中药制剂指纹图谱的目的是控制最终产品中的成分，使批与批之间能保持稳定和一致，以保证成品的质量。

The same Chinese herbal piece plays different roles in different prescriptions, actually because of the different groups of medicinal components in different prescriptions. Therefore, the ideal fingerprint of herbal piece of TCM should be prepared according to the different groups of medicinal components of the herbal pieces to obtain multiple fingerprint. When examining the correlation between the fingerprint of the preparation and the herbal pieces of raw materials, the solvent used to prepare the sample solution should be consistent with the solvent used to extract the preparation. To prepare the solution of the test solution of the extract or intermediate, an appropriate method should be chosen according to the requirements of the physical and chemical properties of the components contained and the detection method, and the preparation process of the preparation and related products. While ensuring that the main chemical components in the extract or intermediate are present, the correlation with the fingerprint of the preparation should be effectively demonstrated. Each kind of preparation according to the specific situation to prepare the sample solution. If the properties of different types of chemical components in the preparation vary widely and are difficult to be reflected in a single map, then different sample solutions can be prepared to obtain the maps of different types of components. The purpose of the establishment of TCM preparation fingerprint is to control the composition of the final product, and maintain the stability and consistency between batches, so as to ensure the quality of the finished product.

（三）对照品（参照物）溶液的制备

### 3. Preparation of Reference Solution

1. 对照品（参照物）的选择　制定指纹图谱必须设立参照物，应根据样品中所含化学成分的性质，选择一个或几个主要的活性成分或指标成分作为参照物（S），以其对照品制备参照物溶液；如果没有适宜的对照品，也可以选择指纹图谱中结构已知、稳定的色谱峰作为参照峰或选择适宜的内标物作为参照物。

**(1) Selection of Reference Materials**　A reference must be set up for the establishment of fingerprint, one or several main active ingredients or index components should be selected as the standard material (S) according to the properties of chemical components contained in the sample, and the reference solution should be prepared with the standard material. If there is no suitable reference, the chromatographic peak with known structure and stability in the fingerprint can be selected as the reference peak or the suitable internal standard can be selected as the reference object.

2. 对照品（参照物）溶液的制备　精密称取参照物对照品适量，以适宜的方法制成标示浓度的参照物溶液（g/ml，mg/ml）。

(2) **Preparation of Reference Solution**　Accurately weigh the appropriate amount of reference substance, and prepare the reference solution with marked concentration (g/ml, mg/ml) by appropriate method.

（四）指纹图谱试验研究

### 4. Fingerprint Study

指纹图谱试验条件应根据指纹图谱的技术要求，以能满足指纹图谱的需要为目的进行试验条件的优化选择，不可直接照搬含量测定方法。

The test conditions of fingerprint shall be in accordance with the technical requirements, and optimizing the experimental conditions according to the needs of fingerprint, can not directly copy the method of content determination.

采用色谱法建立指纹图谱时，需对色谱柱、流动相和检测器进行比较试验，优选最佳条件。建立的最佳色谱条件应使供试品中所含成分尽可能的获得分离，即分得的色谱峰越多越好，使中药的内在特征尽可能多地显现出来，为中药的指纹图谱评价及其鉴别提供足够的信息。

When using chromatographic method to establish fingerprint, chromatographic column, mobile phase and detector should be compared and tested to optimize the best conditions. The optimum chromatographic conditions should be established so that the components contained in the samples can be separated as much as possible, that is, the more chromatographic peaks can be separated and the internal characteristics of TCM can be displayed as much as possible, providing enough information for the fingerprint evaluation and identification of TCM。

由于色谱指纹图谱具有量化的概念，所以从样品的称取、供试液的制备和进行色谱分析时均须定量操作，以保证色谱在整体特征上进行半定量（差异程度或相似程度）的比较，体现色谱指纹图谱量化的特点。

Because chromatographic fingerprint has the concept of quantification, quantitative operations should be carried out during the weighing of samples, preparation of test solution and chromatographic analysis to ensure the semi-quantitative (difference degree or similarity degree) comparison of the overall characteristics of chromatographic, reflecting the quantitative characteristics of chromatographic fingerprint.

采用 HPLC 和 GC 建立指纹图谱，记录时间最少为 1 小时。实验中应记录 2 小时的色谱图，以考察 1 小时以后的色谱峰情况。采用 TLCS 建立指纹图谱，必须提供从原点到溶剂前沿的图谱。

When fingerprint was established by HPLC and GC, the recording time was at least 1 hour. The chromatogram should be recorded for 2 hours to investigate the chromatographic peak after 1 hour. When using TLCS to establish a fingerprint, the map from the origin to the solvent frontier must be provided.

（五）方法学验证

### 5. Methodological Verification

为了验证所建立方法的准确性、可靠性，必须经过严格的方法学考察。中药指纹图谱方法学验证所包含的项目有：稳定性、精密度及重复性等。

In order to verify the accuracy and reliability of the established method, it must pass strict methodological inspection. The verification of TCM fingerprint methodology includes stability, precision and repeatability.

1. 稳定性试验　主要考察供试品溶液的稳定性。取同一供试品溶液，分别在不同时间点检测，考察各共有峰相对保留时间与相对峰面积的一致性，确定检测时间。

**(1) Stability**　The main purpose is to investigate the stability of the sample solution. Take the same sample solution and detect it at different time. The consistency of the retention time and the area of the peak was investigated to determine the detection time.

2. 精密度试验　主要考察仪器的精密度。取同一供试品溶液，连续进样 5 次以上，考察各共有峰的相对峰面积和相对保留时间的相对标准偏差（RSD）。

**(2) Precision**　It mainly studies the precision of the instrument. The relative standard deviation (RSD) of the relative peak area and the relative retention time of each common peak was investigated by sampling the same sample solution for more than 5 consecutive times.

3. 重复性试验　主要考察试验方法的重复性。取同批号的样品 5 份以上，分别照优化的方法制备供试品溶液并检测，考察各共有峰相对保留时间和相对峰面积的一致性。

**(3) Reproducibility**　The main purpose is to examine the repeatability of the test method. More than 5 samples of the same batch number were taken, the sample solution was prepared and detected by the optimized method, and the relative retention time and relative peak area of the chromatographic peak were observed to be consistent.

当采用 HPLC 和 GC 制定指纹图谱时，精密度试验和重复性试验要求，各共有峰峰面积比值的 RSD 应≤3%，其他方法的 RSD 应≤5%，各共有峰的保留时间应在平均保留时间 ±1 分钟内。

Precision and repeatability tests required that, when HPLC and GC were used to established fingerprints, the RSD of the chromatographic peak relative peak area of common peaks should be not more than 3%, the RSD of other method should be not more than 5%, and the retention time of each chromatographic peak should be within an average retention time of ±1 minute.

（六）对照指纹图谱的建立

### 6. Establishment of Reference Fingerprint

根据已确定的试验方法和条件，对所有供试品（10 批次以上）进行检测，根据检测结果，标定其共有峰。在指纹图谱研究中，特征峰的要求是主要特征峰和相邻峰分离度不小于 1.2，其他特征峰也应达到一定的分离，峰尖到峰谷的距离不小于该峰高的 2/3 以上。未达到基线分离的色谱峰，以该组峰作为一个色谱峰，根据参照物的保留时间，计算各共有峰的相对保留时间。

All samples (more than 10 batches) were tested according to the determined test methods and conditions, and the common fingerprint peaks were calibrated according to the test results. In the study of fingerprint spectrum, the requirement of characteristic peak is that the separation degree between the main characteristic peak and the adjacent peak should be greater than or equal to 1.2, other characteristic peaks should also be separated for certain degree, and the distance from peak tip to peak valley should be more than two-thirds of the peak hight. For chromatographic peaks that did not reach the baseline separation, this group of peaks was taken as one peak, according to the retention time of the reference, the relative retention time of each common peak is calculated.

根据 10 批次以上供试品的检测结果及相关参数，制定对照指纹图谱。可选择相似度评价软件中生成的共有模式图谱作为对照指纹图谱，也可选择相似度最高的指纹图谱作为对照指纹图谱。

Establish the reference fingerprint according to the test results and related parameters of more than 10 batches of test products. The common pattern chromatogram in the similarity evaluation software or the fingerprint chromatogram with the highest similarity generated can be selected as the reference fingerprint.

### （七）指纹图谱的辨认和评价
### 7. Identification and Evaluation of Fingerprint

指纹图谱的辨认应注意指纹特征的整体性。辨认和比较时从整体的角度综合考虑，如各共有峰的相对位置、峰面积大小或峰高、各共有峰之间的相对比例等。

The identification of fingerprint should pay attention to the integrity of fingerprint features. Identification and comparison from the overall perspective of comprehensive consideration, such as the relative position of each common peak, size of peak area or peak height, the relative proportion between the peaks.

指纹图谱的评价是指将样品的指纹图谱与该品种建立的对照指纹图谱（共有模式）进行相似性比较。指纹图谱的相似性主要从两个方面考虑，一是色谱的整体"面貌"，即各共有峰的数目、保留时间、各峰之间的大致比例等是否相似。二是样品与对照样品或与所建立的对照指纹图谱之间及不同批次样品指纹图谱之间总积分值进行量化比较，可以用"相似度"表达。相似度是供试品指纹图谱与对照指纹图谱共有模式的相似性的量度。可借助国家药典委员会推荐的"中药指纹图谱计算机辅助相似度评价软件"计算，除个别品种视具体情况而定外，一般情况下相似度大于0.9即认为符合要求。其中采用相似度评价软件计算相似度时，若峰数多于10个，且最大峰面积超过总峰面积的70%；或峰数多于20个，且最大峰面积超过总峰面积的60%，计算相似度时应考虑除去该色谱峰。

The evaluation of fingerprint refers to the comparison of similarity between the fingerprint of the sample and the reference control fingerprint (common pattern) established for the species. Fingerprint similarity is mainly from two aspects, one is the overall "face" of the chromatographic, that is, to observe whether the number of common peaks, retention time, the approximate proportion between the peaks is similar. The second is the quantitative comparison of the total integral value between the sample and the reference or the established reference fingerprint and the fingerprint of different batches of samples, which can be expressed by "similarity". Similarity is a measure of the similarity of the common pattern between the sample fingerprint and the reference fingerprint. It can be calculated with the help of the "computer-aided similarity evaluation software for fingerprint of TCM" recommended by the national pharmacopoeia committee. Except for some varieties, the similarity is more than 0.9 in general, which is considered to meet the requirements. When similarity evaluation software is used to calculate similarity, if the number of peaks is more than 10, and the maximum peak area is more than 70% of the total peak area, or if the number of peaks is more than 20 and the maximum peak area is more than 60% of the total peak product, the chromatographic peak should be considered to remove when calculating similarity.

相似度小于0.9，但直观比较难以否定的样品，可采用主成分分析法等模式识别方法进一步辨识与评价。

For samples whose similarity is less than 0.9, but which are hard to deny intuitively, we can use the pattern recognition method such as principal component segmentation to further check.

#### 四、原料药、提取物和制剂指纹图谱的相关性
### 5.1.4 Correlation of Fingerprints of Raw Materials, Extracts and Preparations

对于复方制剂而言，应同时建立原料药、半成品（提取物）和成品的指纹图谱。半成品的指纹图谱与原料药的指纹图谱应有一定的相关性，而原料药的某些特征峰在制剂指纹图谱中允许因为生产工艺关系等而有规律的丢失。制剂中各特征峰均应能够在原料药及中间体的指纹图谱中得到追溯。

In the case of compound preparation, the fingerprints of the Chinese crude drug, the semi-finished product (extract) and the finished product (preparation) should be established simultaneously. There should be some correlation between semi-crystalline fingerprint and API fingerprint, and some characteristic peaks of compound preparation can be lost regularly due to the production process. Each characteristic peak in the preparation should be traceable in the fingerprint of the Chinese crude drug and intermediate product.

#### 五、应用实例
### 5.1.5 Application Examples

例 5-1 沉香药材及其伪品的指纹图谱鉴别
Example 5-1 Fingerprint Identification of Agarwood and Its Counterfeit

【指纹图谱】色谱条件与系统适用性试验 以十八烷基硅烷键合硅胶为填充剂（250mm×4.6mm，5μm，Diamonsil C$_{18}$ 或 Phenomenex luna C$_{18}$ 色谱柱）；以乙腈为流动相 A，以 0.1% 甲酸溶液为流动相 B，按下表中的规定进行梯度洗脱；流速为每分钟 0.7ml；柱温为 30℃；检测波长为 252nm。理论板数按沉香四醇峰计算应不低于 6000。

**Fingerprint** *Chromatographic system and system suitability* Use octadecylsilane bonded silica gel as stationary phase (250mm×4.6mm, 5μm, Diamonsil C$_{18}$ or Phenomenex luna C$_{18}$ column)and use acetonitrile as mobile phase A, 0.1% solution of formic acid as mobile phase B, elute in gradient as the following. As a column temperature set at 30℃, as detector a spectrophotometer set at 252nm, and the flow rate at 0.7ml per min. The number of theoretical plates of column is not less than 6000, calculated with the reference to the peak of agarotetrol.

| 时间（Time, min） | 流动相 A（Mobile phase A, %） | 流动相 B（Mobile phase B, %） |
|---|---|---|
| 0~10 | 15 → 20 | 85 → 80 |
| 10~19 | 20 → 23 | 80 → 77 |
| 19~21 | 23 → 33 | 77 → 67 |
| 21~39 | 33 | 67 |
| 39~40 | 33 → 35 | 67 → 65 |
| 40~50 | 35 | 65 |
| 50.1~60 | 95 | 5 |

**参照物溶液的制备**　取沉香对照药材约 0.2g，精密称定，置具塞锥形瓶中，精密加入乙醇 10ml，称定重量，超声处理（功率 250W，频率 40kHz）1 小时，放冷，再称定重量，用乙醇补足减失的重量，摇匀，静置，取上清液滤过，取续滤液，作为对照药材参照物溶液。另取沉香四醇对照品适量，精密称定，加乙醇制成每 1ml 含 6μg 的溶液，作为对照品参照物溶液。

*Reference solution*　Weigh accurately about 0.2g of Agarwood reference medicine into a conical flask with a stopper, add 10ml of ethanol, ultrasonicate (power 250W, frequency 40kHz) for 1 hour, cool. Weigh again, replenish the lost weight with ethanol, mix well,filter, use the successive filtrate as the reference solution. And weighed accurately a quantitity of agarotetrol, dissolve in ethanol, to produce solutions containing 6μg to each per ml.

**供试品溶液的制备**　取本品粉末（过三号筛）0.2g，精密称定置具塞锥形瓶中，精密加入乙醇 10ml，称定重量，浸泡 0.5 小时，超声处理（功率 250W，频率 40kHz）1 小时，放冷，再称定重量，用乙醇补足减少的重量，摇匀，静置，取上清液滤过，取续滤液，即得。

*Test solution*　weigh accurately about 0.2g to a conical flask with a stopper, add 10ml of ethanol, ultrasonicate (power 250W, frequency 40kHz) for 1 hour, cool. Weigh again, replenish the lost weight with ethanol, mix well, filter, use the successive filtrate as the test solution.

**测定法**　分别精密吸取参照物溶液与供试品溶液各 10μl，注入液相色谱仪，测定，即得（图 5-1）。

*Procedure*　Inject accurately 10μl of reference solution and test solution into the column, record the chromatograms. As shown in Fig. 5-1.

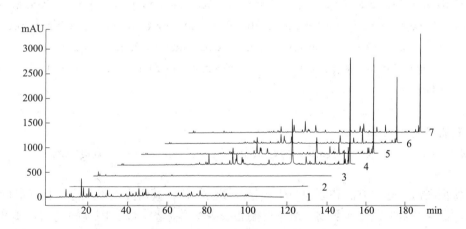

**图 5-1　伪品沉香的指纹图谱**

Fig.5-1　Fingerprint of fake Agarwood

1：沉香对照药材　2~6：沉香伪品

1: the agarwood control medicinal material　2-6: agarwood fakes

# 第二节 中药特征图谱

## 5.2 Characteristic Chromatogram of TCM

PPT

### 一、中药特征图谱的意义

### 5.2.1 Significance of Characteristic Chromatogram of TCM

中药特征图谱是指样品经处理后，采用一定的分析手段，按照指纹图谱原理和方法建立的，得到能够标识该中药各组分群体特征的共有峰图谱。通过不同来源10批以上样品的测定结果，选择特征峰或数个色谱峰组成的具有特征性的色谱峰组合。与中药指纹图谱不同的是，中药特征图谱只要求相对保留时间，而无相似度的要求，是一种定性的中药质量评价方法，在中药鉴别领域发挥重要作用。

The characteristic chromatogram of traditional Chinese medicine refers to the establishment of a common peak chromatogram that can identify the group characteristics of each component of the traditional Chinese medicine after the sample is processed, and it is established according to the principles and methods of fingerprint by a certain analysis method. Through the measurement results of more than 10 batches of samples from different sources, select a characteristic peak or a combination of several chromatographic peaks with characteristic chromatographic peaks. Different from the fingerprint of traditional Chinese medicine, the characteristic chromatogram of traditional Chinese medicine only requires a relative retention time, and no similarity requirement. It is a qualitative evaluation method of traditional Chinese medicine quality and plays an important role in the field of traditional Chinese medicine identification.

### 二、特征图谱的技术要求

### 5.2.2 Technical Requirements of Characteristic Chromatogram

中药特征图谱的建立方法和原理与中药指纹图谱相似，其研究基本程序包括样品的收集、供试品溶液的制备、对照品（参照物）溶液的制备、方法学考察、特征图谱的建立与评价等，其评价采用保留时间或相对保留时间。中药特征图谱只要求相对保留时间，而无相似度的要求，是一种定性的中药质量评价方法。

The method and principle for the establishment of the characteristic chromatogram of TCM is similar to the fingerprint of TCM. The basic research procedures include the collection of samples, the preparation of test solution, the preparation of reference solution (reference material), methodological investigation, establishment and evaluation of characteristic chromatogram etc, and the retention time or relative retention time was used for evaluation. The characteristic chromatogram of traditional Chinese medicine only requires a relative retention time, and no similarity requirement. It is a qualitative evaluation method of traditional Chinese medicine.

### 三、应用实例
### 5.2.3　Application Examples

例 5-2　银黄口服液的特征图谱鉴别

Example 5-2　Identification of Yinhuang Oral Liquid

【特征图谱】色谱条件与系统适用性试验　以十八烷基硅烷键合硅胶为填充剂；以乙腈为流动相 A，以 0.4% 磷酸溶液为流动相 B，按下表中的规定进行梯度洗脱；检测波长为 327nm。理论板数按绿原酸峰计算应不低于 2000。

**Characteristic Chromatogram** *Chromatographic conditions and system suitability* Use octadecylsilane bonded silica gel as stationary phase and acetonitrile(A) and 0.4% solution of phosphoric acid (B) as mobile phase. Elute in gradient as the following. As detector a spectrophotometer set at 327 nm. The number of theoretical plates of column is not less than 2000, calculated with the reference to the peak of chlorogenic acid.

| 时间（Time, min） | 流动相 A（Mobile phase A, %） | 流动相 B（Mobile phase B, %） |
| --- | --- | --- |
| 0~15 | 5 → 20 | 95 → 80 |
| 15~30 | 20 → 30 | 80 → 70 |
| 30~40 | 30 | 70 |

参照物溶液的制备　取绿原酸对照品适量，精密称定，置棕色量瓶中，加 50% 甲醇制成每 1ml 含 40μg 的溶液，即得。

*Reference solution* Weigh accurately a quantity of chlorogenic acid CRS to a brown volumetric flask, add 50% methanol to produce a solution containing 40μg per ml as the reference solution.

供试品溶液的制备　精密量取本品 1ml，置 50ml 棕色量瓶中，加 50% 甲醇稀释至刻度，摇匀，滤过，取续滤液，即得。

*Test solution* Dissolve 1ml in a 50ml volumetric flask with 50% methanol, weighed accurately, shake well, filter, use the successive filtrate as the test solution.

测定法　分别精密吸取参照物溶液与供试品溶液各 10μl，注入液相色谱仪，记录色谱图，即得。

*Procedure* Inject accurately 10μl of reference solution and test solution into the column, record the chromatograms.

供试品色谱中应呈现 7 个特征峰，如图 5-2 所示。与参照物峰相对应的峰为 S 峰，计算各特征峰与 S 峰的相对保留时间，其相对保留时间应在规定值的 ±5% 之内，规定值为：0.76（峰 1）、1.00（峰 2）、1.05（峰 3）、1.80（峰 4）、1.87（峰 5）、2.01（峰 6）、2.33（峰 7）。

It contains 7 characteristic peaks in the test solution, as shown in Fig.5-2. S peak corresponds to the peak of CRS. Calculate the relative retention time of S peak and each of the characteristic peaks, and the deviation of the relative retention time should be not exceed±5%, the specified value: 0.76 (peak 1), 1.00 (peak 2), 1.05 (peak 3), 1.80 (peak 4), 1.87 (peak 5), 2.01 (peak 6), 2.33 (peak 7).

附：金银花提取物对照特征图谱，见图 5-3。

Attachment: Reference chromatogram of Honeysuckle Extract, Fig.5-3.

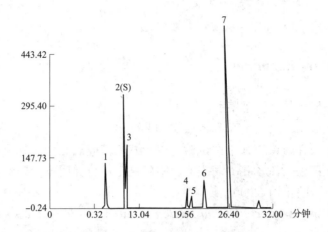

**图 5-2　银黄口服液的对照特征图谱**

**Fig. 5-2　Reference Chromatogram of Yinhuang Oral Liquid**

峰 1：新绿原酸　峰 2：绿原酸　峰 3：隐绿原酸　峰 4：3,4-*O*- 二咖啡酰奎宁酸

峰 5：3,5-*O*- 二咖啡酸奎宁酸　峰 6：4,5-*O*- 二咖啡酰奎宁酸　峰 7：黄芩苷

Peak 1: Neochlorogenic acid　Peak 2: chlorogenic acid　Peak 3: cryptochlorogenic acid

Peak 4: 3,4-O-dicaffeoylquinic acid　Peak 5: 3,5-O-dicaffeic acid, quinic acid

Peak 6: 4,5-O-dicaffeoylquinic acid　Peak 7: Baicalin

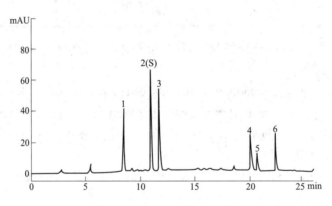

**图 5-3　金银花提取物的对照特征图谱**

**Fig. 5-3　Reference Chromatogram of Honeysuckle Extract**

峰 1：新绿原酸　峰 2：绿原酸　峰 3：隐绿原酸　峰 4：3,4-*O*- 二咖啡酸奎宁酸

峰 5：3,5-*O*- 二咖啡酰奎宁酸　峰 6：4,5-*O*- 二咖啡酰奎宁酸

Peak 1: Neochlorogenic acid　Peak 2: chlorogenic acid

Peak 3: cryptochlorogenic acid　Peak 4: 3,4-O-dicaffeic acid, quinic acid

Peak 5: 3,5-O-dicaffeoylquinic acid　Peak 6: 4,5-O-dicaffeoylquinic acid

供试品色谱中应呈现 6 个特征峰，与参照物峰相对应的峰为 S 峰，计算各特征峰与 S 峰的相对保留时间，其相对保留时间应在规定值的 ±5% 之内。规定值为：0.76（峰 1）、1.00（峰 2）、1.05（峰 3）、1.80（峰 4）、1.87（峰 5）、2.01（峰 6）。

It contains 6 characteristic peaks in the test solution, as shown in Fig. 5-3. S peak corresponds to the peak of CRS. Calculate the relative retention time of S peak and each of the characteristic peaks, and the deviation of the relative retention time should be not exceed ±5%, the specified value: 0.76 (peak 1), 1.00 (peak 2), 1.05 (peak 3), 1.80 (peak 4), 1.87 (peak 5), 2.01 (peak 6).

<h1 style="text-align:center">岗 位 对 接<br>Post Docking</h1>

本章为中药学、中药制药和中药资源专业学生必须掌握的内容，为成为合格的中药学服务人员奠定基础。

This task must be mastered by students majoring in traditional Chinese medicine, traditional Chinese medicine pharmacy and traditional Chinese medicine resources, and lay a solid foundation for becoming qualified Chinese medicine service personnel.

本章内容对应岗位包括中药及相关领域的药品检验与管理的相关工种。

The corresponding positions of this task include traditional Chinese medicine pharmacist, traditional Chinese medicine dispenser, sales representative, QC, QA, product manager, licensed Chinese medicine pharmacist, quality manager and so on.

上述从事中药学服务工作及药品质量监督相关所有岗位的从业人员均需要掌握中药指纹图谱的建立，学会应用本任务开展中药学服务工作。

The above-mentioned practitioners in all positions related to traditional Chinese medicine service and drug quality supervision and management need to master the fingerprint of TCM, and learn to apply this task to carry out traditional Chinese medicine services.

<h1 style="text-align:center">重 点 小 结<br>Summary of Key Points</h1>

中药指纹图谱是一种可量化的中药质量评价方法，用于评价中药质量的均一性和稳定性，其基本属性是"整体性"和"模糊性"。中药指纹图谱强调图谱的相似度，中药特征图谱强调特征峰的相对保留时间。

The fingerprint of traditional Chinese medicine is a quantifiable method for evaluating the quality of traditional Chinese medicine. It is used to evaluate the uniformity and stability of the quality of traditional Chinese medicine. Its basic attributes are "integrity" and "fuzziness". The fingerprint of traditional Chinese medicine emphasizes the similarity of chromatogram, and the characteristic chromatogram of traditional Chinese medicine emphasizes the relative retention time of characteristic peaks.

<h1 style="text-align:center">目 标 检 测</h1>

**一、选择题**

**（一）单项选择题**

1. 中药指纹图谱研究中样品采集应

A. 不少于 10 批      B. 不多于 10 批

C. 不少于 20 批      D. 不多于 20 批

2. 国家药品监督管理局规定，要求建立指纹图谱的中药新药剂型是

A. 丸剂      B. 注射剂

C. 颗粒剂      D. 滴丸剂

题库

127

3. 中药 HPLC 或 GC 指纹图谱进行精密度和重复性考察时，各共有峰相对峰面积的 RSD 不得大于

    A. 1%        B. 2%        C. 3%        D. 4%

4. 下列中药指纹图谱和特征图谱评价指标说法正确的是

    A. 都用相似度评价

    B. 都用相对保留时间评价

    C. 指纹图谱采用相对保留时间评价，特征图谱采用相似度评价

    D. 指纹图谱采用相似度评价，特征图谱采用相对保留时间评价

5. 采用国家药典委员会推荐的"中药指纹图谱计算机辅助相似度评价软件"计算中药指纹图谱的相似度，除个别品种外，一般情况下相似度大于多少即认为符合要求

    A. 0.9        B. 0.6        C. 0.7        D. 0.8

（二）多项选择题

1. 关于中药指纹图谱，下列说法正确的是

    A. 优先考虑色谱法建立中药指纹图谱

    B. 成分复杂时可考虑采用多种检测方法，建立多张指纹图谱

    C. 应根据君臣佐使的组方理论选择有效成分的色谱峰作为共有峰

    D. 可根据供试品中化学成分性质，选择适宜的对照品作为参照物

    E. 应对所有色谱峰进行定性分析

2. 中药指纹图谱的基本属性是

    A. 特征性               B. 整体性               C. 专属性

    D. 模糊性               E. 权威性

3. 中药指纹图谱的方法学验证包括

    A. 线性范围            B. 准确度             C. 精密度

    D. 稳定性            E. 重复性

4. 可用于中药指纹图谱的测定技术有

    A. TLC 法           B. GC 法            C. HPLC 法

    D. MS 法           E. DNA 法

5. 按照研究方法分类，中药指纹图谱可分为

    A. 中药化学指纹图谱            B. 中药生物学指纹图谱

    C. 中药材指纹图谱            D. 中药中间体指纹图谱

    E. 中药成方制剂指纹图谱

## 二、思考题

清开灵注射液收载于《中国药典》一部中，试根据本章所学内容，设计清开灵注射液的指纹图谱研究程序。

# 第六章　中药的含量测定
# Chapter 6　Assay of Chinese Medicine

 **学习目标｜Learning Goal**

知识要求：

**1. 掌握**　紫外－可见分光光度法、高效液相色谱法、气相色谱法在中药分析中的应用及中药含量测定方法学验证的内容和要求。

**2. 熟悉**　薄层色谱法及原子吸收分光光度法在中药分析中的应用。

**3. 了解**　化学分析法、等离子体质谱法在中药分析中的应用。

能力要求：

学会应用紫外－可见分光光度法、高效液相色谱法、气相色谱法等方法和方法学验证的内容与要求解决中药的含量测定。

**Knowledge Requirement**

**1. Master**　The application of ultraviolet-visible spectrophotometry, high performance liquid chromatography, gas chromatography in the analysis of Chinese medicine and validation of content determination method.

**2. Familiar**　The utility of thin-layer chromatography and atomic absorption spectrophotometry in the analysis of Chinese medicine.

**3. Understand**　The application of chemical analysis and inductively coupled plasma mass spectrometry in analysis of Chinese medicine.

**Ability Requirements**

Learn to apply visible-ultraviolet spectrophotometry, high performance liquid chromatography and gas chromatography and the validation of content determination method, to solve the content determination problem of Chinese medicine.

中药的含量测定是指采用化学、物理学或生物学的方法对中药中含有的化学成分（有效成分、指标成分、毒性成分及其他类别性成分等）进行定量分析。中药的含量测定是中药质量控制中的一项重要指标，通过研究中药中某一种或几种成分的含量高低是否符合规定，从而可衡量药物质量的优劣，进而保证中药的质量，以达到临床用药安全、有效的目的。

The content determination of Chinese medicine refers to the quantitative analysis of chemical ingredients (active ingredients, index ingredients, toxic ingredients, and other categories of composition) contained in Chinese medicine by chemical, physical or biological methods. The assay of Chinese medicine, an important indicator in the quality control of Chinese medicine, can be used to measure and guarantee the quality of the Chinese medicine, so as to achieve the purpose of safe and effective clinical medicine by exploring whether the content of one or several ingredients in Chinese medicine meets the requirements.

## 第一节 常用含量测定方法

## 6.1 Common Content Determination Methods

PPT

### 一、化学分析法
### 6.1.1 Chemical Analysis

化学分析法包括重量分析法和滴定分析法，是以物质的化学反应为基础的经典分析方法。化学分析法的特点是仪器简单，结果准确。主要用于测定中药中含量较高的一些成分及矿物药中的无机成分，如总生物碱类、总酸类、总皂苷及矿物药等。但其灵敏度低，不适于微量成分的测定。此外该方法专属性不强，在测定前一般需经提取、分离、净化、浓集（或衍生化）等处理；当被测组分为无机元素时，要经消化破坏其他有机成分后，再选择合适的测定方法；若中药组成简单、干扰成分较少或组方均为无机物时，也可直接测定。

Chemical analysis methods include gravimetric analysis and titration analysis, which are classical analysis methods based on physical chemistry. Chemical analysis is distinguished by simple instruments and accurate results. And it is mainly applied to the determination of some higher content compositions in Chinese medicine and inorganic constitutions in mineral medicine, such as total alkaloids, total acids, total saponins, mineral medicines and so on. However, due to low sensitivity, not suitable for the determination of trace components. In addition, the method is not specific, when measuring the content of ingredients in Chinese medicine with chemical analysis methods, extraction, separation, purification and concentration (or depolarization) are general operation before testing. In addition, measure inorganic elements, it is necessary to select an appropriate method after digesting and destroying other interfered organic components. As for, Chinese medicine with a simple formula, less interference, or pure inorganic, content determination can be performed directly.

### （一）重量分析法
### 1. Gravimetric Analysis

重量分析法是采用适当的方法将待测组分从样品中分离出来，转化成一定的称量形式，根据其重量，计算待测组分含量。可分为挥发法、萃取法和沉淀法。

The gravimetric analysis method uses an appropriate method to separate the measured component from the sample, and calculates the content of the constitutions according to the weight of the weighing form. Gravimetric methods can be generally divided into volatile methods, extraction methods and precipitation methods.

**1. 挥发法** 用于测定试样中具有挥发性或能定量转化为挥发性物质的组分含量。如《中国药典》规定检查项目中干燥失重、水分测定（烘干法）、灰分的测定、炽灼残渣的测定等。

**(1) Volatilization Method** Determine the content of components that are volatile or can be quantitatively converted into volatile substances, such as inspection items in *Chinese Pharmacopoeia*, moisture measurement (drying method), ash content measurement, and so on.

2. 萃取法　是根据被测组分在两种互不相溶的溶剂中溶解度的不同，达到分离的目的。如 2020 年版《中国药典》收载的昆明山海棠片中总生物碱的含量测定。

**(2) Extraction Method**　Achieves the purpose of separation based on the difference in solubility of the measured components in two mutually incompatible solvents. For example, the total alkaloids in Kunming Shanhaitang Tablets are determined by extraction method in 2020 *Chinese Pharmacopoeia*.

3. 沉淀法　是利用某种试剂与被测组分定量转化为难溶性化合物的形式从试样中分离出来，经滤过、洗涤、干燥（烘干或炽灼）、称重，根据称量形式转换，计算其含量的方法。如 2020 年版《中国药典》中西瓜霜润喉片中西瓜霜的含量测定等。

**(3) Precipitation Method**　Utilizes a certain reagent to quantitatively convert the test component into a poorly soluble compound through filtration, washing, drying, and weighing. Then, calculate the content according to the weighing form conversion. The method is appropriate for the determination of higher purity components in Chinese medicine, such as, the determination of the Mirabilitum Praeparatum in the Xiguashuang Runhou tablets in 2020 *Chinese Pharmacopoeia*.

（二）滴定分析法

## 2. Titration analysis

滴定分析法是指将已知准确浓度的标准溶液滴加到待测溶液中，根据标准溶液和待测物完全反应时所消耗的体积，计算待测组分含量的方法。主要分为酸碱滴定、沉淀滴定、配位滴定、氧化还原滴定等。多数滴定分析在水溶液中进行，当被测物质因在水中溶解度小或其他原因不能以水为溶剂时，也采用非水溶剂为滴定介质。

Titration analysis refers to the method of adding a standard solution of known exact concentration to the test solution, and calculating the content of the test component based on the volume consumed when the standard solution and the test object completely react. Titration analysis is mainly divided into acid-base titration, precipitation titration, coordination titration, redox titration, and so on. Most titration analysis is performed in an aqueous solution. However, when the substance to be tested is not soluble in water for low solubility or other reasons, non-aqueous solvents are also used as the titration medium.

1. 酸碱滴定法　适用于测定中药中的生物碱、有机酸类组分的含量。对于 $K \cdot C \geqslant 10^{-8}$ 的酸、碱组分，可在水溶液中直接确定。如 2020 年版《中国药典》收载的北豆根片中总生物碱的含量测定。而对于 $K \cdot C < 10^{-8}$ 的弱有机酸、生物碱或水中溶解度很小的酸碱，采用间接滴定法或非水滴定法测定。

**(1) Acid-base Titration Method**　It is suitable for determining the content of alkaloids and organic acid components in Chinese medicine. For $K \cdot C \geqslant 10^{-8}$, the acid and alkali components can be directly determined in aqueous solution, such as, the determination of total alkaloids in Beidougen tablets contained in 2020 *Chinese Pharmacopoeia*. While weak organic acids, alkaloids, or acids and bases with a low solubility in water with $K \cdot C < 10^{-8}$ can only be determined by indirect titration or non-aqueous titration.

2. 配位滴定法　是以配位反应为基础的一种滴定分析法，主要包括 EDTA 法和硫氰酸铵法等。在中药分析中，主要用于含 $Ca^{2+}$、$Fe^{3+}$、$Hg^{2+}$ 等矿物药的含量测定。如 2020 年版《中国药典》收载的柏子养心片中朱砂的含量测定、复方陈香胃片中氢氧化铝的测定等。

**(2) Coordination Titration Method**　A kind of titration analysis method based on coordination reaction theory, mainly includes EDTA method and ammonium thiocyanate method. In the analysis of

Chinese medicine, it is mainly applied to determine the content of minerals containing $Ca^{2+}$, $Fe^{3+}$, $Hg^{2+}$. In 2020 *Chinese Pharmacopoeia*, the content of cinnabar in Baizi Yangxin Tablets, content of aluminum hydroxide in Compound Chenxiangwei Tablets were measured by coordination titration method.

3. **沉淀滴定法** 是以沉淀反应为基础的滴定方法，包括银量法、四苯硼钠法和亚铁氰化钾法等，在中药分析中主要用于测定生物碱、生物碱的氢卤酸盐及有机卤化物的含量。

**(3) Precipitation Titration Method** A titration method based on the precipitation reaction including the silver method, the sodium tetraphenylborate method, and potassium ferrocyanide, is mainly to determine the content of alkaloids, alkaloids hydrohalide and other organic components containing halogens in the analysis of Chinese medicine.

4. **氧化－还原滴定法** 分为碘量法、高锰酸钾法和亚硝酸钠法等。适用于测定具有氧化还原性的物质，如含酚类、糖类及含 Fe、As 等成分的中药。

**(4) Oxidation-Reduction Titration Method** Including iodometric method, potassium permanganate method and sodium nitrite method, is suitable for the determination of oxidizing or reducing substances, such as Chinese medicines containing phenols, sugars, and Fe, As and other ingredients.

（三）应用实例

3. **Application example**

例 6-1 地奥心血康胶囊中甾体总皂苷的含量测定

Example 6-1 Determination of Total Steriod Saponins in Di'ao Xinxuekang Capsules

【含量测定】甾体总皂苷

*Assay Total steroid saponins*

取装量差异项下的本品内容物，混合均匀，取适量（约相当于甾体总皂苷元 0.12g），精密称定，置 150ml 圆底烧瓶中，加硫酸 40% 乙醇溶液（取 60ml 硫酸，缓缓注入适量的 40% 乙醇溶液中，放冷，加 40% 乙醇溶液至 1000ml，摇匀）50ml，置沸水浴中回流 5 小时，放冷，加水 100ml，摇匀，用 105℃干燥至恒重的 4 号垂熔玻璃坩埚滤过，沉淀用水洗涤至滤液不显酸性，105℃干燥至恒重，计算，即得。

Weigh accurately a quantity of the content equivalent to 0.12g of total steroid sapogenin obtained in the test of packing variation, in a 150ml round flask, add 50ml of a solution of sulfuric acid in 40% ethanol (add 60ml of sulfuric acid to a quantity 40% ethanol, allow to cool, dilute to 1000ml with 40% ethanol, and shake well), heat under reflux on a boiling water bath for 5 hours, allow to cool, add 100ml of water, filter through a NO.4 sintered glass filter, previously dried to constant weight at 105℃, and calculate.

本品每粒含甾体总皂苷以甾体总皂苷元计，不得少于 35mg。

It contains not less than 35mg of total steroid saponins per capsule, calculated as total steroid sapogenins.

二、**紫外－可见分光光度法**

**6.1.2 Ultraviolet-Visible Spectrophotometry**

紫外－可见分光光度法是根据物质分子对波长为 200~800nm 范围内的电磁波的吸收特征建立起来的光谱分析方法，其定量依据是 Lambert-Beer 定律，要求被测成分本身或其显色产物对紫外－可见光具有选择性吸收。紫外－可见分光光度法是中药及其制剂含量测定的一种常用方法，主要用于总成分的含量测定，如总生物碱、总黄酮、总蒽醌、多糖等。

Ultraviolet-visible spectrophotometry is a method to measure the degree of absorption of light between the wavelengths of 200-800nm by substances for assay. Based on Lambert-Beer's law as a quantitative basis, it is required that the measured component itself or its colored product has selective absorption of ultraviolet-visible light. Ultraviolet-visible spectrophotometry is a common method for assaying Chinese medicine and its preparations. It is mainly used for the content determination of total ingredients, such as total alkaloids, total flavones, total anthraquinones, polysaccharides, and so on.

（一）定量方法

## 1. Quantitative Method

由于中药成分复杂，不同组分的紫外吸收光谱彼此重叠，干扰测定，因此在测定前必须经过适当的提取、净化或采用专属的显色反应等来排除干扰，以测定其中某一类总成分或单一成分。测定时通常选用被测成分的 $\lambda_{max}$ 为测定波长，而共存组分在此波长处基本无吸收。一般吸光度值应控制在 0.3~0.7 之间。使用该法时，应注意对仪器波长、空白吸收的校正，吸收度准确度的检定和杂散光的检查，溶剂要符合要求。常用的定量方法有以下三种。

Due to the complex composition of Chinese medicine, the ultraviolet absorption spectra of different components overlap each other and interfere with the determination. Therefore, before the measurement, appropriate extraction, purification, or a dedicated color reaction must be used to eliminate interference to determine one of the total components or single ingredients. For the purpose of assay, the maximum absorption $\lambda_{max}$ of the component to be measured is usually selected as measurement wavelength at which wavelength the coexisting components have almost no absorption. Generally, it is advisable to control the absorbance reading of the test solution at rang of 0.3-0.7. When using this method, attention should be paid to the calibration of the instrument wavelength and blank absorption, the accuracy of the absorbance, the inspection of stray light, and the compliance of the solvent. The three commonly used quantitative methods are as follows:

1. **吸收系数法** 该法是测定供试品溶液在规定波长处的吸收度，根据被测成分的吸收系数（ $E_{1cm}^{1\%}$ ），依据 Lambert-Beer 定律，计算其含量。该方法对仪器的要求严格，优点是无需对照品，方法简便。例如 2020 年版《中国药典》用吸收系数法测定紫草中的羟基萘醌总色素的含量。

**(1) Absorption Coefficient Method** This method is based on Lambert-Beer's law and the absorption coefficient ($E_{1cm}^{1\%}$), determine the absorbance of the test solution at a specified wavelength and calculate its content. The disadvantage of this method is the strict requirements on the instrument, the advantage is that no reference substance is needed and the method is simple. In 2020 *Chinese Pharmacopoeia*, the absorption coefficient method is applied to determine hydroxynaphthoquinone pigments in radix lithospermi.

2. **对照品比较法** 在相同条件下分别配制对照品溶液和供试品溶液，且使对照品溶液中所含被测成分的量应为供试品溶液中被测成分的量的 100%±10%，在规定波长测定二者的吸收度，则可计算出供试品中被测成分的量。例如 2020 年版《中国药典》灯盏细辛注射液中总咖啡酸酯、华山参片中的总生物碱、黄杨宁片中的环维黄杨星 D 的测定。

**(2) Reference Substance Comparison Method** Prepare the reference solution and text solution under the same conditions, the ingredient to be determined in the reference solution should be within 100% ± 10% the ingredient to be determined in the test solution. Determine the absorbance of test solution and reference solution at specified wavelength, calculate the concentration of the ingredient to be determined in test solution. For example, in 2020 edition Chinese Pharmacopoeia, the determination of total caffeoyl ester in Dengzhan Xixin Injection, the determination of total alkaloid in Huashanshen

Tabels and the determination of cyclovirobuxine D in Huangyangning Tablets.

**3. 标准曲线法** 配制一系列不同浓度的对照品溶液（一般为5~7个梯度浓度），在相同条件下分别测定吸收度，绘制吸光度–浓度（A-C）曲线或计算线性回归方程（相关系数 r > 0.999），即得标准曲线。在相同条件下测定供试品溶液的吸收度（要求供试品溶液的吸光度应在标准曲线的线性范围内），通过标准曲线或回归方程即可求得供试品中被测成分的量。如2020年版《中国药典》中小儿七星茶口服液和槐花等中药中总黄酮的测定；金樱子等中金樱子多糖的测定。

**(3) Calibration curve method** Prepare a series of reference substance solutions with different concentrations (usually 5-7 gradient concentrations), determine the absorbance under the same conditions, graphically draw the absorbance versus the concentration or calculate the linear regression equation (correlation coefficient r > 0.999). The calibration curve was obtained. Then, under the same conditions, the absorbance of the test solution is determined (the absorbance of the test solution is required to be within the linear range of the standard curve), and the concentration or content of the tested component can be obtained through the standard curve or regression equation. For example, in 2020 edition *Chinese Pharmacopoeia*, the method can be applied to determine total flavonoids in Xiao' er Qixingcha Koufuye and Sophorae Flos, Rosae Laevigatae Fructus polysaccharide in Fructus Rosae Laevigatae.

（二）应用实例

**2. Application Example**

例 6-2 小儿七星茶口服液中总黄酮的含量测定

Example 6-2 Assay Total Flavonoids in Xiao'er Qixingcha Mixture

**【含量测定】总黄酮**

**Assay *Total flavonoids***

**对照品溶液的制备** 取芦丁对照品50mg，精密称定，置25ml量瓶中，加70%乙醇20ml，置水浴上微热使溶解，放冷，加70%乙醇至刻度，摇匀。精密量取5ml，置50ml量瓶中，加水至刻度，摇匀，即得（每1ml含芦丁0.2mg）。

*Reference solution* Dissolve 50mg of rutin CRS, accurately weighed, in a 25ml volumetric flask, add 20ml of 70% ethanol, dissolve by heating slightly on a water bath, then cool. Dilute to volume with 70% ethanol and mix well. Accurately measure 5ml of the mixture into a 50ml volumetric flask, dilute with water to volume, and mix well (containing 0.2mg of rutin per ml).

**标准曲线的制备** 精密量取对照品溶液1.0ml、2.0ml、3.0ml、4.0ml、5.0ml、6.0ml，分别置25ml量瓶中，各加水至6.0ml，加5%亚硝酸钠溶液1ml，混匀，放置6分钟，加10%硝酸铝溶液1ml，混匀，放置6分钟，加氢氧化钠试液10ml，再加水至刻度，摇匀，放置15分钟；以相应的试剂为空白，照紫外–可见分光光度法（通则0401），在505nm波长处测定吸光度，以吸光度为纵坐标、对照品浓度为横坐标，绘制标准曲线。

*Calibration standard* Transfer accurately 1.0ml, 2.0ml, 3.0ml, 4.0ml, 5.0ml, 6.0ml of the reference solution to a 25ml volumetric flask, respectively. Add water to 6.0ml, then add 1ml of 5% sodium nitrite solution, mix well, and stand for 6 minutes; add 1ml of 10% aluminum nitrate solution, mix well, stand for 6 minutes; add 10ml sodium hydroxide TS, dilute to volume with water, mix well. Stand for 15 minutes. Carry out the method for ultraviolet –visible spectrophotometry <0401>, Using the corresponding solution as the blank, measure the absorbance at 505 nm, and plot the calibration curve with the absorbance as ordinate and the concentration as abscissa.

**测定法** 取装量项下的本品，混匀，精密量取5ml，置50ml量瓶中，加水至刻度，摇匀。精密量取2ml，置25ml量瓶中，照标准曲线制备项下的方法，自"加水至6.0ml"起依法测定吸光度，从标准曲线上读出供试品溶液中芦丁的量，计算，即得。

*Procedure* Mix the mixture well, obtained under the test of packing variation. Measure accurately 5ml to a 50ml volumetric flask, dilute to volume with water, mix well. Measure accurately 2ml of the solution to a 25ml volumetric flask. Carry out the procedure as described in calibration standard, beginning at the words "Add water to 6.0ml", read and calculate the weight (mg), of rutin in the test solution from the calibration curve.

本品每 1ml 含总黄酮以芦丁（$C_{27}H_{30}O_{16}$）计，不得少于 3.0mg。

It contains not less than 3.0mg of total flavonoids per ml, calculated as rutin.

### 三、薄层色谱扫描法
### 6.1.3 TLC Scanning Methods

薄层色谱扫描法（TLCS）简称薄层扫描法，是用一定波长的光照射在薄层板上，对薄层色谱中可吸收紫外光或可见光的斑点，或经激发后能发射出荧光的斑点进行扫描，测定 *A-t* 或 *F-l* 曲线，将扫描得到的图谱及积分数据用于中药的鉴别、杂质检查或含量测定。薄层色谱扫描法可分为薄层吸收扫描法与薄层荧光扫描法。

Thin-layer chromatography scanning (TLCS) method abbreviated as thin-layer scanning irradiate a certain wavelength of light on a thin-layer plate, scan the spots in the thin-layer chromatography that can absorb ultraviolet, visible light or emit fluorescence after excitation and measure the *A-t* or *F-l* curves. The scanned spectrum and integrated data are employed for identification, impurity inspection or content determination of Chinese medicine. Thin-layer chromatography scanning methods can be divided into thin-layer absorption scanning methods and thin-layer fluorescence scanning methods.

（一）基本原理
### 1. Basic Principle
薄层吸收扫描法适用于在可见光或紫外光区有吸收的物质，及通过色谱前或色谱后衍生成上述化合物的样品组分。可分别以钨灯和氘灯为光源，在200~800nm 波长范围内选择合适波长进行测定。薄层荧光扫描法适合于本身具有荧光或经过适当处理后可产生荧光的物质的测定，光源用氙灯或汞灯，采用直线扫描。荧光测定法专属性强，灵敏度比吸收法高1~3 个数量级，最低可测到 10~50pg 样品，但适用范围较窄。对于能产生荧光的物质，可直接采用荧光扫描法测定。对于有紫外吸收，而不能产生荧光的物质，需采用荧光淬灭法测定。

Thin-layer absorption scanning method is suitable for substances that have absorption in the visible or ultraviolet light region, and sample components derived from the above compounds before or after chromatography. Tungsten and deuterium lamps can be applied as light sources, and appropriate wavelengths can be selected for measurement in the wavelength range of 200-800nm. While the thin-layer fluorescence scanning method is suitable for the determination of substances that possess fluorescence or produce fluorescence after proper processing. A xenon lamp or a mercury lamp is set as light source with linear scanning. Fluorescence assay is characterized as strong specificity, and its sensitivity is 1-3 orders of magnitude higher than that of absorption method. The minimum sample detection limit reach to 10-50pg, but the applicable range is narrow. For substances that can produce fluorescence, the fluorescence scanning method can be performed. However, for substances that have ultraviolet absorption and cannot produce fluorescence, the fluorescence quenching method must be used.

薄层色谱扫描法主要操作步骤包括薄层板的制备、活化、点样、展开及检测等。薄层色谱扫描法具有实验成本低、流动相的选择与更换方便等优点，通常作为高效液相色谱法或气相色谱法的补充应用。在 2020 年版《中国药典》中仅收载了清胃黄连丸（水丸）中盐酸小檗碱、牛黄抱龙丸中胆酸、山楂化滞丸中熊果酸及贝羚胶囊中熊去氧胆酸的含量测定等采用薄层扫描法进行。

The main operation steps of TLCS include preparation, activation, spotting, unfolding and detection. TLCS adhere with the advantages of low experimental cost and easy selection and replacement of mobile phases. Therefore, this method is usually applied as a complementary application of high performance liquid chromatography or gas chromatography. In 2020 *Chinese Pharmacopoeia*, only berberine hydrochloride in Qingwei Huanglian Pills (Water Pills), bile acid in Niuhuangbaolong Pills, ursolic acid in Shanzha Huazhi Pills, and ursodeoxycholic acid in Bei Ling capsules assay by TLC.

（二）系统适用性试验

## 2. System suitability test

按各品种项下要求对实验条件进行系统适用性试验，应符合规定的要求。

The system suitability test should be carried out for the experiment conditions according to the requirements specified under the monograph.

1. 比移值（$R_f$） 指从基线至展开斑点中心的距离与从基线至展开剂前沿的距离的比值。除另有规定外，杂质检查时，各杂质斑点的比移值 $R_f$ 以在 0.2~0.8 之间为宜。

**(1) The Retardation Factor ($R_f$)** It is defined as the ratio of the distance from the point of application to the center of the spot and the distance from the point of application to the mobile phase front. Unless otherwise specified,when impurities are tested, for spots of impurities,the retardation factor ($R_f$) should be controlled within 0.2-0.8.

2. 检出限 系指在鉴别或杂质限量检查时，供试品溶液中被测物质能被检出的最低浓度或量。一般采用已知浓度的供试品溶液或对照标准溶液，与稀释若干倍的自身对照标准溶液在规定的色谱条件下，在同一薄层板上点样、展开、检视，显清晰可辨斑点的最小浓度或量作为检出限。

**(2) Detection Limit** It is the minimum concentration or amount of the substance being examined which can be detected in the test solution in limit test or impurity test. Usually the test solution or reference standard solution with known concentration, and series dilute self-control reference standard solution are applied, developed and visualized on the same TLC plate under the prescribed chromatographic conditions. The concentration or amount of the reference standard solution when clear and distinguishable spot is exhibited is the detection limit.

3. 分离度（或称分离效能） 当薄层色谱扫描法用于限量检查和含量测定时，要求定量峰与相邻峰之间有较好的分离度，除另有规定外，分离度应大于 1.0。

**(3) Resolution** For limit test or assay, the peak used for quantification should be well separated with the adjacent peak. Unless otherwise specified, the resolution should be more than 1.0.

4. 相对标准偏差 同一供试品溶液在同一薄层板上平行点样，其待测成分峰面积测量值的相对标准偏差应不大于 5.0%；如需显色，则相对标准偏差应不大于 10.0%。

**(4) Relative Standard Deviation** When the same test solution is applied in parallel on the same thin-layer plate, the relative standard deviation of the peak areas of the ingredients being examined should be not more than 5.0%. The relative standard deviation for those which should be determined after visualization or on different plates should be not more than 10.0%.

（三）定量分析

## 3. Quantitative analysis

薄层色谱扫描法用于含量测定时，通常采用外标两点法计算。供试品溶液和对照标准溶液应交叉点于同一薄层板上，供试品点样不得少于 2 个，标准物质每一浓度不得少于 2 个。扫描时，应沿展开方向扫描，不可横向扫描。

When the TLCS method is used for assay, linear regression two-point method is usually adopted for calculation. The test solution and the reference solution should be applied alternatively on the same TLC plate. The number of the spots of the test solution should not be less than 2 and that of the reference solution should not be less than 2 for each concentration. Scan the plate along the direction of development, but not horizontally.

（四）应用实例

## 4. Application Example

例 6-3　清胃黄连丸（水丸）中盐酸小檗碱的含量测定

Example 6-3　Berberine Hydrochloride in Qingwei Huanglian Pills (Watered Pills)

【含量测定】取装量差异项下的本品，研细（过三号筛），取约 0.1g，精密称定，置具塞锥形瓶中，精密加入盐酸－甲醇（1∶100）的混合溶液 25ml，密塞，称定重量，超声处理（功率 250W，频率 33kHz）45 分钟，放冷，再称定重量，用甲醇补足减失的重量，摇匀，滤过，取续滤液，作为供试品溶液。另取盐酸小檗碱对照品适量，精密称定，加盐酸－甲醇（1∶100）的混合溶液制成每 1ml 含 20μg 的溶液，作为对照品溶液。照薄层色谱法（通则 0502）试验，精密吸取供试品溶液 2~3μl、对照品溶液 2μl 和 4μl，分别交叉点于同一硅胶 G 薄层板上，以环己烷－乙醇乙酯－甲醇－异丙醇－浓氨试液（12∶6∶3∶3∶1）为展开剂，放入展开缸的一侧槽内。另槽加入等体积的浓氨试液，预平衡数分钟后，展开，取出，挥干溶剂后，照薄层色谱法（通则 0502）进行荧光扫描，激发波长 λ = 334nm，测量供试品与对照品荧光强度的积分值，计算，即得。

**Assay** Weigh accurately 0.1g the product under the difference of loading amount, sift (No.3 sieve) to a stoppered conical flask, add accurately 25ml of a mixture of hydrochloric acid and methanol (1∶100), stopper, weigh and stand overnight. Ultrasonicate (power 250W，frequency 33kHz) for 45 minutes, allow to cool, weigh again and replenish the loss of weight with methanol, shake well, filter and use the successive filtrate as the test solution. Dissolve berberine hydrochloride CRS, weighed accurately, in a mixture of hydrochloric acid and methanol (1∶100) to produce a solution containing 20g per ml as the reference solution. Carry out the method for thin layer chromatography (0502)，using silica gel GF254 as the coating substance and a mixture of benzene, ethyl acetate, methanol, isopropanol, and concentrated ammonia TS (12∶6∶3∶3∶1) as the mobile phase, pre equilibrated with concentrated ammonia TS Apply accurately 2-3μl of the test solution, 2μl and 4μl of the reference solutions to the plate. After developing and removal of the plate, dry in air, carry out the method of thin layer chromatography (0502)，scan at the wavelength: λ = 334nm. Measure the integration value of absorbance of the test solution and the reference solution and calculate.

本品每 1g 含黄连、黄柏以盐酸小檗碱（$C_{20}H_{17}NO_4 \cdot HCl$）计，不得少于 5.3mg。

It contains not less than 5.3mg of berberine hydrochloride ($C_{20}H_{17}NO_4 \cdot HCl$) per gram, referred to Rhizoma Coptidis and Cortex Phellodendri.

## 四、气相色谱法
## 6.1.4 Gas Chromatography

在中药分析中，气相色谱法主要用于鉴别及测定中药中挥发油及其他挥发性成分的含量。如冰片、樟脑、麝香酮、桉叶素、丁香酚、薄荷脑、龙脑等；此外，还可用于中药及其制剂中具有良好的挥发性和热稳定杂质的检查，如水分、乙醇量、甲醇量、农药残留量等。中药酒剂和酊剂中甲醇和乙醇量通常采用GC法测定。

In the analysis of Chinese medicine, gas chromatography, as a conventional analysis method, is mainly used to identify and determine the content of volatile oil and other volatile components. Such as borneol, camphor, muscone, eucalyptol, eugenol, menthol, borneol, etc. It can also be applied to the inspection of volatile and thermally stable impurities in Chinese medicine and its preparations, such as the determination of water content, alcohol content, methanol pesticide residues, etc. The content of ethanol and methanol in Chinese medicine medicinal wines and tinctures is usually measured by gas chromatography.

气相色谱法是根据汽化后的试样被载气带入色谱柱，由于各组分在两相间分配系数的不同在色谱柱中移动速度不同，经一定柱长后得到分离，依次被载气带入检测器，将各组分浓度或质量变化转换成电信号变化记录成色谱图。利用色谱峰保留值进行定性分析，利用峰面积或峰高进行定量分析的方法。

The theoretical basis of gas chromatography is the difference in the partition coefficient of each component between the two phases and their discrepancy in the speed of movement in the column. Gas chromatography is a method in which vaporized sample is taken into chromatographic column with carrier gas, separated from each other after passing through a column with a certain column length, and sequentially carried into a detector with carrier gas. Then changes in the concentration or mass of each component are converted into changes in the electrical signal and recorded as a chromatogram. This method uses chromatographic peak retention values for qualitative analysis and peak area or peak height for quantitative analysis.

气相色谱法的两个基本理论是塔板理论和速率理论，分别从热力学观点和动力学观点阐述和归纳出混合物不同组分的层析分离规律。

The two basic theories of gas chromatography are plate theory and rate theory, which explain and summarize the chromatographic separation rules of different components in mixture from the perspective of thermodynamics and kinetics, respectively.

（一）系统适用性试验

### 1. System Suitability Test

色谱系统的适用性试验通常包括理论塔板数、分离度、重复性、灵敏度和拖尾因子等5个参数，其中分离度与重复性尤为重要。按各品种正文项下要求对色谱系统进行适用性试验，即用规定的对照品溶液或系统适用性试验溶液在规定的色谱系统进行试验，必要时，可对色谱系统进行适当调整，以符合要求。

Chromatographic system suitability tests usually include theoretical plate numbers, resolution, repeatability, sensitivity, tailing factors and other parameters. Perform the suitability test on the chromatographic system according to the requirements of the text of each variety, that is, use the specified reference solution or system suitability test solution to perform the test on the specified chromatographic system. If necessary, the chromatographic system can be appropriately adjusted to meet the requirements.

1. **色谱柱的理论塔板数（ $n$ ）** 用于评价色谱柱的效能。由于不同物质在同一色谱柱上的色谱行为不同，采用理论板数作为衡量色谱柱效能的指标时，应指明测定物质，一般为待测物质或内标物质的理论板数。

在规定的色谱条件下，注入供试品溶液或各品种项下规定的内标物质溶液，记录色谱图，量出供试品主成分色谱峰或内标物质色谱峰的保留时间（$t_R$）和峰宽（$W$）或半高峰宽（$W_{h/2}$），按 $n=16（t_R/W）^2$ 或 $n=5.54（t_R/W_{h/2}）^2$ 计算色谱柱的理论塔板数。$t_R$、$W$、$W_{h/2}$ 可用时间或长度计（下同），但应取相同单位。2020 年版《中国药典》中规定使用毛细管柱测定某组分，该组分的 $n$ 一般不低于 10000。

**(1) The number of theoretical plates of the column (*n*)**　The number of theoretical plates is used to evaluate the separation performance of the column. Due to the different chromatographic behavior of different substances on the same chromatographic column, when the number of theoretical plates is used as an index to measure the effectiveness of the column, the measurement substance should be specified, which is generally the number of theoretical plates of the substance to be measured or the internal standard substance.

Under the selected chromatographic conditions, inject the test solution or the internal standard substance solution specified under each variety, record the chromatogram, and measure the retention time ($t_R$), peak width ($W$) or half-peak width ($W_{1/2}$) of the main component or internal standard substance peak of the test substance., calculate the number of theoretical plates of the column according to $n = 16 (t_R/W)^2$ or $n = 5.54 (t_R/W_{h/2})^2$. If the measured number of theoretical plates is lower than the minimum number of theoretical plates specified under each item, certain conditions of the chromatographic column (such as column length, carrier performance, column packing, etc.) *should be modified to meet the required* number of theoretical plates. In 2020 edition *Chinese Pharmacopoeia*, when a capillary column was used to determine a component, the n of the component is generally not less than 10000.

2. **分离度（*R*）**　分离度是衡量色谱系统分离效能的关键指标。无论是定性鉴别还是定量分析，均要求待测峰与其他峰、内标峰或特定的杂质对照峰之间有较好的分离度。定量分析时，除另有规定外，待测物质色谱峰与相邻色谱峰之间的分离度应大于 1.5。

**(2) Resolution (*R*)**　Resolution is a key indicator for evaluating the separation efficiency of chromatographic system. Whether it is qualitative identification or quantitative analysis, it requires a good resolution between the peak to be measured and other peaks, internal standard peaks or specific impurity control peaks. Unless otherwise specified, the resolution between the chromatographic peak of the substance to be measured and the adjacent chromatographic peak should be greater than 1.5.

3. **重复性**　用于评价连续进样时，色谱系统响应值的重复性能。采用外标法时，通常取各品种项下的对照品溶液，连续进样 5 次，除另有规定外，其峰面积测量值的相对标准偏差应不大于 2.0%；采用内标法时，通常配制相当于 80%、100% 和 120% 的对照品溶液，加入规定量的内标溶液，配成 3 种不同浓度的溶液，分别至少进样 2 次，计算平均校正因子，其相对标准偏差应不大于 2.0%。

**(3) Repeatability**　It is used to evaluate the repeatability of the response of the chromatographic system during continuous injection. When the external standard method is used, the reference solution under each variety is usually taken for five consecutive injections. Unless otherwise specified, the relative standard deviation of the peak area measurement value should not be more than 2.0%. When using the internal standard method, usually prepare 80%, 100%, and 120% of the reference solution, add the specified amount of the internal standard solution, and prepare 3 different concentrations of the solution. Inject at least 2 times each to calculate the average correction factor, its relative standard deviation should not be greater than 2.0%.

4. **灵敏度**　用于评价色谱系统检测微量物质的能力，通常以信噪比（S/N）来表示。通过测定一系列不同浓度的供试品溶液或对照品溶液来测定信噪比。定量测定时，信噪比应不小于 10；定性测定时，信噪比应不小于 3。

**(4) Sensitivity** Sensitivity is used to evaluate the ability of a chromatographic system to detect trace substances, and is usually expressed in signal-to-noise ratio (S/N). The signal-to-noise ratio is determined by measuring a series of test solution or reference solution at different concentrations. For quantitative determination, the signal-to-noise ratio should be not less than 10, for qualitative determination, the signal-to-noise ratio should be not less than 3.

5. 拖尾因子（*T*） 用于评价色谱峰的对称性。拖尾因子计算公式为：

**(5) Tailing factor (T)** It is applied to evaluate chromatographic peak symmetry and the tailing factor calculation formula is:

$$T = \frac{W_{0.05h}}{2d_1} \tag{6-1}$$

式中，$W_{0.05h}$ 为 5% 峰高处的峰宽；$d_1$ 为峰顶在 5% 峰高处横坐标平行线的投影点至峰前沿与此平行线交点的距离。

以峰高作定量参数时，除另有规定外，*T* 应在 0.95~1.05 之间。

In the formula: $W_{0.05h}$ is the peak width at 5% of the peak height; $d_1$ is the distance from the projection point of the abscissa parallel line at the peak top at the peak height to the intersection of the parallel line and the parallel line. When the peak height is used as a quantitative parameter, unless otherwise specified, *T* should be within 0.95-1.05.

（二）实验条件的选择

## 2. Selection of Experimental Conditions

GC 用于中药分析，实验条件的优化如下：

The GC method is utilized for the analysis of Chinese medicine. The experimental conditions that need to be optimized are as follows:

1. 固定相 固定液的配比与样品性质有关，高沸点化合物样品，最好采用低配比。采用低配比，可使用较低的柱温，使固定液的选择受最高使用温度的限制较少，可供选择的固定液数目增加。低配比时若保留时间仍过长，可适当再减少。但过低配比，固定液不易涂渍均匀，常会造成色谱峰拖尾。低沸点化合物样品，宜用高配比，以便在分配系数很小的情况下，只有通过增加固定液的量（$V_S$）来增加 *R* 值，以达到良好的分离。

**(1) Stationary Phase** The ratio of the fixing solution is related to the nature of the sample. For samples with high boiling points, it is best to use a low ratio. With a low ratio, a lower column temperature can be used, so that the choice of fixing solution is less limited by the maximum use temperature, and the number of available fixing solutions is increased. If the retention time is too long at low ratios, it can be appropriately reduced. However, if the ratio is too low, the fixative solution is not easy to apply uniformly, which often causes tailing of chromatographic peaks. For low-boiling compound samples, a high ratio should be used, so that when the partition coefficient is small, the *R* value is increased only by increasing the amount of fixed solution ($V_S$), and good separation can be achieved.

中药分析中常用气 – 液色谱法，常用的固定液有甲基聚硅氧烷（非极性）、5% 苯基 –95% 甲基聚硅氧烷（弱极性）、50% 苯基 –50% 甲基聚硅氧烷（中等极性）和聚乙二醇（极性）等，使用时按"相似相溶"的原则选择固定液，此外，也常用气 – 固色谱（固定相大多用高分子多孔微球）用于分离水及含羟基（醇）化合物。

Gas-liquid chromatography is commonly employed to analysis, commonly use a methyl polysiloxane (nonpolar), 50% phenyl-50% methyl polysiloxane and 5% phenyl-95% methyl polysiloxane (medium polarity) and polyethylene glycol (polarity) as stationary phase, and fixed liquids are selected according to similar compatibility principles and main differences. In addition, gas-solid chromatography (mostly, polymer porous microspheres are used for stationary phases) is used to separate water and hydroxyl (alcohol) compounds.

2. 柱温　柱温是改善分离度的重要参数，选择的原则是使难分离物质达到分离度要求的条件下，尽可能采用低柱温。一般根据样品的沸点进行选择：高沸点样品（沸点 300~400℃）采用 1%~5% 低固定液配比，柱温 200~250℃；沸点为 200~300℃ 的样品采用 5%~10% 固定液配比，柱温 150~180℃；沸点为 100~200℃ 的样品采用 10%~15% 固定液配比，柱温选各组分的平均沸点 2/3 左右；气体等低沸点样品采用 15%~25% 高固定液配比，柱温选沸点左右，在室温或 50℃ 下进行分析；对于宽沸程样品，需采用程序升温法。柱温不能超过固定液的最高使用温度。

**(2) Column Temperature** Column temperature is an important parameter to improve the resolution. The principle of selection is to use as low a column temperature as possible on the premise that the difficult-to-separate substances can achieve the required resolution. The column temperature is generally selected based on the boiling point of the sample. For high boiling point samples (boiling point 300-400℃), 1%-5% low fixed solution ratio, column temperature 200-250℃; for samples with boiling point 200-300℃, 5%-10% fixed solution ratio, column temperature150-180℃; for samples with a boiling point of 100-200℃, 10%-15% fixed solution ratio, and the column temperature is selected to be about 2/3 of the average boiling point of each component; for low boiling point samples such as gas, 15%-25% high fixed solution ratio is used, and the column temperature is selected around the boiling point for analysis at room temperature or 50℃. For wide boiling range samples, a programmed temperature method is required. The column temperature must not exceed the maximum use temperature of the fixative.

3. 载气　热导检测器应选用 $H_2$ 或氦气；氢焰检测器、电子捕获检测器一般用 $N_2$；$N_2$ 为最常用载气。常用的载气流速为 20~80ml/min。

**(3) Carrier Gas** The thermal conductivity detector should select $H_2$ or helium as the carrier gas, while hydrogen flame detectors and electron capture detectors generally opt $N_2$ as the carrier gas. $N_2$ is the most commonly used carrier gas. The commonly used carrier gas flow rate is 20~80ml/min.

4. 汽化室（进样口）温度　一般选用样品的沸点或稍高于沸点，以保证瞬间汽化。但一般不要超过沸点 50℃ 以上，以防样品分解。对一般色谱分析，气化温度比柱温高 30~50℃。

**(4) Vaporization Chamber (inlet) Temperature** Generally, the boiling point of the sample or a temperature slightly above the boiling point is used as the temperature of the vaporization chamber (injection port) to ensure the instant evaporation of the sample. But generally do not exceed the boiling point of more than 50℃ to prevent sample decomposition. For general chromatographic analysis, the gasification temperature is 30-50℃ higher than the column temperature.

5. 检测室温度　一般需高于柱温，以免色谱柱的流出物在检测器中冷凝而污染检测器。通常可高于柱温 30℃ 左右或等于汽化室温度。

**(5) Detection Room Temperature** Generally it is higher than column temperature to prevent column effluent from condensing in the detector and contaminating the detector. Usually it can be about 30℃ higher than the column temperature or equal to the temperature of the vaporization chamber.

6. 进样量　对于填充柱，气体样品一般为 0.1~10ml，以 0.5~3ml 为宜；液体样品一般为 0.1~10μl，以最大不超过 4μl 为宜。毛细管柱需用分流器分流进样，分流后的进样量为填充柱的 1/10~1/100。

**(6) Injection Volume** For packed columns, the injection volume of gas samples is generally 0.1-10ml, preferably 0.5-3ml; the injection volume of liquid samples is generally 0.1-10μl, and the maximum is not more than 4μl. Capillary columns need to be injected with a splitter, and the injected volume after the split is 1/10-1/100 of the packed column.

7. 检测器　主要有氢火焰离子化检测器（FID）、热导检测器（TCD）、氮磷检测器（NPD）、火焰光度检测器（FPD）、电子捕获检测器（ECD）、质谱（MS）检测器等。FID 适用于含碳有机物的测定，是中药分析中应用最广泛的质量型检测器；TCD 是通用型检测器，可用于无机物及有机物的分析，如水分的测定；NPD 对含 N、P 有机化合物比较敏感，可用于中药及其制剂中农药残留量的检测；ECD 适用于痕量电负性大的有机物，如含卤素、硫、氧、硝基、羰基、氰基等化合物的分析。MS 检测器可以给出样品某个成分相应的结构信息，可用于结构确证。

**(7) Detector** There are mainly hydrogen flame ionization detectors (FID), thermal conductivity detectors (TCD), nitrogen and phosphorus detectors (NPD), flame photometric detectors (FPD), electron capture detectors (ECD), mass spectrometer (MS) detectors, and so on. FID is suitable for the determination of carbon-containing organic compounds and is the most widely used quality detector in the analysis of Chinese medicine; TCD is a universal detector that can be used for the analysis of inorganic and organic substances, such as the determination of moisture; NPD is more sensitive to organic compounds containing N and P, and can be used to detect pesticide residues in Chinese medicine and its preparations; ECD is suitable for the analysis of trace electronegative organic compounds, such as halogen, sulfur, oxygen, nitro, carbonyl, cyano and other groups. The MS detector can give the corresponding structural information of a component of the sample, which can be used for structural confirmation.

（三）定量分析方法

### 3. Quantitative Analysis Method

气相色谱法主要的定量分析方法包括内标法、外标法、归一化法及标准溶液加入法四种，四种定量分析方法各具不同的适用范围及特点。

The main quantitative analysis methods of gas chromatography include internal standard method, external standard method, normalization method and standard solution addition method. The four quantitative analysis methods have different application scopes and characteristics.

内标法是气相色谱法中最常用的定量方法，选择化学结构相似、物理性质与待测组分相近的纯品作为内标物，通过测量待测成分与内标物质的峰面积（或峰高）差异，通过校正因子的校正来计算待测物质的含量。采用内标法，可避免因进样体积误差对测定结果的影响。

Internal standard method, the most commonly used quantitative method in gas chromatography, selects pure products with similar chemical structure and similar physical properties to test substance. By measuring the peak area (or peak height) difference between the test component and the internal standard substance, correcting the correction factor to calculate the content of the test substance. The internal standard method can be used to avoid the influence of the sample preparation and sample volume errors on the measurement results.

外标法分为标准曲线法和外标一点法。通过测量对照品溶液和供试品溶液中待测物质的峰面积（或峰高），计算待测物质的含量。外标法较为简单，适合大量样品的测定，但要求进样量准确，实验条件恒定。由于微量注射器不易精确控制进样量，当采用外标法测定时，以手动进样器定量环或自动进样器进样为宜。

The external standard method calculating the content of the test substance by measuring the peak area (or peak height) of the test substance in the reference solution and the test solution is divided into a standard curve method and an external standard one-point method. The external standard method is relatively simple and suitable for the determination of a large number of samples, but it requires accurate injection volume and constant experimental conditions. Because it is difficult to accurately control the injection volume of the microinjector, when using the external standard method, it is advisable to use a manual injector loop or an automatic injector to inject.

归一化法要求所有组分在操作时间内都能流出色谱柱，并且检测器对它们都产生信号。通过测量供试品溶液各峰的峰面积和色谱图上除溶剂峰以外的总色谱峰面积，计算各峰面积占总峰面积的百分率。归一化法受测定条件的微小变化影响较小，但由于峰面积归一化法测定误差大，只能用于粗略考察供试品中的杂质含量，一般不适于中药中微量成分的含量测定。

Normalization requires that all components flow out of the column during the operating time and the detector generates signals for them. By measuring the peak area of each peak of the test solution and the total chromatographic peak area except the solvent peak on the chromatogram, the percentage of each peak area to the total peak area is calculated. The normalization method is less affected by small changes in measurement conditions, but due to the large measurement error of the peak area normalization method, it can only be used to roughly check the impurity content in the test product, and is generally not suitable for the determination of trace components in traditional Chinese medicine.

标准溶液加入法指精密称（量）取某个杂质或待测成分对照品适量，配制成适当浓度的对照品溶液，取一定量，精密加入到供试品溶液中，根据外标法或内标法测定杂质或主成分含量，再扣除加入的对照品溶液含量，即得供试品溶液中某个杂质和主成分含量。

The standard solution addition method refers to precisely weighing (quantifying) an impurity or a proper amount of a reference substance of a test component, formulating into a reference solution of appropriate concentration, take a certain amount and precisely add it to the test solution. Determine the content of impurities or main components according to the external standard method or the internal standard method, and then subtract the content of the reference solution added to obtain the content of an impurity and the main component in the test solution.

气相色谱法进行定量分析时，由于进样量较小，为减小进样误差，尤其当采用手工进样时，由于留针时间、室温等条件对进样量也有影响，故以采用内标法定量为宜；当采用自动进样器时，由于进样重复性的提高，在保证分析误差的前提下，也可采用外标法定量。当采用顶空进样时，由于供试品和对照品处于不完全相同的基质中，故可采用标准溶液加入法，以消除基质效应的影响；当标准溶液加入法与其他定量方法结果不一致时，应以标准加入法结果为准。

When performing quantitative analysis by gas chromatography, due to the small injection volume, conditions such as needle retention time and room temperature also affect the injection volume and causes large errors. In order to reduce the injection error, especially when manual injection is used, it is advisable to use the internal standard method for quantification. Using an autosampler, for the repetitiveness of the injection, the external standard method can also be used for quantification under the premise of ensuring the analysis error. Applying headspace injection, because the test and reference materials are not in the same matrix, standard solution addition can be used to eliminate the effect of matrix effects. When the results of the standard solution addition method are inconsistent with other quantitative methods, the results of the standard addition method shall prevail.

（四）应用举例

## 4. Application Examples

例 6-4　十滴水软胶囊中樟脑的含量测定

Example 6-4　Camphor in Shidishui Soft Capsules

【含量测定】色谱条件与系统适用性试验　改性聚乙二醇 20000（PEG-20M）毛细管柱（柱长

为 30m，内径为 0.53mm，膜厚度为 1μm），柱温为程序升温，初始温度为 65℃，以每分钟 2.5℃ 的速率升温至 102℃，再以每分钟 6℃ 的速率升温至 173℃；分流进样。理论板数按桉油精峰计算应不低于 10 000。

**Assay** *Chromatographic system and system suitability* Use modified polyethylene glycol 20000 (PEG-20M) (30m long, 0.53mm) in internal diameter, 1μm in film thickness) as the stationary phase, column temperature gradient: initial temperature at 65 ℃, increase the temperature at 2.5 ℃ per minute to102 ℃, then increase the temperature at 6℃ per minute to 173℃. The number of theoretical plates of the column is not less than 10 000, calculated with the reference to the peak of cineole.

**校正因子测定** 取环己酮适量，精密称定，加无水乙醇制成每 1ml 含 12.5mg 的溶液，作为内标溶液。分别取樟脑对照品约 25mg、桉油精对照品约 10mg，精密称定，置同一 10ml 量瓶中，精密加入内标溶液 1ml，加无水乙醇至刻度，摇匀。吸取 1μl，注入气相色谱仪，计算校正因子。

*Correction factor* Weigh accurately a quantity of cyclohexanone, dissolve in dehydrated ethanol to produce an internal standard solution containing 12.5mg per ml. Weigh accurately 25mg of camphor CRS and 10mg of cineole CRS to a 10ml volumetric flask, add accurately 1ml of the internal standard solution, dilute to volume with dehydrated ethanol, and mix well. Inject accurately 1μl of the solution into the column and calculate the correction factor.

**测定法** 取装量差异项下的本品内容物，混匀，取约 0.8g，精密称定，置具塞试管中，用无水乙醇振摇提取 5 次，每次 4ml，分取乙醇提取液，转移至 25ml 量瓶中，加无水乙醇至刻度，摇匀，精密量取 5ml，置 10ml 量瓶中，精密加入内标溶液 1ml，加无水乙醇至刻度，摇匀，作为供试品溶液。精密吸取 1μl，注入气相色谱仪，测定，即得。

*Procedure* Weigh accurately 0.8g of the content, obtained under the test of weight variation. Extract with five 4ml quantities of, separate the extract, combine and transfer to a 25ml volumetric flask, dilute with dehydrated ethanol to volume, and mix well, measure accurately 5ml to a 10ml volumetric flask, add accurately 1ml of the internal standard solution, dilute with dehydrated ethanol to volume, and mix well as the test solution. Inject accurately 1μl of the solution into the column and calculate the content.

本品每粒含樟脑（$C_{10}H_{16}O$）应为 53.0~71.8mg；含桉油精 ($C_{10}H_{18}O$) 不得少于 15.7mg。

It contains 53.0-71.8mg of camphor ($C_{10}H_{16}O$)and not less than 15.7mg of cineole ($C_{10}H_{18}O$) per capsule.

### 五、高效液相色谱法
### 6.1.5 High Performance Liquid Chromatography

在中药的含量测定方法中，HPLC 法的优势非常突出，2020 年版《中国药典》收载的药材及中成药中，绝大多数采用 HPLC 法进行含量测定。如山茱萸中马钱苷的含量测定，陈皮中橙皮苷的含量测定，黄连上清颗粒中盐酸小檗碱的含量测定，六味地黄丸中丹皮酚的含量测定以及灯盏生脉胶囊中野黄芩苷的含量测定等。HPLC 法也常用于中药的鉴别及检查中，是中药检测中最常用的分析方法。

色谱法的塔板理论和速率理论，也适用于高效液相色谱，但液相色谱与气相色谱的速率理论及影响因素是有差别的。在 HPLC 中流动相为液体，黏度大，柱温低，扩散系数很小，为兼顾柱效与分析速度，一般都采用较低流速，内径 2~4.6mm 的色谱柱多采用流速 1ml/min。

Among the assay methods of Chinese medicine, the advantages of HPLC method are very prominent. Most medicinal materials and proprietary Chinese medicines in 2020 edition *Chinese*

*Pharmacopoeia* are determined by HPLC. Such as the assay of rutin in corni fructus, hesperidin in citri reticulatae pericarpium, berberine hydrochloride in Huanglian Shangqing granules, paeonol in Liuwei Dihuang Pills, wild baicalin in Dengzhan Shengmai capsules and so on. HPLC is also commonly used in the identification and inspection of Chinese medicine. It is the most commonly used analytical method in the detection of Chinese medicine.

The plate theory and rate theory based on gas chromatography are also applicable to high-performance liquid chromatography, but the rate theory and influencing factors of liquid chromatography and gas chromatography are different. In HPLC analysis, the mobile phase is liquid, with high viscosity, low column temperature, and small diffusion coefficient. In order to take into account column efficiency and analysis speed, generally, a lower flow rate is used. For example, Columns with an inner diameter 2~4.6mm usually performed at 1ml/min rate.

（一）HPLC 系统适用性试验

## 1. The System Suitability Test of HPLC

系统适用性试验是为了考察所配置的仪器使用是否正常、设定参数是否适用以及所选实验条件是否合适等。系统适用性测试项目和方法与气相色谱法相同，可参照测定，具体指标应符合品种项下的规定。

The system suitability test is to check whether the configured instrument is used normally, the set parameters are applicable, and the selected experimental conditions are appropriate. The system suitability test items and methods are the same as those of gas chromatography, and can be determined by reference. The specific indicators should meet the requirements under the variety.

（二）HPLC 实验条件的选择

## 2. Selection of Experimental Conditions

1. **色谱柱** 色谱柱按其用途可分为分析型和制备型，含量测定采用分析型色谱柱。固定相是保证色谱柱高柱效和高分离度的关键。大多数药物可用十八烷基硅烷键合硅胶（简称 C18 反相柱，ODS）为固定相进行分离测定。在建立 HPLC 分离方法时可先试用反相柱，有的也可选用辛烷基硅烷键合硅胶或苯基键合硅胶等；亲水性强的可选用正相分配色谱柱（氨基柱、氰基柱）或硅胶吸附色谱柱等；对于解离性药物如生物碱、有机酸等可用离子对色谱、离子抑制色谱或离子交换色谱分离测定；多糖类可选用凝胶色谱。具体选择时应考虑被分离物质的化学结构、极性和溶解度等因素。

**(1) Chromatography Column** Chromatographic columns can be divided into analytical and preparative types according to their functions, and analytical columns are provided for assay. The stationary phase is the key to high column efficiency and high resolution. Most drugs can be separated and determined using octadecylsilane bonded silica gel (C18 reversed-phase column, ODS) as the stationary phase. When establishing an HPLC separation method, a reversed-phase column can be tried first, also octylsilane-bonded silica gel or phenyl-bonded silica gel can be opted. For hydrophilic components, normal phase distribution chromatography column (amino column, cyano column) or silica gel adsorption chromatography column can be selected for separation and determination, for dissociative drugs such as alkaloids, organic acids and other components, ion pair chromatography, ion inhibition chromatography or ion exchange chromatography is used; for polysaccharides, gel chromatography is applied. In addition, factors such as the chemical structure, polarity, and solubility of the material to be separated should be considered in the specific selection.

2. **流动相** 在液相色谱中，可供选择的流动相的范围较宽，且还可组成多元溶剂系统与不同配比；在固定相一定时，流动相的种类、配比、pH值及添加剂等均能显著影响分离效果，因此HPLC中流动相的选择至关重要。

**(2) Mobile Phase**   In liquid chromatography, a wide range of mobile phases can be selected, and multiple solvent systems and different formulation ratios can be formed. When the stationary phase is constant, the types, proportions, pH values, and additives of the mobile phase all significantly affect the separation, so it is crucial to choose mobile phases.

反相键合相色谱的流动相常选用以下三种：①部分含水溶剂：以水为基础溶剂，再加入一定量可与水互溶的有机极性调节剂（如甲醇、乙腈、四氢呋喃等）。适用于分离中等极性、弱极性药物，常用甲醇 – 水、乙腈 – 水系统。②非水溶剂：用于分离疏水性物质，尤其在柱填料表面键合的十八烷基硅烷量较大时，固定相对疏水化合物有异常的保留能力，需用有机溶剂进行洗脱，可在乙腈或甲醇中加入二氯甲烷或四氢呋喃（称非水反相色谱）。③缓冲溶液：适用于可溶于水并具可解离特性的化合物，如蛋白质、肽及弱酸、弱碱类化合物。常用的缓冲液有三乙胺磷酸盐、磷酸盐、醋酸盐溶液等，选用的pH应使溶质尽可能成为非解离形式，使固定相有较大保留能力（如反相离子抑制色谱和反向离子对色谱）。

The mobile phase of reversed-phase bonded phase chromatography is usually selected from the following three: ① Part of the water-containing solvent: Water is used as the base solvent, and a certain amount of organic polar adjuster (such as methanol, acetonitrile, tetrahydrofuran, etc.) that is miscible with water is added. Applicable to the separation of medium-polar and weak-polar drugs, commonly used in methanol-water and acetonitrile-water systems. ② Non-aqueous solvents: Used to separate hydrophobic substances, especially when the amount of octadecylsilane bonded on the column packing surface is large, the fixed relatively hydrophobic compounds have abnormal retention ability, which needs to be eluted with organic solvents. Dichloromethane or tetrahydrofuran is added to acetonitrile or methanol (called non-aqueous reversed-phase chromatography). ③ Buffer solution: Suitable for compounds that are soluble in water and have dissociative properties, such as proteins, peptides, and weak acid and weak base compounds. The commonly used buffers are triethylamine phosphate, phosphate, acetate solutions, etc. The pH should be selected so that the solute is as non-dissociated as possible, so that the stationary phase has a large retention capacity (reverse phase ion suppression chromatography).

正相键合相色谱的流动相通常采用饱和烷烃（如正己烷）中加入一种极性较大的溶剂（无紫外吸收）为极性调节剂，通过调节极性调节剂的浓度来改变溶剂强度。

Usually normal phase bonded phase chromatography selects saturated alkane (such as n-hexane) as mobile phase, and a stronger polar solvent (no UV absorption) as a polarity modifier. The strength of the solvent is modified by adjusting the concentration of the polarity modifier.

3. **洗脱方式**   HPLC按其洗脱方式分为等度洗脱与梯度洗脱。一般样品组分较少、性质差别不大，可采用等度洗脱。对于分析组分数多、性质相差较大的复杂的样品，常采用梯度洗脱。梯度洗脱在液相色谱中所起的作用相当于气相色谱中的程序升温。

**(3) Elution Method**   According to elution category, HPLC is divided into isocratic elution and gradient elution. For general samples with few components and little difference in properties, isocratic elution is applied, for complex samples with many components and large differences in properties, gradient elution is employed. The role of gradient elution in liquid chromatography is equivalent to programmed temperature rise in gas chromatography.

4. **检测器**   HPLC最常用的检测器为紫外检测器（UVD 或 DAD），其他常见的检测器有荧光检测器、蒸发光散射检测器、示差折光检测器、电化学检测器、化学发光检测器和质谱检测器等。

**(4) Detector**　The most commonly used detectors in HPLC are ultraviolet-visible spectroscopic detectors (UVD or DAD). Other common detectors include fluorescence detectors, evaporative light scattering detectors, refractive index detectors, electrochemical detectors, chemiluminescence detectors, mass detectors and more.

紫外检测器是 HPLC 应用最普遍的检测器，具有灵敏度高、线性范围较好、噪音低、对流速和温度波动不灵敏、可用于梯度洗脱等特点，最低检出量可达 $10^{-7}\sim10^{-12}$g，但只能用于检测有紫外吸收的物质。常用的有可变波长型及二极管阵列检测器。

Ultraviolet-visible detector: It is the most commonly used detector in HPLC. It has the characteristics of high sensitivity, good linear range, low noise, insensitivity to flow rate and temperature fluctuation, and can be used for gradient elution. It can reach $10^{-7}$-$10^{-12}$g, but can only be used to detect substances with ultraviolet absorption. Commonly used are variable wavelength type and diode array detectors.

蒸发光散射检测器（ELSD）是一种通用型检测器，特适用于无紫外吸收的样品，要求流动相先于样品挥发，主要用于检测糖类、高分子化合物、高级脂肪酸、维生素、甘油三酯及甾体等。对有紫外线吸收的样品组分检测灵敏度较低。

Evaporative light scattering detector (ELSD): It is a general-purpose detector that is especially suitable for samples without UV absorption. It is mainly used to detect sugars, polymer compounds, higher fatty acids, vitamins, triglycerides, steroids et al. This method of detection is less sensitive to sample components that possess ultraviolet absorption, and is only suitable for chromatographic elution when the mobile phase is volatile.

荧光检测器（FD）具有高灵敏度和选择性，是体内药物分析常用的检测器。但只适用于能产生荧光或其衍生物能发荧光的物质。

Fluorescence detector (FD): It is a common detector for in vivo drug analysis with high sensitivity and selectivity. But it is only applicable to substances themselves or their derivatives that can produce fluorescence.

电化学检测器（ECD）是选择性检测器，包括极谱、库仑、安培和电导检测器，用于能氧化、还原的有机物质的检测。电导检测器主要用于离子色谱；极谱、库仑、安培检测器用于能氧化、还原的有机物质的检测。其中安培检测器的应用最广泛，灵敏度很高，尤其适用于痕量组分的分析。

Electrochemical detector (ECD): It is a selective detector, including polarographic, coulomb, ampere, and conductance detectors, for the detection of organic substances capable of oxidation and reduction. Conductivity detectors are mainly used for ion chromatography, while polarographic, coulomb, and amperometric detectors are used for the detection of organic substances that can be oxidized and reduced. Among them, the amperometric detector is the most widely used and has high sensitivity, and is especially suitable for the analysis of trace components.

示差折光检测器（RID）也是一种通用型检测器，它是利用组分与流动相折射率之差进行检测。该检测器对多数物质的灵敏度低，通常不能用于痕量分析，对少数物质检测灵敏度较高，尤其适合于糖类的检测。

Refractive index detector (RID): It is also a general-purpose detector, which utilize the refractive index disparity between the component and the mobile phase to assay. The detector is of low sensitivity to most substances, and usually cannot be applied to trace analysis. It has high sensitivity to a few substances, and is especially applicable for sugar detection.

化学发光检测器（CLD）是高选择性、高灵敏度的新型检测器。化学发光反应常用酶为催化剂，将酶标记在待测物、抗原或抗体上，可进行药物代谢分析及免疫发光分析。

Chemiluminescence detector (CLD): It is a new type of detector with high selectivity and sensitivity.

Enzymes commonly used in chemiluminescence reactions can be labeled on a test object, an antigen or an antibody as catalyst to perform drug metabolism analysis and immunoluminescence analysis.

### （三）HPLC 定量分析方法
### 3. Quantitative analysis method by HPLC

高效液相色谱法测定是常用的定量分析方法，包括外标法、内标法及面积归一化法，其具体内容同气相色谱法项下的规定。

High performance liquid chromatography is a commonly used quantitative analysis method including external standard method, internal standard method and area normalization method. The specific content is the same as that specified under gas chromatography.

当采用 HPLC 定量测定中药化学成分时，由于 HPLC 以手动进样器定量环或自动进样器进样，进样量重复性高，常以外标法计算含量。当采用 HPLC 进行体内药物分析时，由于生物样品的基质干扰较大、样品前处理过程繁杂等因素，常以内标法计算含量。另外，可采用面积归一化法粗略计算杂质含量。

HPLC is usually equipped with a manual sampler loop or an automatic sampler to inject, the injection volume is highly repeatable, so external standard methods is commonly applied to calculated the content when quantitative the chemical composition of Chinese medicine using HPLC. When HPLC is used for drug analysis in vivo, due to the large matrix interference of biological samples and the complicated process of sample pretreatment, the internal standard method is often used to calculate the content. In addition, the area normalization method can be utilized to roughly measure the impurity.

### （四）应用实例
### 4. Application Examples

例 6-5　牛黄解毒丸中黄芩苷的含量测定

Examples 6-5　Baicalin in Niuhuang Jiedu Pills

【含量测定】色谱条件与系统适用性试验　以十八烷基硅烷键合硅胶为填充剂；以甲醇 – 水 – 磷酸（45: 55:0.2）为流动相；检测波长为 315nm。理论板数按黄芩苷峰计算应不低于 3000。

**Assay** *Chromatographic system and system suitability*　Use octadecylsilane bonded silica gel as the stationary phase and a mixture of methanol, water and phosphoric acid (45:55:0.2) at the mobile phase. As detector, a spectrophotometer set at 315nm. The number of theoretical plates of the column is not less than 3000，calculated with the reference of the peak of baicalin.

**对照品溶液的制备**　取黄芩苷对照品适量，精密称定，加甲醇制成每 1ml 含 30μg 的溶液，即得。

*Reference solution*　Weigh accurately a quantity of baicalin CRS, dissolve it in methanol to produce a reference solution containing 30μg per ml.

**供试品溶液的制备**　取重量差异项下的本品大蜜丸，剪碎，混匀，取约 1g，精密称定；或取本品水蜜丸，研碎，取约 0.6g，精密称定，加 70% 乙醇 30ml，超声处理 30 分钟，放冷，滤过，滤液置 50ml 量瓶中，用少量 70% 乙醇分次洗涤容器和残渣，洗液滤入同一量瓶中，加 70% 乙醇至刻度，摇匀；精密量取 2ml，置 10ml 量瓶中，加 70% 乙醇至刻度，摇匀，即得。

*Test solution*　Take the big honey pill of this product under the weight difference, cut it and mix well, take about 1g, accurately weigh. Or, take about 0.6g weighed accurately, add 30ml of 70% ethanol, ultrasonicate for 30 minutes, allow to cool and filter. Transfer the filtrate to a 50ml of volumetric flask, wash the container and the residue with small quantity of 70% ethanol in portions, combine the washings to the same volumetric flask, dilute to volume with 70% ethanol and shake well. Measure accurately 2ml of the solution to a 10ml volumetric flask, dilute to volume with 70% ethanol and shake well.

**测定法**　分别精密吸取对照品溶液与供试品溶液各 10μl，注入液相色谱仪，测定，即得。

*Procedure*　Inject accurately 10μl each of the test solution and the reference solution into the column, and calculate the content.

本品含黄芩以黄芩苷（$C_{21}H_{18}O_{11}$）计，水蜜丸每 1g 不得少于 10.0mg；大蜜丸每丸不得少于 20.0mg。

It contains not less than 10.0mg of baicalin ($C_{21}H_{18}O_{11}$) per 1g honey pill, or 20.0mg per big tablet, referred to Radix Scutellariae.

### 六、原子吸收分光光度法
### 6.1.6　Atomic Absorption Spectrophotometry

原子吸收分光光度法（AAS）测定对象是呈原子状态的金属元素和部分非金属元素，适合低含量矿物药及重金属元素测定。该法灵敏度高、选择性好、操作简便、测定范围广，但线性范围窄、测定不同元素需要不同光源。

Atomic absorption spectrophotometry is used in the determination of metal elements and some non-metal elements in atomic state. It is suitable for the determination of low content mineral Chinese medicine and heavy metal elements. The method has the advantages of high sensitivity, good selectivity, simple operation and wide range of determination, but the linear range is narrow and different light sources are needed for the determination of different elements.

（一）基本原理
### 1. Basic Principle

待测元素灯（空心阴极灯）发出的特征谱线通过供试品经原子化产生的原子蒸气时，被蒸气中待测元素的基态原子吸收，通过测定辐射光强度减弱的程度，可求出供试品中待测元素的含量。当原子蒸气的厚度固定时，吸光度 $A$ 和被测组分的浓度 $C$ 呈线性关系，即：

The light of characteristic wavelength emitted from a cathodic discharge lamp is absorbed when it passed through the atomic vapor generated from sample containing the element being examined atomized to the ground state. The assay of the element being examined is tested by determing the decreased degree of light intensity of radiation. When the thickness of the atomic vapor is fixed, there is a linear relationship between the absorbance and the concentration of the tested component.

$$A=K'C \qquad\qquad (6\text{-}2)$$

该式是原子吸收分光光度法的定量依据，$K'$ 为比例系数。

The formula is the quantitative basis of atomic absorption spectrophotometry and $K'$ is the ratio coefficient.

（二）定量方法
### 2. Determination Method

原子吸收分光光度法定量的方法有标准曲线法和标准加入法。

Atomic absorption spectrophotometric methods include standard curve method and standard addition method.

**1. 标准曲线法**　标准曲线法是应用最多的一种定量方法。在仪器推荐的浓度范围内，配制含待测元素的对照品溶液至少 5 份，浓度依次递增，并分别加入各品种项下制备供试品溶液的相应试剂，同时以相应试剂制备空白对照溶液。将仪器按规定启动后，依次测定空白对照溶液和各浓度对照品溶液的吸光度，以每一浓度 3 次吸光度读数的平均值为纵坐标，以相应浓度为横坐标，绘制标准曲线。然后测定供试品溶液的吸光度，取 3 次读数的平均值，从标准曲线上查得相应的浓度，计算元素的含量。

**(1) Standard Curve Method** Direct calibration method is the most widely used quantitative method. Unless otherwise specified, prepare not fewer than 5 reference solutions of the element being examined of different concentrations, coving the range recommended by the instrument manufacturer and add separately the corresponding reagents as that for the test solution and prepare the blank reference solution with corresponding reagents. Measure the absorbances of the blank reference solution and each reference solution of different concentrations separately, prepare a calibration curve with the average value of 3 readings of each concentration on the ordinate and the corresponding concentration on the abscissa. Measure the absorbance of the test solution 3 times, and calculated the average value. Interpolate the mean value of the readings on the calibration curve to determine the concentration of the element.

2. **标准加入法** 取同体积按各品种项下规定制备的供试品溶液 4 份，分别置于 4 个同体积的量瓶中，除 1 号量瓶外，其他量瓶分别精密加入不同浓度的待测元素对照品溶液，分别用去离子水稀释至刻度，制成从零开始递增的一系列溶液。按标准曲线法中操作，测定吸光度并记录数据。将吸光度读数与相应的待测元素加入量作图，延长此直线与含量轴的延长线相交，此交点与原点的距离即相当于供试品溶液取用量中待测元素的含量，如图 6-1 所示。再以此计算供试品中待测元素的含量。此法适用于试样基体干扰较大，又没有纯净的基体空白，或者测定纯物质中极微量的元素时。

**(2) Standard addition method** Place equal volume of the test preparation prepared as specified in the individual monograph in each of 4 similar volumetric flasks, add to all but the first one of the flasks an accurately measured amount of the reference solution containing increasing amounts of the element being determined. Dilute the contents of each flask to volume with deionized eater and proceed as described in the direct calibration. Measure the absorbances and record the readings. Plot the mean values of each group of absorbances against the corresponding concentration of the element contributed by the reference solution, and extrapolate the straight line to intersect with the axis of zero absorbance. The interception represents the concentration of the element contributed by the test preparation. Calculate the concentration of the element in the test preparation from the result so obtained.

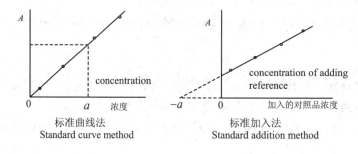

图 6-1　AAS 各定量方法的图示

Fig 6-1　Diagram of quantitative methods in AAS

### 七、电感耦合等离子体质谱法
### 6.1.7　Inductively Coupled Plasma Mass Spectrometry

电感耦合等离子体质谱法（ICP-MS）是一种无机质谱技术，分析对象为绝大多数的金属元素和部分非金属元素，适合于各类药品中从痕量到常量的元素分析，尤其适合于重金属元素分析，具有分析速度快、灵敏度高、可以同时测定多种元素等优点。

Inductively coupled plasma mass spectrometry (ICP-MS) is a kind of inorganic mass spectrometry technology, and is used in the determination of the vast majority of metal elements and some non-metal elements. The method is applicable for analysis of elements from trace to macro quantities. It is especially suitable for determination of trace heavy metal elements. It has the advantages of fast analysis speed, high sensitivity and simultaneous determination of multiple elements.

（一）基本原理
### 1.　Basic Principle

ICP-MS 由等离子体离子源、接口装置和质谱仪三部分组成。样品在等离子体离子源中转化成带正电荷的正离子，通过接口装置进入质谱仪，在质谱的质量分析器中按照质荷比不同分离，根据元素质谱峰强度测定样品中相应元素的含量。定量计算公式如下。

ICP-MS consists of inductively coupled plasma ion source, interface device and mass spectrometer. The sample is converted into positively charged ions in inductively coupled plasma ion source, and enters the mass spectrometer through the interface device. The mass spectrometer separates the ions according to mass-to-charge ratio, and the quantity of corresponding elements in the sample can be determined by referring to the intensity of the elemental mass peak. The quantitative formula is as follows.

$$I = aC + b \qquad (6\text{-}3)$$

式中，$I$ 为信号强度，$C$ 为元素浓度，$a$ 为校正系数，$b$ 为截距。

Where $I$ is the intensity of the element, $C$ is concentration of the element, $a$ is the correction coefficient and $b$ is intercept.

（二）定量方法
### 2.　Quantitative Method

对于待测元素，目标同位素的选择一般需根据待测样品基体中可能出现的干扰情况，选取干扰少、丰度高的同位素进行测定。某些同位素需采用干扰方程校正，对于干扰不确定的情况可选择多个同位素测定，常用的方法包括标准曲线法（分内标法和外标法）和标准加入法。

For each elements to be measured, selection of the preferred isotope is usually simply based on the most abundant isotope that is free from direct isobaric overlap. It is also necessary to consider the potential for interferences that might occur in the sample matrix. Isotopes with least interference and highest abundance should be selected for determination. Commonly used methods for test element calibration and quantitation include:

1.　**外标标准曲线法**　在选定的分析条件下，测定不同浓度的标准系列溶液，以待测元素的响应值为纵坐标、浓度为横坐标，绘制标准曲线，计算回归方程。在同样的分析条件下，测定样品，并进行空白试验，根据仪器说明书要求扣除空白后按标准或回归方程计算待测元素含量。

**(1) Standard curve method**　Under the analysis conditions selected for the samples, measure a series of solutions containing different known concentrations of the elements. Draw a standard curve with response value as Y-axis and concentration as X-axis to calculate regression equations. Measure the response value of the sample under the same analysis condition, and subtract the blank, calculate the corresponding concentrations and content of test element in the sample from standard curve or regression equation.

2. **内标校正的标准曲线法**　在每个样品（包括供试品溶液、标准溶液和空白溶液）中，添加相同浓度的内标元素，以待测元素响应值比内标元素响应值为纵坐标、浓度为横坐标，绘制标准曲线，计算回归方程。利用待测元素分析峰响应值与内标响应值比值，扣除试剂空白后，从标准曲线或回归方程获得相应的浓度，计算待测元素的含量。内标校正的标准曲线法是最常用的方法。

**(2) Internal standard corrected calibration standard curve method**　Prepare a solution of internal standard elements and add a spike at the same concentration in every sample (including standard solution, sample solution and blank solution). Draw a standard curve for each test element with the ration of response value of test elements in standard solutions to that of internal standard elements as Y-axis and concentration as X-axis. Calculate regression equations. Obtain the ratio of response value of analysis peak in sample solution to that of internal standard elements reference peak, subtract blank, determine the corresponding concentrations from standard curve or regression equation, and calculate the content of test elements in the sample.

3. **标准加入法**　当试样组成比较复杂，存在基体效应或者杂质干扰严重时，可采用标准加入法进行定量，具体定量方法同原子吸收法中标准加入法。

**(3) Standard addition method**　Standard addition method can be used for quantitative analysis when the sample composition is relatively complex, such as serious matrix effect or interference of impurities. The specific quantitative method is the same as that of the standard addition method in the atomic absorption spectrophotometry.

## 第二节　含量测定方法的验证
## 6.2　Validation of Content Determination Methods

### 一、含量测定方法选择
### 6.2.1　Selection of Content Determination Methods

在进行中药含量测定时，通常根据分析对象的组成、化学性质、含量高低等性质选择相应的含量测定方法。

In the analysis of Chinese medicine, the content determination method is usually selected according to the composition, chemical properties, content and properties of the analysis object.

（一）根据分析对象的组成多少选择
#### 1. According to the Composition of the Analysis Object
中药成分复杂，根据需要可对某一类成分进行分析，也可对某一个或几个成分进行分析。如果对某一类成分进行分析，如总生物碱、总黄酮、总有机酸、总多糖等，可以选择化学分析法或紫外-可见分光光度法。如果对某一个或几个成分进行分析，通常采用色谱法进行分离，然后对待测成分进行含量测定。

The components of Chinese medicine are complex. A certain kind of components or several specific components can be analyzed according to specific conditions. If a certain kind of components are analyzed, such as total alkaloids, total flavonoids, total organic acids, total polysaccharides, etc., chemical analysis or ultraviolet-visible spectrophotometry can be selected. If several specific components are analyzed, it is usually separated by chromatography first, and then the content determination is performed.

### （二）根据分析对象的化学性质选择
### 2. According to the Chemical Properties of the Analysis Object

中药含量测定的对象可以分为有机物和无机物。有机物可采用气相色谱法、液相色谱法或化学分析法。无机物分析可采用化学分析法、原子吸收法等。

The analysis object in Chinese medicine can be divided into organic and inorganic matter. Mostly organic compounds are analyzed by chromatography, such as gas chromatography, liquid chromatography, sometimes chemical analysis is also used. Chemical analysis and atomic absorption can be used for inorganic analysis.

### （三）根据分析对象的含量高低选择
### 3. According to the Content of Analysis Object

根据分析对象含量的高低，可选择不同灵敏度的分析方法。常量分析和微量分析可选用化学分析法和色谱分析法。对于痕量分析，可选用高灵敏度的质谱分析法，如 HPLC-MS、GC-MS、ICP-MS。

According to the content of the analysis object, different sensitivity methods can be selected. Chemical analysis and chromatography can be used for constant analysis and microanalysis. For trace analysis, high sensitive mass spectrometry can be used, such as HPLC-MS, GC-MS, ICP-MS.

### 二、含量测定方法验证
### 6.2.2　Verification of the Content Determination Methods

为保证测定的可靠性、可重现性等，在对样品进行测定时，必须对采用的方法进行方法学验证，证明所采用的方法适合于相应的检测要求。方法学验证的内容有：专属性、准确度、精密度（包括重复性、中间精密度和重现性）、检测限、定量限、线性、范围和耐用性。

The purpose of verification of an analytical method is to ensure that the adopted method meets the requirements for the intended analytical applications. The validation indexes include: specificity, accuracy, precision (including repeatability, intermediate precision and reproducibility), detection limit, quantitation limit, linearity, range and robustness.

### （一）专属性
### 1. Specificity

专属性系指在其他成分（如杂质、辅料等）可能存在的情况下，采用的方法能正确测定被测物的能力。鉴别试验、杂质检查、含量测定等方法均应考察其专属性。如该方法专属性不强，则应用原理不同的其他方法。

The specificity of an analytical method is the ability to measure the analyte accurately and specifically in the presence of components that may be expected to be present in the sample matrix, such as impurities, degradation products and excipients. Specificity should be investigated on identification, impurity test and content determination. If the specificity of the method is not enough, other methods with different principles should be adopted for supplementation.

### （二）准确度
### 2. Accuracy

准确度系指用所建立方法测定的结果与真实值或参考值接近的程度，一般用回收率（%）表示。准确度应在规定的线性范围内实验。准确度也可由所测定的精密度、线性和专属性推算出来。

The accuracy of an analytical method is the closeness of test results obtained by that method to the true value or the reference value. Accuracy is often represented as prevent recovery and should be determined in the specified range. Accuracy can also be calculated from the measured precision, linearity and specificity.

1. **测定方法** 可用已知纯度的对照品进行加样回收率测定，即向已知被测成分含量的供试品中再精密加入一定量的已知纯度的被测成分对照品，依法测定。用实测值（$C$）与供试品中含有量（$A$）之差，除以加入对照品量（$B$）计算回收率，见式（6-4）。

**(1) Test methods** Reference substances can be used for the determination of the recovery of added sample, e. g. certain amount of the reference substance of test substance is precisely added into the test sample with known content of analyte to be examined. The recovery ratio is calculated by margin of the determined value and the amount of the substance being examined divided by the amount of added reference.

$$回收率（Recovery\ Ratio，\%）= \frac{C-A}{B} \times 100\% \tag{6-4}$$

在加样回收试验中须注意对照品的加入量与供试品中被测成分含有量之和必须在标准曲线线性范围之内；加入的对照品的量要适当，过小则引起较大的相对误差，过大则干扰成分相对减少，真实性差；为减小误差，加入的对照品一般配制成一定浓度的溶液，再精密量取适量的体积。

In the test of the recovery of added samples, the sum of the added amount of the reference substance and the amount of the analyte in the substance being examined must be in the linearity range of the standard curve. The amount of the added reference substance should be proper. A very low amount of reference substance will cause a large relative error while a high amount of reference substance will reduce the relative amount of the interference substances, so the authenticity is poor. In order to reduce the error, the added reference substance is generally configured as a solution of a certain concentration, and then the appropriate volume is accurately measured.

2. **数据要求** 在规定范围内，设计3种不同浓度，每种浓度分别制备3份供试品溶液进行测定，用9份样品的测定结果进行评价。对于中药，应报告供试品取样量、供试品中含有量、对照品加入量、测定结果和回收率（%）计算值，以及回收率（%）的相对标准偏差（RSD%）或置信区间。

**(2) Requirement for the data** In the specified range, the accuracy should be evaluated by using results 9 samples with 3 different concentrations of test substance and 3 test solutions at each concentration. The amount of sample used, the content of test substance in the sample, the amount of reference substance added, the testing result and calculated percent recovery, and the relative standard deviation (RSD, %) or confidence interval of percent recovery should be reported.

样品中待测成分含量越高，回收率限度要求就越严格，在基质复杂、组分含量低于0.01%及多成分等分析时，回收率限度可适当放宽。样品中待测成分含量和回收率限度关系可参考表6-1。

Table 6-1 can be used as a reference for the relation between the content of test substance in sample and the limit of percent recovery. The limit of prevent recovery can be broadened in some conditions, such as complex matrix, the content of component lower than 0.01% and multi-components analysis.

表 6-1 样品中待测成分含量和回收率限度
Table 6-1 The content of test substance in sample and the limit of percent recovery

| 待测成分含量（Content of Test Substance in Sample） | | | 待测成分质量分数（Mass Fraction of Test Substance in Sample） | 回收率限度（Limit of Percent Recovery, %） |
|---|---|---|---|---|
| （%） | （ppm or ppb） | （mg/g or μg/g） | （g/g） | |
| 100 | — | 1000mg/g | 1.0 | 98~101 |
| 10 | 100000ppm | 100mg/g | 0.1 | 95~102 |
| 1 | 10000ppm | 10mg/g | 0.01 | 92~105 |
| 0.1 | 1000ppm | 1mg/g | 0.001 | 90~108 |
| 0.01 | 100ppm | 100μg/g | 0.0001 | 85~110 |
| 0.001 | 10ppm | 10μg/g | 0.00001 | 80~115 |
| 0.0001 | 1ppm | 1μg/g | 0.000001 | 75~120 |
| | 10ppb | 0.01μg/g | 0.00000001 | 70~125 |

From AOAC *Guidelines for Single Laboratory Validation of Chemical Methods for Dietary Supplements and Botanicals.*

（三）精密度

## 3. Precision

精密度系指在规定的测试条件下，同一个均匀供试品，经多次取样测定所得结果之间的接近程度。精密度一般用偏差、标准偏差或相对标准偏差表示。精密度验证内容包含重复性、中间精密度和重现性。

The precision of an analytical method is the closeness of agreement between a series of measurements obtained from multiple sampling of the same homogeneous sample under the prescribed conditions. The precision of an analytical method is usually expressed as deviation, standard deviation or relative standard deviation. The precisions includes repeatability, intermediate precision and reproducibility.

1. **重复性** 在规定范围内，取同一浓度（分析方法拟定的样品测定浓度，相当于 100% 浓度水平）的供试品，用至少测定 6 份的结果进行评价；或设计 3 种不同浓度，每个浓度各分别制备 3 份供试品溶液进行测定，用 9 份样品的测定结果进行评价。采用 9 份测定结果进行评价时，浓度的设定应考虑样品的浓度范围。

**(1) Repeatability** In specified range, the repeatability of the precision study should be evaluated using results from at least 6 samples of test substance at the same concentration (equivalent to 100% concentration level), or 9 samples with 3 different concentrations of test substance and 3 test solutions at each concentration. When the repeatability is evaluated by 9 testing results, the concentrations should be designed according to the test substance.

2. **中间精密度** 为考察随机变动因素，如不同日期、不同分析人员、不同设备对精密度的影响，应进行中间精密度试验。

**(2) Intermediate-precision** A scheme should be designed to inspect the effect of random variable factors on the precision. The variable factors include different dates, different analysts and different equipments.

3. **重现性** 当分析方法将被法定标准采用时，应进行重现性试验。例如，建立药典分析方法时，通过协同检验得出重现性结果。协同检验的目的、过程和重现性结果均应记载在起草说明中。应注意重现性试验用样品质量的一致性及贮存运输中的环境对该一致性结果的影响，以免影响重现性结果。

**(3) Reproducibility** Reproducibility should be tested when an analytical method is adopted as the national drug quality standard, for example, reproducibility should be inspected by different laboratory studies. Both the process of the collaborative study and result of the reproducibility should be recorded in the description of draft file. Where a reproducibility testing is to be conducted, the sample should be uniform, properly stored and transported to obtain reliable result.

**4. 数据要求** 均应报告偏差、标准偏差、相对标准偏差或置信区间。样品中待测成分含量和精密度 RSD 可接受范围见表 6-2（计算公式，重复性：$RSD_r = C^{-0.15}$；重现性：$RSD_R = 2C^{-0.15}$，其中 $C$ 为待测成分含量），可接受范围可在给出数值 0.5~2 倍区间。在基质复杂、含量低于 0.01% 组分的分析中，精密度可接受范围可适当放宽。

**(4) Requirements for Data** Deviation, standard deviation, relative standard deviation and confidence interval should be reported. Table 6-2 can be used as a reference for the content of test substance in sample and acceptable range of the RSD for the precision (calculation formula, repeatability: $RSD_r = C^{-0.15}$; reproducibility: $RSD_R = 2C^{-0.15}$, and $C$ is the content of the tested ingredient), acceptable range is 0.5-2 times of the given value. Acceptable range of the RSD for the precision can be broadened in some conditions, such as complex matrix, the content of component lower than 0.01% and multi-components analysis.

表 6-2　样品中待测成分的含量与精密度可接受范围

Table 6-2　The content of test substance in sample and acceptable range of the RSD for precision

| 待测成分含量（Content of Test Substance in Sample） | | | 待测成分质量分数（Mass Fraction of Test Substance in Sample） | 重复性（Repeatability, $RSD_r$%） | 重现性（Reproducibility, $RSD_R$%） |
|---|---|---|---|---|---|
| （%） | （ppm or ppb） | （mg/g or μg/g） | （g/g） | | |
| 100 | — | 1000mg/g | 1.0 | 1 | 2 |
| 10 | 100000ppm | 100mg/g | 0.1 | 1.5 | 3 |
| 1 | 10000ppm | 10mg/g | 0.01 | 2 | 4 |
| 0.1 | 1000ppm | 1mg/g | 0.001 | 3 | 6 |
| 0.01 | 100ppm | 100μg/g | 0.0001 | 4 | 8 |
| 0.001 | 10ppm | 10μg/g | 0.00001 | 6 | 11 |
| 0.0001 | 1ppm | 1μg/g | 0.000001 | 8 | 16 |
| | 10ppb | 0.01μg/g | 0.00000001 | 15 | 32 |

引自 AOAC *Guidelines for Single Laboratory Validation of Chemical Methods for Dietary Supplements and Botanicals*.

## （四）检测限

## 4. Limit of Detection

检测限（LOD）系指试样中被测物能被检测出的最低量。检测限仅作为限度试验指标和定性鉴别的依据，无需准确定量。常用的方法如下。

Limit of detection is the lowest concentration of the analyte in a sample that can be detected. The limit of detection can only be used as the reference for limit test and qualitative identification, which is not quantitative meaning. The methods in common use are as follows.

**1. 直观法** 用已知浓度的被测物质，试验出能被可靠地检测出的最低浓度或量。

**(1) Noninstrumental Method**　The detection limit is generally determined by the analysis of samples with known concentrations of analyte and by establishing the minimum level at which the analyte can be reliably detected.

2. **信噪比法**　用于能显示基线噪声的分析方法，即把已知低浓度供试品测出的信号与空白样品测出的信号进行比较，计算出能被可靠地检测出的最低浓度或量。一般以信噪比为 3:1 或 2:1 时相应浓度或注入仪器的量确定检测限。

**(2) Signal-to-noise Ratio Method**　For the instrumental method recording the noise at the baseline, the lowest concentration or content of test substance that is reliably detected can be calculated by comparing the signal of sample at a known low concentration and the signal of the blank. The concentration or the amount injected into the instrument corresponding to the signal-to-noise ratio of 2:1 or 3:1 is generally accepted.

3. **基于响应值标准偏差和标准曲线斜率法**　按照 LOD=3.3$\delta$/S 公式计算。式中，LOD 为检测限；$\delta$ 为响应值的偏差；S 为标准曲线的斜率。$\delta$ 可以通过下列方法测得：①测定空白值的标准偏差；②采用标准曲线的剩余标准偏差或截距的标准偏差来代替。

**(3) Method of Standard Deviation and Slope of Standard Curve Based on Response Value**　The detection limit is calculated by the following formula: LOD=3$\delta$/S. In the formula, LOD is the detection limit, $\delta$ is the standard deviation of response value, and S is the slope of standard curve. $\delta$ can be determined by following method: ① determining the standard deviation of blank;② substituting by the residue standard deviation or the standard deviation of intercept of standard curve.

4. **数据要求**　上述计算方法获得的检测限数据须用含量相近的样品进行验证。应附测试图谱，说明测试过程和检测限结果。

**(4) Requirment for Data**　Detection limit obtained by above methods must be validated by samples with similar content of test substance. The test graphs should be attached and the test procedures and the results of detection limit should be reported.

（五）定量限

## 5. Limit of Quantitation

定量限（LOQ）系指试样中被测成分能被定量测定的最低量，其测定结果应符合准确度和精密度要求。对微量或痕量药物分析、定量测定药物杂质和降解产物时，应确定方法的定量限。常用的方法如下。

Limit of quantitation is the lowest concentration of the analyte in a sample that can be determined with acceptable precision and accuracy under the stated experimental conditions. The limit of quantitation should be determined for the analytical method of micro or trace substance or the quantitative determination for impurities and degraded products. The methods in common use are as follows.

1. **直观法**　用已知浓度的被测物质，试验出能被可靠地定量测定的最低浓度或量。

**(1) Noninstrumental Method**　Limit of quantitation is generally determined by the minimum concentration or content of the analyte in a known concentration of sample that can be reliably detected.

2. **信噪比法**　用于能显示基线噪声的分析方法，即将已知低浓度供试品测出的信号与空白样品测出的信号进行比较，计算出能被可靠地检测出的最低浓度或量。一般以信噪比为 10∶1 时相应浓度或注入仪器的量确定定量限。

**(2) Signal-to-noise Ratio Method**　For the instrumental method recording the noise at the baseline, the lowest concentration or content of test substance that is reliably detected can be calculated by comparing the signal of sample at a known low concentration and the signal of the blank. The concentration or the amount injected into the instrument corresponding to the signal-to-noise ratio of 10:1 is generally accepted.

3. 基于响应值标准偏差和标准曲线斜率法　按照 LOQ=10 $\delta$/$S$ 公式计算。式中，LOQ 为定量限；$\delta$、$S$ 的含义与 $\delta$ 的获得方法同检测限。

**(3) Method of Standard Deviation and Slope of Standard Curve Based on Response Value**　The limit of quantitation is calculated by the following formula: LOQ=10 $\delta$/$S$. In the formula, LOQ is the quantitation limit, $\delta$ and $S$ are the same as LOD.

4. 数据要求　上述计算方法获得的定量限数据须用含量相近的样品进行验证。应附测试图谱，说明测试过程和检测限结果，包括准确度和精密度验证数据。

**(4) Requirment for Data**　Limit of quantitation obtained by above methods must be validated by samples with similar content of test substance. The test graphs should be attached and the test procedures and the results of quantitation limit, including validation data of precision and accuracy, should be reported.

（六）线性

## 6. Linearity

线性系指在设计的范围内，测试结果与试样中被测物浓度或质量直接呈正比关系的程度。应在设计的范围内测定线性关系。可用同一对照品贮备液经精密稀释，或分别精密称取对照品，制备一系列对照品溶液的方法进行测定，至少制备 5 份梯度浓度的对照品溶液。以测得的响应信号作为被测物浓度的函数作图，观察是否呈线性。数据要求列出回归方程、相关系数（$r$）和线性图（或其他数学模型）。

The linearity of an analytical method is its ability to elicit test results that are directly proportional to the concentration of analyte in samples within a given range. Linear relationship should be determined over the claimed range of the method. The samples with varying concentrations of analyte for linearity determination are prepared by diluting accurately a stock solution, or by measuring accurately an amount of analyte separately. At least 5 portions of samples should be prepared. Requirement for data: regression equation, correlation coefficient and the linear graph should be listed (or other mathematical models).

（七）范围

## 7. Range

范围系指分析方法能达到一定精密度、准确度和线性要求时的高低限浓度或量的区间。范围应根据分析方法的具体应用及其线性、准确度、精密度结果及要求确定。原料药和制剂含量测定，范围一般为测定浓度的 80%~120%；制剂含量均匀度检查，范围一般为测定浓度的 70%~130%，特殊剂型，如气雾剂和喷雾剂，范围可适当放宽；溶出度或释放度中的溶出量测定，范围一般为规定限度的 ±20%，如规定了限度范围，则应为下限的 −20% 至上限的 +20%；杂质测定，范围应根据初步实际测定数据，拟定为规定限度的 ±20%。如果含量测定与杂质检查同时进行，用峰面积归一化法进行计算，则线性范围应为杂质规定限度的 −20% 至含量限度（或上限）的 +20%。在中药分析中，对于有毒的、具特殊功效或药理作用的成分，其验证范围应大于被限定含量的区间。

The range of an analytical method is the concentration or quantity interval between the upper and lower levels of analyte (including these levels) that have been demonstrated to be determined with precision, accuracy, and linearity using the method as written. The range of the analytical method should be determined based on specific application of the method, its linearity, accuracy and precision, and related requirement. For content determination of drug substance and preparation, the range should be 80%-120% of the test concentration. For content uniformity of preparation, the range should be 70%-130% of test concentration and this range may be widened appropriately for special dosage forms, such as aerosols and sprays. For dissolution test and drug release test, the range should be ±20% of the limit. If the range of limit is provided, it should be -20% of lower limit to +20% of upper limit. For impurity determination, the range should be stipulated from -20% to +20% of the provided limit on the basis of preliminary actual determination. If the content determination and impurities test are performed simultaneously with the peak area normalization method, the linear range should be -20% of the provided limit of impurity to +20% of the provided limit of content (or upper limit). For toxic ingredients or those with unique efficacy or pharmacological effect in Chinese medicine, the range to be validated should be wider than the range of content.

（八）耐用性

### 8. Robustness

耐用性系指在测定条件有小的变动时，测定结果不受影响的承受程度，为所建立的方法用于常规检验提供依据。开始研究分析方法时，就应考虑其耐用性，如果测试条件要求苛刻，则应在方法中写明，并注明可以接受变动的范围，可以先采用均匀设计确定主要影响因素，再通过单因素分析等确定变动范围。典型的变动因素有：被测溶液的稳定性、样品提取次数、时间等。高效液相色谱法中典型的变动因素有：流动相的组成和 pH、不同品牌或不同批号的同类型色谱柱、柱温、流速等。气相色谱法变动因素有：不同品牌或批号的色谱柱、固定相，不同类型的担体、载气流速、柱温、进样口和检测器温度等。经试验，应说明测定条件小的变动能否满足系统适用性试验要求，以确保方法有效。

Robustness of an analytical method is the degree of tolerance that the determination result is not affected when there is small change in the operational condition. The robustness of the method should be taken into account at the beginning to develop an analytical method. If the requirement for test condition is strict, it should be recorded clearly in the method and the acceptable range of variations should be indicated. Uniform design can be used for determination of primary influencing factor then the changing range can be confirmed by single factor analysis. The typical variable factors are stability of the test solution, times and duration of sample extraction, and so on. The variable factors of liquid chromatography are composition and pH value of the mobile phase, same type of chromatographic column from different manufactures or batches, column temperature, flow rate, etc. The variable factors of GC are column and stationary phase with different brands or batches, different types of support, carrier gas flow rate, column temperature, temperature of injection port and detector, etc. To ensure reliability of the method, the testing conditions with slight change should be confirmed to meet the requirements for system suitability.

### 三、验证项目的选择
### 6.2.3　Selection of Validation Parameters

验证的分析项目有：鉴别试验、杂质测定（限度或定量分析）、含量测定（包括特性参数和含量/效价测定，其中特性参数有药物溶出度、释放度等）。

一种分析方法的验证，并非需要对所有指标全面验证，应视具体对象拟定验证内容。选择验证项目应足以证明采用的方法适合于相应的分析要求。验证内容的选择一般遵循下列原则：

The analysis items of verification include: identification test, impurity determination (limit or quantitative analysis), and content determination (including characteristic parameters and content/potency determination, in which characteristic parameters such as drug dissolution, release, etc.).

In the dissolution test and drug release test of pharmaceuticals, the analytical method of dissolution amount must also be validated. The parameters to be validated should be decided depending on specific analytical method involved. The selection of validation parameters generally follows the following principles:

**1. 非定量分析** 鉴别实验，一般需验证专属性和耐用性两项；杂质的限度检查一般需验证专属性、检测限和耐用性三项。

**(1) Non-Quantitative Analysis** Usually, the specificity and robustness should be validated in identification experiment. Specificity, detection limit and robustness should be validated in limit of impurity test.

**2. 定量分析** 如中药中主成分或有效成分的含量测定及溶出度的测定，除检测限与定量限外，其余均须验证。

**(2) Quantitative Analysis** For content determination and dissolution determination of main or active ingredient in Chinese medicine, all the parameters should be validated except detection limit and quantitative limit.

**3. 微量定量分析** 如杂质限量的测定，除检测限视情况而定外，其他均须验证。需验证的具体内容见表6-3。

**(3) Micro Quantitative Analysis** For the quantitation of impurity test, all the parameters should be validated except detection limit. The analytical items and the corresponding parameters to be validated are listed in Table 6-3, which can be used as a reference.

表6-3 分析方法验证项目的选择

| 项目内容 | 鉴别 | 杂质测定 | | 含量测定及溶出量测定 |
| --- | --- | --- | --- | --- |
| | | 定量 | 限度 | |
| 专属性[1] | + | + | + | + |
| 准确度 | − | + | − | + |
| 精密度 | | | | |
| 重复性 | − | + | − | + |
| 中间精密度 | − | +[2] | − | +[2] |
| 检测限 | − | −[3] | + | − |
| 定量限 | − | + | − | − |
| 线性 | − | + | − | + |
| 范围 | − | + | − | + |
| 耐用性 | + | + | + | + |

1：如果一种方法专属性不够，可采用其他分析方法补充；2：已有重现性验证，不需中间精密度验证；3：视具体情况予以验证。

**Table 6-3　List of validation characteristics required to be evaluated in test of each type**

| Parameters | Identification | Impurity test | | Determination of content or release |
| --- | --- | --- | --- | --- |
| | | Quantitation | Limit of test | |
| Specificity[1] | + | + | + | + |
| Accuracy | – | + | – | + |
| Precision | | | | |
| Repeatability | – | + | – | + |
| Intermediate precision | – | +[2] | – | +[2] |
| Detection Limit | – | –[3] | + | – |
| Quantification Limit | – | + | – | – |
| Linearity | – | + | – | + |
| Range | – | + | – | + |
| Robustness | + | + | + | + |

1: Lack of specificity of an individual analytical method may be compensated by other supporting analytical methods; 2: It is not necessary to validate the intermediate precision when the reproducibility has been developed; 3: It depends on the specific condition

# 岗 位 对 接
# Post Docking

本章为中药学、中药制药、中药资源类专业学生必须掌握的内容，为成为合格的中药学服务人员奠定坚实的基础。

This task is a content that must be mastered by students majored in Traditional Chinese Medicine to lay a solid foundation for becoming a qualified traditional Chinese medicine service staff.

本章内容对应岗位包括中药分析、中药质量控制、中药检验、中药新药研究与开发等相关工种。

The corresponding positions for this task include Chinese medicine analysis, Chinese medicine quality control, Chinese medicine inspection and other related jobs.

上述从事药学服务及药品质量监督管理相关所有岗位的从业人员均需要掌握化学分析法、紫外－可见分光光度法、高效液相色谱法、气相色谱法、薄层色谱法等用于中药含量测定的原理和方法，以及方法学验证内容，能熟记上述分析方法的定量公式、方法学验证的内容和方法，学会应用含量测定方法开展中药学服务工作。

All employees in positions related to the above-mentioned pharmaceutical services and drug quality supervision and management need to master the principles and methods for measuring traditional Chinese medicine content with chemical analysis method, UV-visible spectrophotometry method, high performance liquid chromatography method, gas chromatography and thin layer chromatography method, to memorize the quantitative formulas of the above analysis methods, the content and methods of methodological verification, to learn to apply content determination methods to pharmaceutical service work.

# 重 点 小 结
# Summary of Key Points

中药的含量测定是中药质量控制中的一项重要指标，通过研究中药中某一种或几种成分的含量高低是否符合规定，从而可衡量药物质量的优劣，保证中药的质量。中药的含量测定常用的方法有紫外－可见分光光度法、高效液相色谱法、气相色谱法、原子吸收分光光度法、电感耦合等离子体质谱法等。为保证测定的可靠性、可重现性等，在对样品进行测定时，必须对采用的方法进行方法学验证。方法学验证的内容有：专属性、准确度、精密度（包括重复性、中间精密度和重现性）、检测限、定量限、线性、范围和耐用性等。

The determination of the content of traditional Chinese medicine is an important indicator in the quality control of traditional Chinese medicine. By studying whether the content of one or several ingredients in traditional Chinese medicine meets the regulations, it can measure the quality of the medicine and ensure the quality of the Chinese medicine. Commonly used methods for the determination of traditional Chinese medicine include ultraviolet−visible spectrophotometry, high performance liquid chromatography, gas chromatography, atomic absorption spectrophotometry, inductively coupled plasma mass spectrometry, etc. In order to ensure the reliability and reproducibility of the measurement, the method used must be validated when the sample is measured. The contents of methodological verification are: specificity, accuracy, precision (including repeatability, intermediate precision and reproducibility), detection limit, quantification limit, linearity, range and durability.

# 目 标 检 测

题库

## 一、选择题
（一）单项选择题

1. 化学分析法主要适用于测定中药中
   A. 含量较高的一些成分及矿物药中的无机成分
   B. 微量成分
   C. 多糖类
   D. 生物碱类

2. 薄层色谱扫描法最常用的定量方法是
   A. 内标法                     B. 外标法
   C. 标准加入法           D. 回归曲线定量法

3. 气相色谱法用于中药的定量分析主要适用于
   A. 含挥发油成分及其他挥发性组分的中药
   B. 含生物碱类成分的中药
   C. 含三萜皂苷类成分的中药
   D. 含黄酮类成分的中药

4. 采用气相色谱法或高效液相色谱法用于中药的含量测定时，定量的依据一般是
   A. 分离度                     B. 保留时间

医药大学堂
WWW.YIYAODXT.COM

C. 峰面积　　　　　　　　　　　　　D. 拖尾因子

5. 采用气相色谱法进行中药成分含量测定时，最常用的定量方法是

　　A. 外标法　　　　　　　　　　　　B. 标准加入法

　　C. 归一化法　　　　　　　　　　　D. 内标法

6. 采用 HPLC 法测定中药中某化学成分含量时，最关键的实验条件是

　　A. 洗脱方式　　　　　　　　　　　B. 流速

　　C. 流动相　　　　　　　　　　　　D. 检测器

7. 回收率试验是在已知被测物含量（$A$）的试样中加入一定量（$B$）的被测物对照品进行测定，得总量（$C$），则

　　A. 回收率（％）=$C/(A+B)\times100\%$　　　　B. 回收率（％）=$(C-A)/B\times100\%$

　　C. 回收率（％）=$B/(C-A)\times100\%$　　　　D. 回收率（％）=$A/(C-B)\times100\%$

8. 采用 HPLC 法进行中药成分含量测定时，最常用的定量方法是

　　A. 内标法　　　　　　　　　　　　B. 外标一点法

　　C. 外标二点法　　　　　　　　　　D. 内加法

9. 中药分析中，在可见、紫外区有吸收的组分通常采用下列哪种检测器检测

　　A. 紫外检测器（UVD）　　　　　　B. 示差折光检测器（RID）

　　C. 蒸发光散射检测器（ELSD）　　　D. 荧光检测器（FD）

10. ICP-MS 在中药分析中主要用于哪些成分的含量测定

　　A. 挥发油　　　　　　　　　　　　B. 甾体皂苷类

　　C. 有机酸类　　　　　　　　　　　D. 重金属元素及微量元素

**（二）多项选择题**

1. 中药中成分含量测定常用的方法有

　　A. 高效液相色谱法　　　　B. 气相色谱法　　　　　C. 紫外－可见分光光度法

　　D. 薄层色谱扫描法　　　　E. 原子吸收分光光度法

2. 化学分析法主要用于测定中药哪些成分的含量

　　A. 总酸类　　　　　　　　B. 总生物碱类　　　　　C. 总皂苷

　　D. 矿物药　　　　　　　　E. 黄芩苷

3. 中药中皂苷类成分的含量测定方法通常有

　　A. 化学分析法　　　　　　B. 紫外－可见分光光度法　　C. 薄层扫描法

　　D. 气相色谱法　　　　　　E. 高效液相色谱法

4. 采用色谱法建立中药成分含量测定方法时，需要对仪器进行系统适用性试验，该试验内容包括

　　A. 分离度　　　　　　　　B. 色谱柱的理论塔板数　　C. 灵敏度

　　D. 拖尾因子　　　　　　　E. 重复性

5. 采用气相色谱法进行中药分析时，应对哪些实验条件进行选择

　　A. 固定相　　　　　　　　B. 柱温　　　　　　　　C. 载气

　　D. 检测室温度　　　　　　E. 进样量

6. 属于考察 HPLC 的耐用性的变动因素包括以下哪几项内容

　　A. 流动相的组成比例或 pH　　　　　B. 不同厂牌或不同批号的同类型色谱柱

　　C. 不同检测波长　　　　　　　　　D. 不同流速

　　E. 不同的供试品溶液

7. 高效液相色谱法常用的检测器主要有
   A. 紫外检测器　　　　　　　B. 氢火焰离子化检测器　　　C. 荧光检测器
   D. 蒸发光散射检测器　　　　E. 示差折光检测器

8. 含量测定方法选择的原则主要有
   A. 根据分析对象的组成多少
   B. 根据分析对象的化学性质
   C. 根据分析对象的含量高低
   D. 根据分析对象的灵敏度
   E. 根据分析对象的分子量大小

9. 在建立中药质量标准时，分析方法需要进行验证，方法验证的内容包括
   A. 专属性　　　　　　　　　B. 准确度　　　　　　　　　C. 精密度
   D. 线性　　　　　　　　　　E. 耐用性

10. 在含量测定方法验证的内容中，重现性考察的因素是
    A. 不同实验室　　　　　　　B. 不同分析人员　　　　　　C. 不同分析环境
    D. 不同测试时间　　　　　　E. 不同批次样品

## 二、思考题

对中药中成分进行含量测定时，分析方法验证的项目有哪些？各有什么要求？

## 三、计算题

1. 内标法测某样品中薄荷脑含量。以萘为内标物测得薄荷脑相对校正因子为 1.30。精密称取样品 0.5208g，萘 0.1152g，置于 10ml 容量瓶中，用乙醚稀释至刻度，进行气相色谱测定。测得薄荷脑峰面积为 55360，萘峰面积为 54785，试计算样品中薄荷脑的百分含量（29.06%）。

2. 用外标法测定槐米中芦丁的含量。称取槐米粗粉 0.1036g，用甲醇提取后定容于 250ml 容量瓶中，作为样品溶液。分别吸取样品溶液和芦丁标准品溶液（$C$: 0.1mg/ml）各 10μl，注入液相色谱仪，测得 $A_样$=6320，$A_标$=6930。计算槐米中芦丁的含量（22.01%）。

# 第七章　中药各类化学成分分析

# Chapter 7　Analysis of Various Chemical Components in Chinese Medicine

**学习目标 | Learning Goal**

知识要求：

**1. 掌握**　中药中生物碱类、黄酮类、蒽醌类、三萜皂苷类成分的分析方法。

**2. 熟悉**　中药中挥发油类、有机酸类成分和动物药、矿物药的分析方法。

**3. 了解**　其他成分（香豆素类、木脂素类、环烯醚萜类、鞣质类、多糖类、氨基酸类、核苷类、色素类）的分析方法。

能力要求：

学会应用中药各类成分分析解决中药的质量控制与评价。

**Knowledge Requirements**

**1. Master**　The analysis methods of alkanoids, flavonoids, quinoids and triterpenod saponins.

**2. Familiar**　The analysis methods of volatile components, organic acids and some mineral medicines, animal medicines.

**3. Understand**　The analysis methods of other phytochemicals (coumarins, lignans, iridoids, tannins, polysaccharides, amino acids, nucleosides and pigments).

**Ability Requirements**

Learn to apply the analysis methods of various chemical components, to solve the quality control and evaluation of Chinese medicine.

## 第一节　生物碱类成分分析

## 7.1　Analysis of Alkanoids

### 一、概述

### 7.1.1　Overview

生物碱是中药中分布较广的一类化学成分，结构中具有未共用孤对电子的氮原子而显碱性，大多具有显著的生物活性。因此，中药中的生物碱类成分常被作为定性、定量分析的指标成分。

Alkanoid is a kind of natural products spreading widely in lots of common Chinese medicinal materials，and appear alkaline due to the trogen atoms without sharing lone pair electrons in the chemical structures. Many alkanoids demonstrate the definite biological effects, Thus, alkanoids are often used as the chemical markers for qualitative and quantitative analysis of Chinese medicines.

### 二、定性鉴别
### 7.1.2　Qualitative Analysis

中药中生物碱类成分的定性鉴别方法主要有化学反应法、薄层色谱法、气相色谱法及高效液相色谱法。

The methods for qualitative analysis of alkanoids in Chinese medicines include chemical reaction method, TLC, GC and HPLC.

（一）化学反应法
#### 1．Chemical Reaction Method
利用生物碱的沉淀反应法进行鉴别，常用的生物碱沉淀试剂有碘化铋钾、碘化汞钾、磷钼酸、苦味酸等。但专属性较差，如有些成分如蛋白质、多肽和鞣质等也可与沉淀试剂反应出现假阳性结果。此外，有些生物碱（如麻黄碱）不与沉淀试剂反应，易出现假阴性结果；中药制剂中有两种或两种以上药味含有生物碱时，难以对其中某一味药进行鉴别。

For physical and chemical identification of Chinese medicine, chemical reaction method is frequently used with some precipitation agents, such as bismuth potassium iodide, mercury potassium iodide, phosphmolybic acid, picric acid, etc. Chemical reaction method is characterized with poor specificity. The false-positive results would happen to some components like proteins, polypeptides and tannins while the false-negative results would happen to some alkanoids such as ephedrine and caffeine. For some Chinese medicine preparations with two or more medicine material crude slices containing alkanoids, chemical reaction method is not suitable for individual identification.

（二）色谱法
#### 2．Chromatography
鉴别中药中生物碱类成分可用薄层色谱法、纸色谱法、高效液相色谱法和气相色谱法等，其中以薄层色谱法最常用。

TLC, PC, HPLC and GC are the common methods for qualitative analysis of alkanoids in Chinese medicines. TLC is the most commonly used one.

1．**薄层色谱法**　生物碱薄层色谱鉴别时常用硅胶或氧化铝为吸附剂，多以三氯甲烷、苯、乙酸乙酯等低极性溶剂为主为展开剂，再根据被检成分的极性加入其他溶剂调节极性。由于硅胶的硅醇基显弱酸性，能与强碱性生物碱成盐，导致 $R_f$ 值很小或拖尾，甚至形成复斑，因此常用碱性板、碱性展开剂系统或在碱性环境下展开。氧化铝略显碱性，吸附性强，适合分离亲脂性较强的生物碱，一般采用中性展开剂。

(1) **TLC**　For TLC of alkanoids, silica gel and alumina are the commonly used adsorbents. The developing system consists of some weak polarity solvents mainly such as chloroform, benzene, ethyl acetate and other solvents as a supplement to adjust the general polarity. Due to weakly acidic of the silanol groups, it can form a salt with a strong alkaline alkaloid, resulting in a small $R_f$ value or tailing, or even the formation of complex spots, silica gel plates should be developed with the alkaline developing

agents or in the alkaline environment to avoid above phenomenon. Alumina is often used with the neutral developing agents to isolate the strongly lipophilic alkanoids because alumina appears weak alkalinity and strong adsorbability.

除少数生物碱可直接于日光下或紫外光灯下检视外，大多数生物碱需显色后方可检视。最常用的显色剂是改良碘化铋钾试剂，有时可再喷硝酸钠试剂，消除背景的颜色，使样品斑点突显易于观察。也可利用某些生物碱特殊的颜色反应（如麻黄碱与茚三酮试剂反应）或碘蒸气熏等显色后检视。

Except that the minority of alkanoids are observed through the colours of the spots in daylight and those of the fluorescent spots in the ultraviolet light, the majority are observed through some chromogenic reactions. Improved bismuth potassium iodide TS is the mostly used chromogenic reagent. To light the blank background, sodium nitrate TS is often sprayed later. Sometimes, alkanoids are also observed through iodine vapor fumigation or through some other special chromogenic reactions.

2. **纸色谱法**　纸色谱法可用于生物碱盐或游离生物碱的鉴别。鉴别生物碱盐时，一般以滤纸中所含的水为固定相，用极性强的酸性溶剂为展开剂，最常用的是正丁醇 – 醋酸 – 水（BAW）系统。如果用一定 pH 值的酸性缓冲液为固定相，则应选用极性较小的溶剂系统为展开剂。鉴别游离生物碱时，常以极性溶剂如甲酰胺为固定相，以甲酰胺饱和的亲脂性有机溶剂，如三氯甲烷、乙酸乙酯等为展开剂。生物碱纸色谱的显色剂和薄层色谱的基本相同，但不能用含有硫酸等强腐蚀性的试剂。

**(2) PC**　Both free alkanoids and their salts could be also identified by PC. As for identification of free alkanoids, water in the filter paper is the stationary phase and the strong polarity acidic solvents are the mobile phase, especially BAW system (*n*-butanol-acetic acid-water). If some acidic buffer solution is used as the stationary phase, the weak polarity solvent system should be used as the mobile phase. As for identification of alkanoid salts, formamide usually is the stationary phase and the lipophilic solvents (chloroform，ethyl acetate) saturated by formamide usually are the stationary phase. The chromogenic reagents containing concentrated sulphuric acid should not be used in PC.

3. **高效液相色谱法**　高效液相色谱法也常用于生物碱类成分的鉴别，大多采用对照品、对照提取物随行对照法。在一定色谱条件下各种生物碱均有一定的保留时间，可作为定性鉴别的依据。

**(3) HPLC**　HPLC is also an effective used for identification of alkanoids. Under certain chromatographic conditions, each alkanoid emerges at its specific retention time, corresponding to that of its reference substance or extract, which provide the identification basis.

例 7-1　颠茄流浸膏中生物碱的鉴别

Example 7-1　Identification of Alkanoids in Belladonna Liquid Extract

取本品 1ml，加水 5ml、浓氨试液 5ml，用乙醚振摇提取 3 次，每次 10ml，合并乙醚液，蒸干，残液加乙酸乙酯 1ml 使溶解，作为供试品溶液。另取硫酸阿托品对照品，加甲醇制成每 1ml 含 2mg 的溶液，作为对照品溶液。照薄层色谱法（通则 0502）试验，吸取供试品溶液 1μl、对照品溶液 5μl，分别点于同一硅胶 G 薄层板上，以乙酸乙酯 – 甲醇 – 浓氨试液（17∶2∶1）为展开剂，展开，取出，晾干，喷以稀碘化铋钾试液。供试品色谱中，在与对照品色谱相应的位置上，显相同颜色的斑点。

To 1ml, add 5ml each of water and concentrated ammonia TS, extract with three 10ml quantities of ether, combine the ether solutions, and evaporate to dryness. Dissolve the residue in 1ml of ethyl acetate, and use it as the test solution. Dissolve atropine sulfate CRS in methanol to produce a solution containing 2mg per ml as the reference solution. Carry out the method for thin layer chromatography (General rule 0502), using silica gel G as the coating substance and a mixture of ethyl acetate, methanol and concentrated ammonia TS (17 : 2 : 1) as the mobile phase. Apply separately 1μl of the test solution and 5μl of the reference solution to the plate. After developing and removal of the plate, dry in air, and spray with dilute potassium iodobismuthate TS. The spot in the chromatogram obtained with the test solution corresponds in colour and position to the spot in the chromatogram obtained with the reference solution.

### 三、含量测定
### 7.1.3 Quantitative Analysis

总生物碱的含量测定常用分光光度法和化学分析法，单体生物碱的含量测定常用高效液相色谱法、气相色谱法和薄层扫描法。

Assay methods of total alkanoids include spectrophotometry and chemical analysis method, assay methods of monomer alkanoids include HPLC, GC and TLCS.

（一）总生物碱的含量测定
### 1. Assay of Total Alkanoids

1. **化学分析法** 根据生物碱的性质选择水溶液或非水溶液酸碱滴定法。滴定终点的确定可用电位法或指示剂法。采用滴定法测定总生物碱时，通常采用返滴定法，即先将生物碱溶于定量过量的标准酸溶液，反应完全后再用标准碱溶液滴定剩余的酸。强碱滴定生物碱盐时，在70%~90%乙醇中终点比在水中明显，所以常将生物碱盐溶于90%乙醇，再用标准碱乙醇液滴定。

**(1) Chemical Analysis Method** Aqueous titration and nonaqueous titration could be selected according to the property of alkanoids. Titration end point is usually determined by potential method or indicator method. The common method is back titration: alkanoids are dissolved in the excessive and known volume of standard solution of some acid, then another standard solution of some alkali is used to titrate the residual acid. When alkanoid salt is titrated by some alkali, titration end point is more easily to be observed in 70%-90% ethanol than in water. So alkanoid salt is firstly dissolved in 90% ethanol and then is titrated by some alkali standard solution in ethanol.

重量分析法测定总生物碱可采用萃取法和沉淀法。萃取法是以适宜溶剂将生物碱从原溶液中萃取出来，蒸去溶剂后干燥，直接称重。沉淀法是加入沉淀剂与生物碱生成具有固定组成的不溶性盐沉淀，经洗涤、干燥后称重，按照换算因数计算生物碱的含量。

Both extraction method and precipitation method are the two gravimetric methods to determine total alkanoids. Extraction method is carried out as follows: total alkanoids are extracted with some suitable solvent from the initial alkanoid extract and dried to remove the solvent, then the dry residual is weighed. Precipitation method is carried out as follows: some precipitation reagent is added to alkanoid to obtain the precipitate with solid composition, which is filtered, washed, dried and weighed. Calculated content based on conversion factor.

2. **比色法** 总生物碱的分光光度法含量测定大多采用比色法，单波长测定，主要有酸性染料比色法和雷氏盐比色法，苦味酸盐比色法和异羟肟酸铁比色法也有一定应用。

**(2) Colorimetry** Colorimetry with a certain individual wavelength is the dominant method for quantitative analysis of alkanoids. The fundamental quantitative methods include acid dye colorimetry and Reinecke's salt colorimetry. Sometimes, picrate colorimetry and iron hydroxamate colorimetry are also used.

**（1）酸性染料比色法** 在适当的 pH 介质中，生物碱（B）可与氢离子（H⁺）结合成盐，成为阳离子（BH⁺），而酸性染料（HIn）在此条件下解离为阴离子 In⁻，BH⁺ 与 In⁻ 定量地结合成有色的离子对（BH⁺·In⁻）。该离子对可被某些有机溶剂定量萃取，在一定波长下测定其吸光度，即可测定生物碱的含量。本法的关键在于介质的 pH、酸性染料的种类、有机溶剂的选择和微量水分的干扰，尤以介质的 pH 最为重要。

*Acid dye colorimetry* In the solution of proper pH, an alkanoid (B) combines with a hydrogen ion (H⁺) to obtain a compound positive ion (BH⁺) while a negative ion (In⁻) separates from acidic dye (HIn). Then, BH⁺ and In⁻ are combined quantitatively to produce a colored ion pair (BH⁺·In⁻). This ion pair could be extracted from the test solution quantitatively by some organic solvents. The content of total alkanoids could be determined with the absorbance of the ion pair in the organic phase under the certain wavelength. The keys to this method lie in the solution pH value, types of acid dye and organic solvent, interference of trace water. pH value is the most important

酸性染料选择的依据是：①染料阴离子可与生物碱阳离子定量结合；②生成的离子对易溶于有机溶剂；③离子对在最大吸收波长处有较高的灵敏度；④染料阴离子在有机相中不溶或少溶。常用的酸性染料有溴麝香草酚蓝、甲基橙、溴甲酚绿、溴酚蓝和溴甲酚紫等。

What are the rules to select an acid dye? ① BH⁺ could combine with In⁻ quantitatively. ②BH⁺·In⁻ could be easily dissolved in the organic solvent. ③ BH⁺·In⁻ is detected with higher sensitivity at the wavelength of maximum absorption. ④ In⁻ is not or hardly dissolved in the organic phase. Thus, bromothymol blue, methyl orange, bromo cresol green, bromphenolam, and bromine cresol violet are frequently used as the acid dyes.

选择有机溶剂的原则是根据离子对与有机相能否形成氢键以及形成氢键能力的强弱而定，三氯甲烷、二氯甲烷可与离子对形成氢键。微量水分可使三氯甲烷出现浑浊，并导致过量染料带入有机相，影响测定结果。通常加入适量脱水剂（如无水硫酸钠）或经干燥滤纸滤过除去微量的水分。

Selection of the proper organic solvent depends on whether hydrogen bond could be formed between BH⁺·In⁻ and the solvent and even the capacity of forming hydrogen bond. Chloroform and dichloromethane are the appropriate.Trace water could cause turbidity and bring excessive acid dye in chloroform, which would affect the result. To avoid the unfavorable situation, some dehydrating agent like anhydrous sodium sulfate should be added into the organic phase and dry filter paper should be used to remove the trace water.

**（2）雷氏盐比色法** 雷氏盐在酸性条件下可与生物碱定量生成难溶于水的有色配合物。该沉淀易溶于丙酮，因此，可将沉淀滤过洗净后溶于丙酮直接测定；也可以精密加入定量过量的雷氏盐试剂，滤除生成的沉淀后，测定滤液中的过量雷氏盐，间接计算生物碱的含量。

*Reinecke's salt colorimetry* In the acidic solution, Reinecke's salt could be quantitatively combined with alkanoid to obtain the colored complex, which is hardly soluble in water and easily soluble in acetone. Therefore, alkanoid could be directly determined after the complex precipitate is filtered, washed and dissolved in acetone. On the other hand, some excessive and known amount of Reinecke's salt is added into the test solution. After the complex precipitate is filtered, unreacted Reinecke's salt could be determined and the content of alkanoid could be calculated indirectly.

进行雷氏盐比色法测定时，需注意：雷氏盐的水溶液在室温可分解，故用时应新鲜配制，沉淀也需在低温进行；雷氏盐丙酮溶液的吸光度，随时间而有变化，应尽快测定。

It is noted that Reinecke's salt is stable neither in water nor in acetone. So Reinecke's salt TS should be freshly prepared before use. Precipitation reaction should go on at lower temperature and determination should be completed in a short time.

（3）苦味酸盐比色法　苦味酸在弱酸性或中性溶液中可与生物碱定量生成苦味酸盐沉淀，该沉淀可溶于三氯甲烷等有机溶剂。测定方法有三种：①将生物碱苦味酸盐沉淀过滤，洗涤，加碱使沉淀解离，以有机溶剂萃取游离出的生物碱，测定碱性水溶液中的苦味酸，换算出生物碱的含量；②在生物碱的缓冲溶液（pH=7）中加苦味酸试剂生成沉淀，加三氯甲烷萃取并溶解，再用缓冲溶液（pH=11）使其解离，苦味酸转容到碱水液中进行测定，再换算出生物碱的含量；③在缓冲溶液（pH=4-5）中加三氯甲烷萃取并溶解该沉淀，直接测定生物碱的含量。

*Picrate colorimetry*　In the weak acidic solution and neutral solution, picric acid could be quantitatively combined with alkanoid to obtain the picrate precipitate, which is soluble in acetone. There are three quantitative method: ① filter, wash and add some alkali solution to decompose the picrate precipitate, extract the free alkanoid with some organic solvent, determine picric acid in the aqueous solution and calculate the content of alkanoid; ② add picric acid TS into alkanoid buffer solution (pH=7) to produce the precipitate, dissolve it with chloroform, decompose it with the alkaline buffer solution (pH=11), determine picric acid in the alkaline solution and calculate the content of alkanoid; ③ add chloroform to dissolve the precipitate in the buffer solution (pH=4-5), determine and calculate the content of alkanoid directly.

（4）异羟肟酸铁比色法　含有内酯键结构的生物碱，在碱性介质中加热使酯键水解，产生的羧基与盐酸羟胺反应生成异羟肟酸，该成分会与 $Fe^{3+}$ 生成紫红色的异羟肟酸铁配合物，可以在最大吸收波长 530nm 处测定。由于含有酯键（包括内酯）结构的成分均能与试剂反应，因此用该法测定时，供试品溶液中必须不存在其他具有内酯键的成分。

*Iron hydroxamate colorimetry*　For the alkanoid with ester bond, in the alkaline solution, heating could hydrolyze the ester bond to produce free carboxyl group. Hydroxylamine hydrochloride could react with carboxyl group to produce hydroxamic acid, which could combine with ferric ion to produce the violet-red iron hydroxamate complex. This complex could be determined at 530nm, the wavelength of maximum absorbance. Since the similar reaction could happen to any component with ester bond, there should not be any ester in the test solution when this method is used.

例 7-2　川贝母中总生物碱的测定

Example 7-2　Assay of sipeimine in Fritillariae Cirrhosae Bulbus

**对照品溶液的制备**　取西贝母碱对照品适量，精密称定，加三氯甲烷制成每 1ml 含 0.2mg 的溶液，即得。

*Reference solution*　Dissolve a quantity of sipeimine CRS, accurately weighed, in chloroform to prepare a solution containing 0.2mg per ml.

**标准曲线的制备**　精密量取对照品溶液 0.1ml、0.2ml、0.4ml、0.6ml、1.0ml，置 25ml 具塞试管中，分别补加三氯甲烷至 10.0ml，精密加水 5ml、再精密加 0.05% 溴甲酚绿缓冲液 2ml，密塞，剧烈振摇 1 分钟，转移至分液漏斗中，放置 30 分钟。取三氯甲烷液，用干燥滤纸滤过，取续滤液，以相应的试剂为空白，照紫外 – 可见分光光度法（通则 0401），在 415nm 的波长处测定吸光度，以吸光度为纵坐标、浓度为横坐标，绘制标准曲线。

*Calibration standard*　Measure accurately 0.1ml, 0.2ml, 0.4ml, 0.6ml and 1.0ml of the reference solution, respectively, each into a 25ml stopper test tube, replenish chloroform to 10.0ml, add accurately 5ml of water and 2ml of a 0.05% buffer solution of bromocresol green, tightly stopper and strongly shake, transfer to a separating funnel, stand for 30 minutes and separate the chloroform solution. Filter with a piece of dry filter paper, use the successive filtrate as the test solution. Carry out the method for ultraviolet spectrophotometry and colourimetry (General Chapters 0401), with the corresponding solvent solution as the blank, measure the absorbance at 415nm and plot the standard curve, using absorbance as ordinate and concentration as abscissa.

**测定法**　取本品粉末（过三号筛）约 2g，精密称定，置具塞锥形瓶中，加浓氨试液 3ml，浸润 1 小时，加三氯甲烷 – 甲醇（4∶1）混合溶液 40ml，置 80℃ 水浴加热回流 2 小时，放冷，滤过，滤液置 50ml 量瓶中，用适量三氯甲烷 – 甲醇（4∶1）混合溶液洗涤药渣 2~3 次，洗液并入同一量瓶中，加三氯甲烷 – 甲醇（4∶1）混合溶液至刻度，摇匀。精密量取 2~5ml，置 25ml 具塞试管中，水浴上蒸干，精密加入三氯甲烷 10ml 使溶解，照标准曲线的制备项下的方法，自 "精密加水 5ml" 起，依法测定吸光度，从标准曲线上读出供试品溶液中西贝母碱的重量（mg），计算，即得。

*Procedure*　Weigh accurately 2g of the powder (through No.3 sieve) to a stopper conical flask, macerate for 1 hour with 3ml of ammonia concentrated TS, add 40ml of a mixture of chloroform and methanol (4∶1), heat under reflux on a water bath for 2 hours at 80℃, cool and filter to a 50ml volumetric flask, wash the residue with a quantity of the above mixture for 2-3 times, combine the washings to the same flask, dilute with the same mixture to the volume and mix well. Measure accurately 2-5ml to a 25ml stopper test tube, evaporate to dryness on a water bath and add accurately 10ml of chloroform, carry out the procedure as described under *Calibration standard*, beginning at the words "add accurately 5ml of water ...". Measure the absorbance and read out the weight of sipeimine (mg) in the test solution from the standard curve.

本品按干燥品计算，含总生物碱以西贝母碱（$C_{27}H_{43}NO_3$）计，不得少于 0.050%。

It contains not less than 0.050 per cent of total alkaloids, calculated as sipeimine ($C_{27}H_{43}NO_3$) with reference to the dried drug.

**（二）单体生物碱的含量测定**

### 2. Assay of Monomer Alkanoid

中药单体生物碱的含量测定一般采用高效液相色谱法、气相色谱法、薄层色谱扫描法等色谱法。

HPLC, GC, TLCS are usually used for assay of monomer alkanoid in Chinese medicine.

**1. 高效液相色谱法**　高效液相色谱法测定单体生物碱含量时，通常采用 $C_{18}$ 柱反相色谱法。$C_{18}$ 柱残存游离硅醇基容易引起生物碱色谱峰保留时间延长、峰形变宽、拖尾等。为避免这些情况，可采取以下措施：①在流动相中加入硅醇基抑制剂，如二乙胺、三乙胺等；②在合适的 pH 下，流动相中加入低浓度离子对试剂掩蔽生物碱的碱性基团，如辛烷磺酸钠或十二烷基磺酸钠；③可在流动相中加入季铵盐试剂，如溴化四甲基胺，能在较短的保留时间内得到很好的分离，色谱峰重现性好，也不拖尾；④可在流动相中加入电解质缓冲盐，可以改变离子强度、稳定 pH 值及促进离子对相互作用，从而改善峰形及分离效果。

**(1) HPLC**　Reversed chromatography on $C_{18}$ column is the mostly used method. Residual free silanol groups in $C_{18}$ column would induce retention time prolonging, shape widening and trailing of alkanoid peak. To avoid the above situations, the following actions should be taken: ① Silanol group inhibitor could be added into mobile phase, such as diethylamine and triethylamine; ② At the proper pH, ion pair reagent of low concentration (sodium octane sulfonate and sodium dodecyl sulfonate) could be added into mobile phase to shelter alkaline group of alkanoid; ③ Quaternary ammonium salt like tetramethylamine bromide could be added into mobile phase to obtain satisfactory separation in a short time and repeatable and symmetry shapes of alkanoid; ④ Electrolyte buffer salt could be added into mobile phase to change ionic strength, stabilize pH value, activate interaction of ion pair and improve peak shape and separation.

高效液相色谱法测定中药中生物碱成分时，大多采用紫外检测器，根据待测生物碱成分的性质，也可用化学发光检测器或荧光检测器。

Ultraviolet detector is the commonly used detector for HPLC analysis of alkanoids. Sometimes, chemiluminescence detector and fluorescent detector are also used.

**2. 气相色谱法**　气相色谱法适用于测定挥发性、热稳定性好的生物碱成分，如麻黄碱、槟榔碱、石斛碱和颠茄类生物碱等。

**(2) GC**　Some volatile and thermostable alkanoids could be determined by GC, such as ephedrine, arecoline, dendrobine and Belladonna alkaloids.

**3. 薄层色谱扫描法**　采用薄层色谱扫描法测定生物碱含量所选用的吸附剂、展开剂及显色方法与鉴别相似，但要求更严格。

**(3) TLCS**　The adsorbents, developing agents and chromogenic methods in TLCS determination are similar to those in TLC identification. However, the requirements are stricter.

例 7-3　延胡索中延胡索乙素的测定

Example 7-3　Assay of Tetrahydropalmatine in Corydalis Rhizoma

**色谱条件与系统适用性试验**　以十八烷基硅烷键合硅胶为填充剂；以甲醇 -0.1% 磷酸溶液（三乙胺调 pH 值至 6.0）（55 : 45）为流动相；检测波长为 280nm。理论板数按延胡索乙素峰计算应不低于 3000。

*Chromatographic system and system suitability*　Use octadecylsilane bonded silica gel as the stationary phase and a mixture of methanol and 0.1% solution of phosphoric acid (adjust to pH 6.0 with triethylamine) (55 : 45) as the mobile phase. As detector a spectrophotometer set at 280nm. The number of theoretical plates of the column is not less than 3000, calculated with reference to the peak of tetrahydropalmatine.

**对照品溶液的制备**　取延胡索乙素对照品适量，精密称定，加甲醇制成每 1ml 含 46μg 的溶液，即得。

*Reference solution*　Weigh accurately a quantity of tetrahydropalmatine CRS, dissolve in methanol to produce a solution containing 46μg per ml.

**供试品溶液的制备**　取本品粉末（过三号筛）约 0.5g，精密称定，置平底烧瓶中，精密加入浓氨试液 – 甲醇（1 : 20）混合溶液 50ml，称定重量，冷浸 1 小时后加热回流 1 小时，放冷，再称定重量，用浓氨试液 – 甲醇（1 : 20）混合溶液补足减失的重量，摇匀，滤过。精密量取续滤液 25ml，蒸干，残渣加甲醇溶解，转移至 5ml 量瓶中，并稀释至刻度，摇匀，滤过，取续滤液，即得。

*Test solution*　Weigh accurately 0.5g of the powder (through No.3 sieve) to a flat bottom flask, accurately add 50ml of a mixture of strong ammonia TS and methanol (1 : 20), weigh, macerate for 1 hour and then heat under reflux for 1 hour, cool and weigh again, replenish the loss of solvent with the above mixture, mix well and filter. Evaporate accurately 25ml of the successive filtrate to dryness, dissolve the residue in methanol, transfer to a 5ml volumetric flask, dilute with methanol to volume and mix well.

**测定法**　分别精密吸取对照品溶液与供试品溶液各 10μl，注入液相色谱仪，测定，即得。

*Procedure*　Accurately inject 10μl of each of the reference solution and the test solution, respectively, into the column, and calculate the content.

本品按干燥品计算，含延胡索乙素（$C_{21}H_{25}NO_4$）不得少于 0.050%。

It contains not less than 0.050 per cent of tetrahydropalmatine ($C_{21}H_{25}NO_4$), calculated with reference to the dried drug.

# 第二节 黄酮类成分分析
# 7.2 Analysis of Flavonoids

## 一、概述
## 7.2.1 Overview

多数黄酮类成分的结构中具有桂皮酰基与苯甲酰基组成的交叉共轭体系，因此在 200~400nm 范围内有较强的紫外吸收。 大多数黄酮类成分在日光下具有颜色。黄酮类成分作为中药中一类重要的化学成分，具有多种多样的生理活性，因此，常作为中药的质量评价指标。

For most flavonoids, their ultraviolet absorptions in 200-400nm are observed strong, attributing to their cross conjugated systems consisting of cinnamoyl group and benzoyl group. As an important part of phytochemicals, flavonoids exhibit multiple bioactivities, Thus, flavonoids are often used as the chemical markers for quality evaluation of Chinese medicines.

## 二、定性鉴别
## 7.2.2 Qualitative Analysis

中药中黄酮类成分的定性鉴别常采用化学反应法和薄层色谱法，其中薄层色谱法为主要的鉴别方法。

Chemical reaction method and TLC are often adopted for identification of flavonoids in Chinese medicines. TLC is the dominant identification method of flavonoids.

（一）化学反应法
### 1. Chemical Reaction Method

**1. 盐酸－镁粉（或锌粉）反应** 取 5~10ml 经过提取分离制成的供试品溶液，加入数滴盐酸，再加入少量镁粉或锌粉（必要时加热）。如果有黄酮、黄酮醇、二氢黄酮或二氢黄酮醇存在，数分钟后出现红～紫红色。

**(1) Hydrochloric Acid-magnesium Powder (or Zinc Powder) Reaction** To 5-10ml filtered test solution, add several drops of hydrochloric acid and a small quantity of magnesium powder or zinc powder successively. If there are flavonoes, flavonols, dihydroflavonoes or dihydroflavonols, the solution would turn to red or violet red in a few minutes.

**2. 与金属盐类试剂的配位反应** 黄酮类化合物分子中存在游离的 3-OH、5-OH 或邻二酚羟基时，可与 $Al^{3+}$、$Zr^{4+}$、$Pb^{2+}$、$Sr^{2+}$ 等形成配位化合物使溶液发生颜色的变化或者生成沉淀，利用此性质进行黄酮类成分的定性鉴别。

**(2) Coordination Reaction with Metal Salt Reagent** There are 3-hydroxyl group, 5-hydroxyl group or two neighbouring phenolic hydroxyl groups existing in some flavonoids. They could react with $Al^{3+}$, $Zr^{4+}$, $Pb^{2+}$, $Sr^{2+}$ to produce some complexes, which are fluorescent, colour deepening or insoluble. These reactions could be employed for qualitative analysis of these flavonoids.

例 7-4　莲房的鉴别

Example 7-4　Identification of Nelumbinis Receptaculum

取本品粉末 0.5g，加乙醇 5ml，温热浸泡数分钟，滤过，滤液加镁粉少量与盐酸 1~2 滴，溶液渐变为红色。

Macerate warmly 0.5g of the powder in 5ml of ethanol for several minutes and filter. To the filtrate add a small quantity of magnesium powder and 1-2 drops of hydrochloric acid; the solution turns to red gradually.

（二）薄层色谱法

2. TLC

黄酮类成分最常用的定性分析方法是吸附薄层法，常用的吸附剂有硅胶与聚酰胺。

Adsorption TLC is the common method for qualitative analysis of alkanoids with silica gel and polyamide as the adsorbents.

1. 硅胶薄层色谱法　硅胶色谱分离弱极性黄酮类成分较好，遵循正相色谱规律。硅胶除对黄酮类成分产生吸附外，还与游离酚羟基生成氢键产生拖尾现象。在制备硅胶薄层板时加入适量的氢氧化钠或醋酸钠溶液，可有效减少黄酮类成分的拖尾现象。此外，也可在展开剂中加入少量的有机酸。

(1) Silica Gel TLC　Silica gel TLC is suitable to separate those low polarity flavonoids in line with the rules of normal phase chromatography. However, there would be trailing spots attributing to the hydrogen bands between silica gel and free hydroxyl groups. To effectively avoid this phenomenon, moderate amount of sodium hydroxide solution or sodium acetate solution could be added into silica gel when preparing TLC plates. Additionally, small amount of organic acid could be added into developing agent.

黄酮类成分大多具有荧光，薄层展开后可在紫外灯（365nm）下检识。由于黄酮类成分与铝盐反应生成的配合物具有较强的荧光，也可喷三氯化铝乙醇溶液显色后在紫外灯（365nm）下检识。具有游离酚羟基的黄酮类成分，可与三氯化铁溶液发生显色反应。根据酚羟基的位置及数目，可呈现紫、绿、蓝等不同颜色。

Most flavonoids are fluorescent and could be directly observed under ultraviolet light at 365nm after development. In addition, flavonoids could react with $Al^{3+}$ to produce the fluorescent complexes. So, these flavonoids could be observed under ultraviolet light at 365nm after spraying aluminium chloride TS. Some flavonoids with free hydroxyl groups could also react with ferric trichloride TS to obtain purple, green or blue products according to the positions and numbers of the phenolic hydroxyl groups.

2. 聚酰胺薄层色谱法　黄酮类成分的酚羟基与聚酰胺分子中的酰胺基可以形成氢键，而且不同黄酮的酚羟基数目和位置不同，与聚酰胺形成氢键的能力有所差异。因此，聚酰胺薄层色谱法用于分离含游离酚羟基的黄酮苷和苷元。聚酰胺色谱需要的展开剂极性较强，一般来说，大多含有醇、酸或水。

(2) Polyamide TLC　Phenolic hydroxyl groups of flavonoids usually combine with of amide groups of polyamide to form hydrogen bonds. Due to different numbers and positions of hydroxyl groups in different flavonoids, abilities to combine with amide groups experience difference. So, polyamide TLC

is suitable for separation of flavonoid aglycones and glycosides with some free phenolic hydroxyl groups. It would be best to adopt the developing agents containing acid, alcohol or water in polyamide TLC, due to their strong polarity.

3. **高效液相色谱法**　高效液相色谱法用于定性鉴别一般为（多）成分鉴别或化学特征谱鉴别。2020 年版《中国药典》采用高效液相色谱法鉴别清开灵片中黄芩苷、灯盏细辛和灯盏花素中野黄芩苷、槐角中槐角苷等。中药成分复杂，采用高效液相色谱法鉴别时，供试品溶液制备大多参照含量测定项下方法。

**(3) HPLC**　Qualitative analysis by HPLC generally refers to identification of compound (s) or characteristic spectrum. In *Chinese Pharmacopoeia* (2020 Edition), HPLC is used for identification of baicalin in Qingkailing Tablets, scutellarin in Erigerontis Herba and Breviscapine, sophorin in Sophorae Fructus, and so on. For identification of flavonoids by HPLC, the test solution is the same as that for assay.

例 7-5　小儿百部止咳糖浆中黄芩的鉴别

Example 7-5　Identification of Scutellariae Radix in Xiao'er Baibu Zhike Syrup

取本品 5ml，加 75% 乙醇 15ml，超声处理 20 分钟，滤过，滤液作为供试品溶液。另取黄芩苷对照品，加 75% 乙醇制成每 1ml 含 0.2mg 的溶液，作为对照品溶液。照薄层色谱法（通则 0502）试验，吸取上述两种溶液各 1~3μl，分别点于同一聚酰胺薄膜上，以醋酸为展开剂，展开，取出，晾干，置紫外光灯（365nm）下检视。供试品色谱中，在与对照品色谱相应的位置上，显相同颜色的荧光斑点。

To 5ml of the syrup, add 15ml of 75% ethanol, ultrasonicate for 20 minutes, filter, use the filtrate as the test solution. Dissolve baicalin CRS in 75% ethanol to produce a solution containing 0.2mg per ml as the reference solution. Carry out the method for thin layer chromatography (General rule 0502), using polyamide as the coating substance and acetic acid as the mobile phase. Apply separately 1-3μl of each of the test solution and the reference solution to the plate. After developing and removal of the plate, dry in air. Examine under the ultraviolet light at 365nm. The fluorescent spot in the chromatogram obtained with the test solution corresponds in position and colour to the spot in the chromatogram obtained with the reference solution.

## 三、含量测定
### 7.2.3　Quantitative Analysis

（一）总黄酮的含量测定

### 1. Assay of Total Flavonoids

1. **紫外 – 可见分光光度法**　黄酮类化合物的 I 带在 300~40nm，II 带在 240~285nm 均有最大吸收。含黄酮类化合物的中药经提取纯化后，可直接于最大吸收波长处测定其吸收度，以吸收系数法或对照品对照法计算含量。该法适用于干扰小的中药或单方制剂。

**(1) Ultraviolet-Visible Spectrophotometry**　Flavonoid could be examined with the maximum absorbance during 300-40nm ( I belt) and 240-285nm ( II belt). Therefore, the test solution of Chinese medicine containing flavonoids could be determined at the wavelength of maximum absorbance and the content of total flavonoids could be calculated by absorption coefficient method or by comparing with the reference substance. Ultraviolet spectrophotometry is only suitable to Chinese medicine with little interference.

若供试液中其他组分形成干扰，可采用亚硝酸钠－硝酸铝－氢氧化钠比色法或者三氯化铝－醋酸钾比色法测定。前者以芦丁为对照品，利用黄酮类成分 3-OH、5-OH、邻二酚羟基与铝盐反应生成的配合物在 500nm 附近有最大吸收，且与背景最大吸收波长差别较大，可消除背景的干扰，显著提高选择性，而后者显色后的化合物最大吸收波长与配位反应位置、数量有关，因此，最好用所含黄酮作对照品，确定反应产物的最大吸收波长后再进行测定。

If there exists the interference from other components in the test solution, the sodium nitrite-aluminum nitrate-sodium hydroxide colorimetric method or aluminum trichloride-potassium acetate colorimetric method can be used for determination. The former uses rutin as a reference substance, and the complex produced by the reaction of the flavonoids 3-OH, 5-OH, catechol hydroxyl group and aluminum salt has a maximum absorption near 500nm, and has a large difference from the background maximum absorption wavelength. Eliminate background interference and significantly improve selectivity. The maximum absorption wavelength of the latter compound after coloration is related to the coordination reaction position and quantity. Therefore, it is best to use the flavonoids in sample as a reference substance to determine the maximum absorption wavelength of the reaction product.

**2. 铝盐配位比色法** 采用分光光度法测定总黄酮，若供试液中其他组分形成干扰，可进行比色测定。该法利用黄酮类成分 3-OH、5-OH、邻二酚羟基与铝盐反应生成的配合物与背景最大吸收波长差别较大，可消除背景的干扰，显著提高选择性。由于目前还没有黄酮类化合物的专属反应，因此，必须明确每种测定方法的原理、适用范围和可能存在的干扰。

(2) Aluminium salt coordination colourimetry As for assay of total flavonoids by spectrophotometry, colorimetry should be employed if there exists the interference from other components in the test solution. 3-hydroxyl group, 5-hydroxyl group or two neighbouring phenolic hydroxyl groups in flavonoid could react with $Al^{3+}$ to obtain a complex differing from the background in terms of $\lambda_{max}$, which could eliminate the interference from the background and increase the selectivity. At present, there is no exclusive reaction for flavonoids. So, we must make clear the principle and application scope of each assay method and possible interference.

（1）亚硝酸钠 - 硝酸铝 - 氢氧化钠比色法 该法常用芦丁作为对照品，显色生成的红色配合物在 500nm 附近测定。如上所述，这并非黄酮类化合物的专属反应，具有类似结构的非黄酮类化合物也可发生此反应，而不具有类似结构的黄酮类成分则不能发生此反应。因此，误差较大。

1) *Sodium nitrite-aluminum nitrate-sodium hydroxide colourimetry* In this method, rutin is usually used as the reference substance and chromogenic product is red and could be determined at near 500 nm. As mentioned above, this is not a exclusive reaction.It is positive for those non-flavonoids with the similar structures while it is negative for those flavonoids without the similar structures, which would bring some errors.

（2）三氯化铝 - 醋酸钾比色法 本法常用芦丁为对照品，采用三氯化铝 - 醋酸钾为显色剂，显色后在 420nm 波长处测定。值得注意的是，反应产物的最大吸收波长并不一定都在 420nm 处，与配位反应位置、数量有关。因此，最好用所含黄酮作对照品，确定反应产物的最大吸收波长后再进行测定。

2) *Aluminium trichloride-potassium acetate colourimetry* In this method, rutin is usually used as the reference substance, aluminium trichloride and potassium acetate are used as chromogenic reagents and chromogenic product is determined at 420nm. It is noted that $\lambda_{max}$ of each flavonoid is not always at 420nm, which in fact depends on the position and number of chromogenic reactions.

Thus, it would be best to use a flavonoid in the test solution as the reference substance and to reconfirm $\lambda_{max}$.

例 7-6 消咳喘糖浆中总黄酮的测定

Example 7-6 Assay of Total Flavonoids in Xiaokechuan Syrup

**对照品溶液的制备** 取芦丁对照品适量，精密称定，加 60% 乙醇制成每 1ml 含芦丁 60μg 的溶液，即得。

*Reference solution* Dissolve a quantity of rutin CRS, weighed accurately, in 60% ethanol to produce a solution containing 60μg per ml.

**标准曲线的制备** 精密量取对照品溶液 0.5ml、1ml、2ml、3ml、4ml 与 5ml，分别置 10ml 量瓶中，各加 0.1mol/L 三氯化铝溶液 2ml、1mol/L 醋酸钾溶液 3ml，加 60% 乙醇至刻度，摇匀，放置 30 分钟；以相应试剂为空白。照紫外 – 可见分光光度法，在 420nm 波长处测定吸光度，以吸光度为纵坐标、浓度为横坐标，绘制标准曲线。

*Calibration curve* Measure accurately 0.5ml, 1ml, 2ml, 3ml, 4ml and 5ml of the reference solution in 10ml volumetric flask separately, add 2ml of 0.1mol/L solution of aluminium chloride, 3ml of 1mol/L solution of potassium acetate to each flask, dilute with 60% ethanol to volume, mix well and allow to stand for 30 minutes. Carry out the method for spectrophotometry, using the corresponding solvent as blank, measure the absorbance at 420nm, plot the calibration curve, using absorbance as ordinate and concentration as abscissa.

**测定法** 精密量取本品 2ml，置 50ml 量瓶中，加 60% 乙醇至刻度，摇匀，精密量取 1ml，置 10ml 量瓶中，照标准曲线的制备项下的方法，自"加 0.1mol/L 三氯化铝溶液"起依法操作，制成供试品溶液。另精密量取本品 2ml，置 50ml 量瓶中，加 60% 乙醇稀释至刻度，精密量取 1ml，置 10ml 量瓶中，加 60% 乙醇至刻度，摇匀，作空白，依法测定吸光度，从标准曲线上读出供试品溶液中芦丁的重量，计算，即得。

*Procedure* Measure accurately 2ml of the syrup to a 50ml volumetric flask, add 60% ethanol, dilute to volume, and mix well. Measure accurately 1ml of the solution to a 10ml volumetric flask, carry out the procedure as described under *Calibration curve*, beginning at the words "add 2ml of 0.1mol/L aluminium chloride solution" to prepare the test solution. In addition, transfer 2ml of the syrup, dilute with 60% ethanol to 50ml. Measure accurately 1ml of the ethanol solution, add 60% ethanol to 10ml as the blank. Measure the absorbance, read out the weight of rutin (μg) in the test solution from the calibration curve and calculate.

本品每 1ml 含总黄酮以芦丁（$C_{27}H_{30}O_{16}$）计，不得少于 2.0mg。

It contains not less than 2.0mg of total flavonoids per ml, calculated as rutin ($C_{27}H_{30}O_{16}$).

**（二）单体黄酮的含量测定**

## 2. Assay of Monomer Flavonoid

**1. 高效液相色谱法** 多采用反相高效液相色谱法，固定相多用 $C_{18}$ 柱，流动相常用加入酸的甲醇 – 水体系或乙腈 – 水体系，大多采用紫外检测器。

**(1) HPLC** In Chinese Pharmacopoeia (2015 Edition), assay of monomer flavonoid usually adopt RP-HPLC, C18 column as the stationary phase and methanol-water or acetonitrile-water with containing moderate amount of some acid as the mobile phase.

**2. 薄层色谱扫描法** 样品经提取后，分离净化制成供试品，采用硅胶薄层板或聚酰胺薄膜进行薄层色谱展开，再在薄层扫描仪上进行测定。

**(2) TLCS** Similar to TLC analysis, flavonoids in the test solution are separated by silica gel or polyamide as stationary phase. Then, the developed spots are scanned by the instrument.

例 7-7　银黄口服液中黄芩苷的测定

Example 7-7　Assay of baicalin in Yinhuang Mixture

**色谱条件与系统适用性试验**　以十八烷基硅烷键合硅胶为填充剂；以甲醇 – 水 – 磷酸（50∶50∶0.2）为流动相；检测波长为 274nm。理论板数按黄芩苷峰计算应不低于 2500。

*Chromatographic system and system suitability*　Use octadecylsilane bonded silica gel as the stationary phase and a mixture of methanol, water and phosphoric acid (50 : 50 : 0.2) as the mobile phase. As detector a spectrophotometer set at 274nm. The number of theoretical plates of the column is not less than 2500, calculated with the reference to the peak of baicalin.

**对照品溶液的制备**　取黄芩苷对照品适量，精密称定，加 50% 甲醇制成每 1ml 含 50μg 的溶液，即得。

*Reference solution*　Weigh accurately a quantity of baicalin CRS, dissolve in 50% methanol to product a solution containing 50μg of baicalin per ml.

**供试品溶液的制备**　精密量取本品 1ml，置 50ml 量瓶中，加水稀释至刻度，摇匀，精密量取 3ml，置 25ml 量瓶中，加 50% 甲醇稀释至刻度，摇匀，滤过，取续滤液，即得。

*Test solution*　Measure accurately 1ml of the mixture in a 50ml volumetric flask, dilute with water to volume, and mix well. Measure accurately 3ml in a 25ml volumetric flask, dilute with 50% methanol to volume, mix well, filter, and use the successive filtrate as the test solution.

**测定法**　分别精密吸取对照品溶液与供试品溶液各 10μl，注入液相色谱仪，测定，即得。

*Procedure*　Inject accurately 10μl of each of the reference solution and the test solution into the column, and calculate the content.

本品每 1ml 含黄芩提取物以黄芩苷（$C_{21}H_{18}O_{11}$）计，不得少于 18.0mg。

It contains not less than 18.0mg of baicalin ($C_{21}H_{18}O_{11}$) per ml, referred to Extractum Scutellariae.

## 第三节　醌类成分分析

## 7.3　Analysis of Quinoids

### 一、概述
### 7.3.1　Overview

醌类成分主要有苯醌、萘醌、菲醌和蒽醌四种类型，中药中以蒽醌及其衍生物最为多见。蒽醌类成分在中药中既有游离形式，也有蒽醌苷形式。含蒽醌类成分的常用中药有大黄、决明子、虎杖、茜草等。萘醌类化合物分为 1，2- 萘醌和 1，4- 萘醌两种类型，常见于紫草。菲醌类化合物被认为是影响丹参质量和颜色的标志物。醌类化合物具有显著的生物活性，因此，中药中含醌类成分时，常选择醌类成分作为质量评价的指标。

Quinoids include benzoquinones, naphthoquinones, phenanthraquinones and anthraquinones. Anthraquinones and the derivatives are usually found as aglycones and as glycosides in many common Chinese medicinal materials, such as Rhei Radix et Rhizoma, Cassiae Semen, Polygoni Cuspidati Rhizoma et Radix, Rubiae Radix et Rhizoma. Naphthoquinones are grouped into two subtypes, 1,2-naphthoquinone and 1,4-naphthoquinone and are often observed in Arnebiae Radix. Phenanthraquinones are considered as the key chemical markers responsible for quality and colour of Salviae Miltiorrhizae Radix et Rhizoma. Quinoids have been investigated to have some notable activities, they are often used as the index phytochemical for quality evaluation of those Chinese medicines containing quinoids.

## 二、定性鉴别
## 7.3.2　Qualitative Analysis

中药中醌类成分的鉴别常采用化学反应法、升华法和薄层色谱法。后者是醌类主要的鉴别方法。

Chemical reaction method, sublimation method and TLC could be employed for identification of quinoids. TLC is the main identification method for quinones.

（一）化学反应法
### 1.　Chemical Reaction Method
羟基蒽醌类化合物在碱性溶液中多呈橙色、红色、紫红色或蓝色；在醋酸镁甲醇溶液中呈红色。因此，利用此性质可对中药中的羟基蒽醌类成分进行鉴别。蒽酮、蒽酚、二蒽酮类化合物需经过氧化形成蒽醌后方能发生此反应。

Hydroxyanthraquinones often appear orange, red, violet-red or blue in alkaline solutions and appear red in methanol solution of magnesium acetate. So, identification of hydroxyanthraquinones in Chinese medicines could be performed on this chemical property. However, for anthrones, anthrols and dianthrones, the chemical reactions could be realized only after they are oxidized to anthraquinones.

（二）升华法
### 2.　Sublimation Method
一些游离蒽醌及醌类衍生物多具有升华性。对于在中药中含量较大的此类成分，可以通过显微镜下观察升华物的晶型或显色反应进行定性鉴别。

Due to sublimability of some anthraquinones and quinone derivatives, identification could be carried out through examining crystalline shapes and chromogenic reactions under microscope if they exist in Chinese medicines with high contents.

（三）薄层色谱法
### 3.　TLC
薄层色谱法是中药中醌类成分最主要的定性鉴别方法。吸附剂多用硅胶，不同的醌类选择不同的展开系统。乙酸乙酯－甲醇－水系统适用于分离蒽醌苷及蒽醌苷元；正丙醇－乙酸乙酯－水系统适用于分离二蒽酮苷；石油醚－甲酸乙酯－甲酸系统适用于分离蒽醌苷元。检视方法包括喷碱性试剂或醋酸镁甲醇液、氨气熏及在紫外灯下观察荧光或在可见光下直接观察。

TLC is the dominant identification method for anthraquinones in Chinese medicines. Silica gel is mostly used stationary phase. Developing systems vary according to different quinoids. Ethyl acetate-methanol-water system is suitable for separation of anthraquinone glycosides and aglycones; n-propanol-ethyl acetate-water is suitable for separation of dianthrone glycosides; petroleum ether-ethyl formate-formic acid system is suitable for separation of anthraquinone glycosides. Quinoid spots could be examined under daylight or under ultraviolet light after ammonia fumigation or spraying alkaline agents or magnesium acetate TS.

例 7-8　大黄的鉴别

Example 7-8　Identification of Rhei Radix et Rhizoma

取本品粉末 0.1g，加甲醇 20ml，浸泡 1 小时，滤过，取滤液 5ml，蒸干，残渣加水 10ml 使溶解，再加盐酸 1ml，加热回流 30 分钟，立即冷却，用乙醚分 2 次振摇提取，每次 20ml，合并乙醚液，蒸干，残渣加三氯甲烷 1ml 使溶解，作为供试品溶液。另取大黄对照药材 0.1g，同法制成对照药材溶液。再取大黄酸对照品，加甲醇制成每 1ml 含 1mg 的溶液，作为对照品溶液。照薄层色谱法试验，吸取上述三种溶液各 4μ1，分别点于同一以羧甲基纤维素钠为黏合剂的硅胶 H 薄层板上，以石油醚（30~60℃）- 甲酸乙酯 – 甲酸（15：5：1）的上层溶液为展开剂，展开，取出，晾干，置紫外光灯（365nm）下检视。供试品色谱中，在与对照药材色谱相应的位置上，显相同的五个橙黄色荧光主斑点；在与对照品色谱相应的位置上，显相同的橙黄色荧光斑点，置氨蒸气中熏后，斑点变为红色。

Macerate 0.1g of the powder in 20ml of methanol for 1 hour, and filter. Evaporate 5ml of the filtrate to dryness, dissolve the residue in 10ml of water, add 1ml of hydrochloric acid, heat under reflux on a water bath for 30 minutes and cool immediately. Extract by shaking with two 20ml quantities of ether, combine the ether extracts, evaporate to dryness and dissolve the residue in 1ml of chloroform as the test solution. Prepare a solution of Rhei Radix et Rhizoma reference drug in the same manner as the reference drug solution, Dissolve rhein CRS in methanol to produce a solution containing 1mg per ml as the reference solution. Carry out the method for thin layer chromatography, using silica gel H mixed with sodium carboxymethylcellulose as the coating substance and the upper layer of a mixture of petroleum ether (30-60℃), ethyl formate and formic acid (15 : 5 : 1) as the mobile phase. Apply separately 4μl of each of the above three solutions to the plate. After developing and removal of the plate, dry in air, and examine under ultraviolet light at 365nm. The five orange fluorescent spots in the chromatogram obtained with the test solution correspond in position and colour to the spots in the chromatogram obtained with the reference drug solution; the orange fluorescent spot in the chromatogram obtained with the test solution corresponds in position and colour to the spot in the chromatogram obtained with the reference solution. The spot becomes red on exposure to ammonia vapour.

### 三、含量测定
### 7.3.3　Quantitative Analysis

（一）总蒽醌的含量测定
### 1. Assay of Total Anthraquinones

蒽醌类化合物常以游离型和结合型的形式同时存在于中药中，因此蒽醌类成分的含量测定包括游离蒽醌含量测定、结合蒽醌含量测定和总蒽醌含量测定。测定时，均以所含的某几种蒽醌类化合物为对照计算它们在中药中的总含量。

In Chinese medicines, anthraquinones exist in free form and in combined form simultaneously. Thus, assay is grouped into assay of FAQ, assay of combined anthraquinones (CAQ) and assay of total anthraquinones (TAQ). In most cases, the reference substances of two or more anthraquinones are prepared for the mixed reference solution to calculate their sum content in the samples.

**1. 游离蒽醌的测定**　测定游离蒽醌时，可用三氯甲烷或乙醚提取，提取液蒸干后，经适当方法净化，再加甲醇溶解定容，作为供试品溶液。

**(1) Assay of FAQ**　The test solution is prepared as follows: extract the Chinese medicine with chloroform or ethyl ether, evaporate the extract to dryness, dissolve it with methanol to some volume after purification.

**2. 结合蒽醌的测定**　测定结合蒽醌时，可以将测定游离蒽醌中的药渣加甲醇提取，提取液蒸干后再用酸水（6mol/L 盐酸或 2.5mol/L 硫酸溶液）加热水解，再用三氯甲烷或乙醚萃取，将三氯甲烷或乙醚液蒸干后加甲醇溶解定容作为供试品溶液；也可将样品中总蒽醌含量减去游离蒽醌含量计算得到。

**(2) Assay of CAQ**　The test solution is prepared as follows: extract the decoction dregs in "Assay of FAQ" with methanol, evaporate the extract to dryness, heat and hydrolyze it with acid solution, extract with chloroform or ethyl ether, evaporate the organic phase to dryness, dissolve with methanol to some volume. CAQ content is also obtained by subtracting FAQ content from TAQ content.

**3. 总蒽醌的测定**　测定总蒽醌时，可先用甲醇提取，提取液蒸干后加酸水加热水解，再用三氯甲烷或乙醚萃取，蒸干萃取液，加甲醇溶解定容作为供试品溶液。

**(3) Assay of TAQ**　The test solution is prepared as follows: extract the Chinese medicine with methanol, evaporate the extract to dryness, heat and hydrolyze it with acid solution, extract with chloroform or ethyl ether, evaporate the organic phase to dryness, dissolve with methanol to some volume.

（二）单体蒽醌的含量测定

## 2. Assay of Monomer Anthraquinones

进行游离蒽醌类单体成分测定时，通常选用适宜的溶剂提取后直接测定。当测定其成分游离态与结合态的总量时，一般样品需要水解后测定，测定方法主要是 HPLC，固定相采用十八烷基键合硅胶，流动相多选用甲醇 – 水（常加少量的酸），检测器为紫外检测器。

When measuring the composition of free anthraquinone monomers, a suitable solvent is usually selected for extraction and then directly measured. When measuring the composition of anthraquinone monomers, the main measurement method is HPLC. The stationary phase uses octadecyl bonded silica gel. The mobile phase is mostly methanol-water (a small amount of acid is often added). The detector is an ultraviolet detector.

例 7-9　何首乌中结合蒽醌的测定

Example 7-9　Assay of Combined Anthraquinones in Polygoni Multiflori Radix

**色谱条件与系统适用性试验**　以十八烷基硅烷键合硅胶为填充剂；以甲醇 –0.1% 磷酸溶液（80∶20）为流动相；检测波长为 254nm。理论板数按大黄素峰计算应不低于 3000。

*Chromatographic system and system suitability*　Use octadecylsilane bonded silica gel as the stationary phase and a mixture of methanol and 0.1% solution of phosphoric acid (80:20) as the mobile phase. As detector a spectrophotometer set at 254nm. The number of theoretical plates of the column is not less than 3000, calculated with the reference to the peak of emodin.

**对照品溶液的制备**　取大黄素对照品、大黄素甲醚对照品适量，精密称定，加甲醇分别制成每 1ml 含大黄素 80μg、大黄素甲醚 40μg 的溶液，即得。

*Reference solution*　Weigh accurately emodin CRS and physcion CRS, respectively, and dissolve in methanol to produce a mixture containing 80μg and 40μg of each per ml as the reference solution.

**供试品溶液的制备**　取本品粉末（过四号筛）约 1g，精密称定，置具塞锥形瓶中，精密加入甲醇 50ml，称定重量，加热回流 1 小时，取出，放冷，再称定重量，用甲醇补足减失的重量，摇匀，滤过，取续滤液 5ml 作为供试品溶液 A（测游离蒽醌用）。另精密量取续滤液 25ml，置具塞锥形瓶中，水浴蒸干，精密加 8% 盐酸溶液 20ml，超声处理（功率 100W，频率 40kHz）5 分钟，加三氯甲烷 20ml，水浴中加热回流 1 小时，取出，立即冷却，置分液漏斗中，用少量三氯甲烷洗涤容器，洗液并入分液漏斗中，分取三氯甲烷液，酸液再用三氯甲烷振摇提取 3 次，每次 15ml，合并三氯甲烷液，回收溶剂至干，残渣加甲醇使溶解，转移至 10ml 量瓶中，加甲醇至刻度，摇匀，滤过，取续滤液，作为供试品溶液 B（测总蒽醌用）。

*Test solution*   Weigh accurately 1g of the powder (through No.4 sieve) to a stoppered conical flask, accurately add 50ml of methanol and weigh. Heat under reflux for 1 hour, cool and weigh again, replenish the loss of the solvent with methanol and mix well, filter, use the successive filtrate as the test solution A (for determination of FAQ). Measure accurately another more 25ml of the successive filtrate to a stoppered conical flask, evaporate to dryness on a water bath, add accurately 20ml of 8% solution of hydrochloric acid, ultrasonicate (power, 100W; frequency, 40kHz) for 5 minutes, add 20ml of chloroform, heat under reflux for 1 hour and cool immediately, then transfer to a separating funnel, wash the container with a small quantity of chloroform and combine the washings to the same separating funnel, separate the chloroform solution and extract the acidic solution again by shaking with three 15ml quantities of chloroform, combine the chloroform solutions and evaporate to dryness. Dissolve the residue in methanol and transfer to a 10ml volumetric flask, dilute with methanol to volume, mix well, filter and use the successive filtrate as the test solution B (for determination of TAQ).

**测定法**   分别精密吸取对照品溶液与上述两种供试品溶液各 10μl，注入液相色谱仪，测定，即得。

*Procedure*   Inject accurately 10μl of each of the reference solution and the above two test solutions, respectively, into the column, and calculate the content.

$$结合蒽醌含量 = 总蒽醌含量 - 游离蒽醌含量$$

$$\text{Content of CAQ} = \text{content of TAQ} - \text{content of FAQ}$$

本品按干燥品计算，含结合蒽醌以大黄素（$C_{15}H_{10}O_5$）和大黄素甲醚（$C_{16}H_{12}O_5$）的总量计，不得少于 0.10%。

It contains not less than 0.10 per cent of CAQ, calculated as the total amount of emodin ($C_{15}H_{10}O_5$) and physcion ($C_{16}H_{12}O_5$) with reference to the dried drug.

（三）萘醌、菲醌类成分的含量测定

### 3. Assay of Naphthoquinones and Phenanthraquinones

紫草及其制剂的含量测定常以其中所含的萘醌类成分紫草素、乙酰紫草素为指标。丹参及其制剂的含量测定常以其中所含的丹参酮Ⅰ、丹参酮ⅡA 等菲醌类成分为指标。

Shikonin and acetylshikonin are often used as quality indicators in Arnebiae Radix and related preparations while tanshinone Ⅰ and tanshinone ⅡA are often used as quality indicators in Salviae Miltiorrhizae Radix et Rhizoma and related preparations.

例 7-10   复方丹参颗粒中丹参酮ⅡA 的测定

Example 7-10   Assay of Tanshinone IIA in Fufang Danshen Granules

**色谱条件与系统适用性试验**   以十八烷基硅烷键合硅胶为填充剂；以甲醇 – 水（73：27）为流动相；检测波长为 270nm。理论板数按丹参酮ⅡA 峰计算应不低于 2000。

*Chromatographic system and system suitability*   Use octadecylsilane bonded silica gel as the stationary phase and a mixture of methanol and water (73:27) as the mobile phase. As detector a spectrophotometer set at 270nm. The number of the theoretical plates is not less than 2000, caculated with the reference to the peak of tanshinone ⅡA.

**对照品溶液的制备**   取丹参酮ⅡA 对照品适量，精密称定，置棕色量瓶中，加甲醇制成每 1ml 含 20μg 的溶液，即得。

*Reference solution*   Dissolve a quantity of tanshinone ⅡA CRS, weighed accurately, in an amber volumetric flask to prepare a solution containing 20μg per ml as the reference solution.

**供试品溶液的制备** 取装量差异项下的本品，混匀，取适量，研细，取约 0.2g，精密称定，置具塞棕色瓶中，精密加入甲醇 25ml，密塞，称定重量，超声处理（功率 250W，频率 33kHz）15 分钟，放冷，再称定重量，用甲醇补足减失的重量，摇匀，滤过，取续滤液，即得。

*Test solution* Weigh acccurately 0.2g, obtained in the test of Weight variation, to a stoppered conical flask add 25ml of methanol, tightly stopper and weigh accurately. Ultrasonicate for 15 minutes (power, 250W; frequency, 33kHz), cool, weigh accurately again, and replenish the lost weight with methanol, stir well and filter, use the successive filtrate as the test solution.

**测定法** 分别精密吸取对照品溶液与供试品溶液各 10μl，注入液相色谱仪，测定，即得。

*Procedure* Inject accurately 10μl of each of the reference solution and test solution into the column, and calculate the content.

本品每袋含丹参以丹参酮 $II_A$（$C_{19}H_{18}O_3$）计，不得少于 1.3mg。

It contains not less than 1.3mg of tanshinone $II_A$ ($C_{19}H_{18}O_3$) per pack, referred to Salviae Miltiorrhizae Radix et Rhizoma.

---

## 第四节 三萜皂苷类成分分析
## 7.4 Analysis of Triterpenoid Sapogenins

PPT

### 一、概述
### 7.4.1 Overview

三萜类成分在植物中分布广泛，具有抗肿瘤、增强免疫功能、消炎、抗菌、抗病毒等多方面的生物活性，所以常用作为相关中药质量评价的重要指标。

Triterpenoids have been found widely in many plants. Due to their antitumour, improving immunity, antibacterial, anti-inflammation and antivirus activities, triterpenoids are always employed as the chemical markers for quality evaluation of the related Chinese medicines.

### 二、定性鉴别
### 7.4.2 Qualitative Analysis

中药中三萜皂苷类成分鉴别可采用泡沫反应、显色反应和薄层色谱法。其中薄层色谱法应用最广泛，鉴别专属性较强；而泡沫反应、显色反应专属性较差。

In Chinese medicines, triterpenoid saponins could be identified by foaming reaction, chromogenic reaction and TLC. Due to the different specificities, TLC is extensively used and the other two are rarely applied for identification of triterpenoid saponins.

三萜皂苷类成分的薄层色谱通常以硅胶为吸附剂，展开剂的极性一般较大，常用三氯甲烷 - 甲醇 - 水（13:7:2，10℃以下放置，下层）、正丁醇 - 乙酸 - 水（4:1:5，上层）、正丁醇 -3mol/L 氢氧化铵 - 乙醇（5:2:1）、三氯甲烷 - 甲醇（7:3）等。对于分层的展开剂，控制展开剂饱和的温度和时间非常重要。三萜皂苷元的极性较小，需用亲脂性较强的展开系统，如环己烷 - 乙酸乙酯、

三氯甲烷 - 乙醚、三氯甲烷 - 丙酮、三氯甲烷 - 乙酸乙酯等。

Silica gel is the common adsorbent. Developing systems with high polarity are often adopted, including the lower layer of chloroform-methanol-water (13:7:2) under 10℃, the upper layer of *n*-butanol-acetic acid-water (4:1:5), *n*-butanol-ammonium hydroxide solution (3mol/L)-ethanol (5:2:1), chloroform-methanol (7:3). For those layered mobile phases, it is important to control the saturation temperature and time. However, triterpenoid sapogenins are characterized with low polarity and lipophilic developing agents should be adopted, such as cyclohexane-ethyl acetate, chloroform-ethyl ether, chloroform-acetone, chloroform-ethyl acetate.

三萜皂苷类成分可选用 25% 三氯醋酸乙醇溶液、香草醛硫酸溶液、磷钼酸、浓硫酸 - 醋酐、碘蒸气等显色剂显色，也可在紫外光灯（365nm）下观察斑点荧光。

There are many chromogenic reagents for identification of triterpenoid saponins, including 25% solution of trichloroacetic acid in ethanol, the solution of vanillin in sulfuric acid, phosphmolybic acid, concentrated sulfuric acid-acetic anhydride and iodine vapour. The component spots could be examined under daylight or under ultraviolet light at 365nm.

### 三、含量测定
### 7.4.3  Quantitative Analysis

（一）总皂苷的含量测定
#### 1.  Assay of Total Saponins
1. 比色法　三萜皂苷类成分多为末端吸收，因此通常采用比色法测定。常用显色剂有香草醛 - 硫酸、香草醛 - 高氯酸、醋酐 - 硫酸等。皂苷类成分的显色反应专属性虽较差，但反应比较灵敏，方法简便、易行。

（1）**Colourimetry**　Triterpenoid saponins are characterized with end absorption in ultraviolet region. So, colourimetry is suitable for determination with following chromogenic reagents：vanillin-sulphuric acid，vanillin-perchloric acid，acetic anhydride-sulfuric acid. The specificity of chromogenic reaction is poor. These chromogenic reactions are sensitive and easy to operate.

2. 重量法　采用适当方法提取、纯化后得总皂苷，恒重，称量并计算样品中总皂苷含量。当中药制剂处方中含皂苷类成分药味较多时，常用正丁醇作溶剂，测定正丁醇浸出物，计算总皂苷含量。

（2）**Gravimetric Method**　Total triterpenoid saponins could be obtained after extracting, purification and dried to constant weight prior to content calculation. If there are several Chinese medicinal materials containing triterpenoid saponins in the preparations, total saponins could be calculated by weighting *n*-butanol extract.

（二）三萜皂苷类单体成分的含量测定
#### 2.  Assay of Monomer Saponins
三萜皂苷单体的测定方法主要有高效液相色谱法和薄层色谱扫描法，其中以高效液相色谱法最为常用。

The determination methods of triterpene saponin monomers mainly include HPLC and TLCS methods, of which HPLC is the most commonly used.

1. 高效液相色谱法　高效液相色谱法是单体皂苷类成分最常用的含量测定方法，常用十八烷基键合硅胶作固定相，不同比例的乙腈 - 水或甲醇 - 水为流动相。若三萜皂苷类成分本身具有较强的紫外吸收，如甘草酸、远志皂苷等，可用 HPLC 分离并用紫外检测器检测。若仅有末端吸收，亦可采用 HPLC 分离并用蒸发光散射检测器测定，如黄芪甲苷等。

**（1）HPLC**　HPLC is the mostly used determination method for monomer saponins with octadecylsilane bonded silica gel as the stationary phase and acetonitrile-water or methanol-water as the mobile phase。HPLC-UV method could be applied for those saponins with strong ultraviolet absorption, such as glycyrrhizic acid and onjisaponins。HPLC-ELSD method could be applied for those saponins with end absorption, such as astragaloside Ⅳ。

**2. 薄层色谱扫描法**　样品经提取纯化后经薄层色谱扫描法分离，用 10% 硫酸乙醇溶液显色后采用双波长薄层色谱扫描法测定。

**（2）TLCS**　TLCS with double-wavelength is often applied after spraying with 10% ethanol solution of sulphuric acid。

# 第五节　挥发性成分分析
# 7.5　Analysis of Volatile Components

## 一、概述
## 7.5.1　Overview

挥发性成分是指一类气味芳香且易挥发的成分，主要包括挥发油和制剂中的冰片、麝香酮等其他小分子易挥发的化合物。挥发性成分极性较小，常用极性小的有机溶剂提取，对于挥发油还可采用水蒸气蒸馏法提取，对某一有升华性的成分还可选用升华法提取。挥发油组成复杂，包括萜类化合物、小分子芳香族化合物和小分子脂肪族化合物，具有止咳平喘等多种生物活性，因此，分析含有挥发性成分的中药时，常选择该中药所含有的挥发性成分作为定性、定量的评价指标。

Volatile components refer to a class of aromatic and volatile components, mainly including volatile oil and other small molecule volatile compounds such as borneol and muscone in preparations. The polarities of volatile components are small, and organic solvents with small polarities are commonly used for extraction. Distillation of water steam can also be used for the extraction of volatile oil, and sublimation method can also be used for extraction of a sublimated component. The composition of volatile oil is complex, including terpenoids, small molecular aromatic compounds and small molecular aliphatic compounds, which have various biological activities such as suppress cough and relieve wheezing. Therefore, when analyzing Chinese medicines containing volatile components, often choose the volatiles contained in the Chinese medicines as qualitative and quantitative evaluation indicators.

## 二、定性分析
## 7.5.2　Qualitative Analysis

中药中挥发油类成分可采用化学反应法、薄层色谱法、气相色谱法、气相色谱 - 质谱（GC-MS）联用及气相色谱 - 红外光谱（GC-FTIR）联用进行定性分析，其中薄层色谱法最常用。

Chemical reaction, thin layer chromatography, gas chromatography, gas chromatography-mass spectrometry (GC-MS) and gas chromatography-infrared spectroscopy (GC-FTIR) were used for qualitative analysis of volatile oils in traditional Chinese medicine, of which TLC is the most commonly used.

（一）化学反应法

## 1. Chemical Reaction Method

利用中药所含挥发油各组分的化学结构或主要官能团的化学性质进行鉴别。如酚类化合物可与三氯化铁的乙醇溶液反应；醛、酮类化合物与 2,4- 二硝基苯肼、氨基脲、羟胺等试剂产生结晶性衍生物沉淀；不饱和萜类成分可被高锰酸钾氧化；挥发油中的内酯类化合物可用亚硝酰铁氰化钠及氢氧化钠溶液鉴别；薁类化合物可用溴的三氯甲烷溶液或浓硫酸鉴别；此外大多数挥发油类成分还可采用香草醛 - 浓硫酸反应进行鉴别等。但由于中药成分复杂、干扰因素多，化学反应法的灵敏度不高、专属性不强。

The chemical structure or chemical properties of the main functional groups of the volatile oil contained in traditional Chinese medicine were used for identification. For example, phenolic compounds can react with the ethanol solution of ferric trichloride; Aldehydes, ketones and 2, 4-dinitrophenylhydrazine, semicarbazide, hydroxylamine produced crystalline derivatives precipitation; Unsaturated terpenoids can be oxidized by potassium permanganate. Lactones in volatile oil can be identified as natrium nitroferrocyanatum and sodium hydroxide solution. Azulene compounds can be identified by bromine trichloromethane solution or concentrated sulfuric acid. In addition, most volatile oil components can also be identified by vanillin-concentrated sulfuric acid reaction. However, the sensitivity and specificity of the chemical reaction method are not high due to the complexity of the ingredients and interference factors.

（二）薄层色谱法

## 2. Thin Layer Chromatography

挥发油成分复杂，各类化合物的极性大小不同，其极性大小顺序为：烃（萜）＜醚＜酯＜醛、酮＜醇、酚＜酸。因此，可根据不同组分的极性差异进行分离，吸附剂常用硅胶 G，对于难分离且含不同双键的萜类化合物，可用硝酸银薄层分离，吸附剂中硝酸银含量 2.5%。不含氧的烃类常以正己烷（或石油醚）作展开剂，含氧烃类用正己烷（或石油醚）- 醋酸乙酯混合溶剂展开。对于组成特别复杂的挥发油，可根据具体情况选择双向展开或二次展开。挥发油类成分 TLC 鉴别常用的显色剂有 0.5%~1.0% 茴香醛（香草醛）- 浓硫酸试剂、2% 高锰酸钾水溶液、三氯化铁试剂、2,4- 二硝基苯肼、0.05% 溴酚蓝乙醇溶液等。

The components of the volatile oil are complex, and the polarity of various compounds is different. The order of polarity is as follows: hydrocarbon (terpene) < ether < ester < aldehyde, ketone < alcohol, phenol < acid.Therefore, It can be separated according to the polarity of different components, silica gel G or Ⅱ - Ⅲ level neutral aluminum oxide commonly used as adsorbent, oxygen-free hydrocarbons are often developed with *n*-hexane (or petroleum ether), oxygenated hydrocarbons are developed in a mixed solvent of *n*-hexane (or petroleum ether) - ethyl acetate. According to the number and position of the double bond in the volatile oil composition, and the difference of the difficulty and stability of π-complex formed with silver nitrate, the appropriate content of silver nitrate in the adsorbent is 2.5%. For volatile oils with particularly complex composition, it is better to choose the same or different developing agent for orthogonal or twice development.0.5%-1.0% anisaldehyde (vanillin)-concentrated sulfuric acid, 2% potassium permanganate solution, ferric trichloride, 2,4-dinitrophenylhydrazine, 0.05% bromophenol blue ethanol solution are commonly used as a color reagent for volatile oil components.

### （三）气相色谱法
### 3. Gas Chromatography

气相色谱法现已广泛应用于挥发油的定性和定量分析。用于定性分析主要解决挥发油中已知成分的鉴定，常用对照品对照法，即在相同的色谱条件下，利用已知成分对照品与供试品色谱峰的相对保留时间确定挥发油中的某一成分的存在与否，或通过指纹图谱对中药材或提取物进行整体定性鉴别。

Gas chromatography has been widely used in the qualitative and quantitative analysis of volatile oil. Used for qualitative analysis to solve the identification of known components in volatile oil, commonly used reference substance control method. Under the same conditions, the relative retention time of the chromatographic peak of the reference and the sample was the same, the Chinese medicinal materials or extracts can also be qualitatively identified by fingerprint.

### （四）GC-MS 联用与 GC-FTIR 联用
### 4. GC-MS and GC-FTIR

由于中药挥发油组成非常复杂，而且许多都是未知成分，此时可选用 GC-MS 联用或 GC-FTIR 联用进行定性鉴别，这两种方法还具有预测未知成分相对分子量、快速定性和推断分子结构的鉴别能力，特别适合多组分混合物中未知成分的定性鉴别，可提高定性鉴别的准确性和可靠性。

Because the composition of the volatile oil of traditional Chinese medicine is very complex, and many of them are unknown components and no reference substances for contrast, GC-MS or GC-FTIR can be used for qualitative identification, These two methods can also correct the wrong judgment of chromatographic analysis, they can predict the relative molecular weight of unknown components and determine the molecular structure quickly, especially suitable for qualitative identification of unknown components in multicomponent mixtures to improve the accuracy and reliability of qualitative identification.

### 三、定量分析
### 7.5.3 Quantitative Analysis

中药中总挥发油的含量测定常用水蒸气蒸馏法。挥发油单一成分的含量测定，气相色谱法应用最广泛。此外，高效液相色谱法亦有应用。

The total content of volatile oil in plants is determined by steam distillation. Because the volatile oils contained in traditional Chinese medicine are volatile and all are mixtures with complex composition, gas chromatography is the most widely used method to determine the content of a single component. Besides, high performance liquid chromatography also has applications.

### （一）总挥发油的含量测定
### 1. Determination of the Content of Total Volatile Oil

常采用挥发油测定器以水蒸气蒸馏法测定，仪器装置见图 7-1。

The volatile oil detector and steam distillation method are often used for determination. The apparatus is shown in Fig. 7-1.

（1）相对密度在 1.0 以下的挥发油含量测定　取供试品适量（相当于含挥发油 0.5~1.0ml），称定重量（准确至 0.01g），置烧瓶中，加水 300~500ml（或适量）与玻璃珠数粒，振摇混合后，连接挥发油测定器与回流冷凝管。自冷凝管上端加水使充满挥发油测定器的刻度部分，并溢流入烧瓶时为止。置电热套中或用其他适宜方法缓缓加热至沸，并保持微沸约 5 小时，至测定器中油量不再增加，停止加热，放置片刻，开启测定器下端的活塞，将水缓缓放出，至油层上端到达刻度 0 线上面 5mm 处为止。放置 1 小时以上，再开启活塞使油层下降至其上端恰与刻度 0 线平齐，读取挥发油量，并换算成供试品中挥发油的含量（%）。

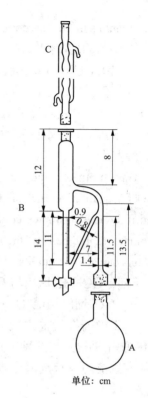

**(1)** *This method is used for the determination of volatile oils of which the relative density is less than 1.0* Weigh a quantity of the sample to be examined accurately to 0.01g (equivalent to 0.5-1.0ml of volatile oil) into flask A. Add 300-500ml of water and a few glass beads, followed by shaking to mix it well. Connect flask A to volatile oil determination tube B and then connect B to reflux condenser C. Add water through the top of reflux condenser C until the graduated tube of B is filled and the water overflows to flask A. Heat the flask gently to boiling in an electric heating jacket or other appropriate methods, and continue heating for about 5 hours until the volume of oil does not increase. Stop heating, allow to stand for a few minutes, open the stopcock at the lower part of B, and run off the water layer slowly until the oil layer reaches 5mm above the zero marks. Allow to stand for more than 1 hour, then open the stopcock again and run off the remaining water layer carefully until the oil layer is just on the zero marks. Read the volume of volatile oil in the graduated portion of the tube and calculate the content of volatile oil in the sample to be examined, expressed as percentage (%).

单位：cm

图 7-1  **挥发油测定仪器装置**
Fig.7-1  Apparatus for Determination of Volatile Oil
A. flask    B. volatile oil determination tube    C. reflux conderser

（2）**相对密度在 1.0 以上的挥发油含量测定** 取水约 300ml 与玻璃珠数粒，置烧瓶中，连接挥发油测定器。自测定器上端加水使充满刻度部分，并溢流入烧瓶时为止，再用移液管加入二甲苯 1ml，然后连接回流冷凝管。将烧瓶内容物加热至沸腾，并继续蒸馏，其速度以保持冷凝管的中段呈冷却状态为度。30 分钟后停止加热，放置 15 分钟以上，读取二甲苯的容积。然后将称定重量的供试品加入烧瓶中依照上法进行蒸馏，从油层量减去二甲苯量，即为挥发油量，再换算成供试品中挥发油的含量（%）。

**(2)** *This method is used for the determination of volatile oils of which the relative density is more than 1.0* Add 300ml of water and a few glass beads to flask A. Connect flask A to volatile oil determination assembly B. Add water through the top of B until the graduated tube of B is filled and the water overflows to flask A. Add 1ml of xylene with a pipette and then connect the reflux condenser C to B.Heat the flask to boiling and keep distilling at a rate that will keep the middle part of the condenser cold. Stop heating after 30 minutes, and allow to stand for at least 15 minutes. Read the volume of xylene in the graduated portion of the tube. Carry out the procedure described under Method 1, beginning at the words "Weigh a quantity of the sample to be examined accurately to 0.01g".Subtract the volume of xylene previously observed from the volume of the oil layer, and the remainder is taken to be the volume of volatile oil. Calculate the content of volatile oil in the sample to be examined, expressed as percentage (%).

（二）挥发性单一成分的含量测定

## 2. Determination of the Content of a Single Volatile Component

1. **气相色谱法** 测定单一挥发性成分含量时，气相色谱法最常用，多采用弹性石英毛细管柱，也可用硅藻土或高分子多孔小球为载体的填充柱。根据待测组分的极性，可选择角鲨烷、阿皮松、硅酮类、甲基硅油等非极性的饱和烃润滑油类或聚乙二醇类、聚酯类等极性固定液。定量时采用内标法或者外标法，但常用内标法。

**(1) Gas Chromatography** Gas chromatography is the most common method for the determination of volatile oils, mostly using a quartz capillary column. In the early days, packed columns supported by acid-washed and silanized diatomite or porous polymer beads were commonly used. According to the polarity of the components to be tested, the stationary liquid shall be non-polar saturated hydrocarbon lubricating oil such as squalane, apiezon, silicone and methyl silicone oil, or polar stationary liquid such as polyethylene glycol and polyester. The internal standard method or external standard method is used for quantification, but the internal standard method is commonly used.

常用的检测器有氢火焰离子化检测器（FID）或质谱检测器（MS）。也可采用闪蒸气相色谱法或顶空气相色谱法，以克服气相色谱分析中药成分操作复杂，周期长所导致的成分破坏或损失。

Flame ionization detector (FID) or mass spectrometry detector (MS) are commonly used. Due to the complicated operation and long cycle of gas chromatography in the analysis of traditional Chinese medicine components, some components may be damaged or lost, flash vapor chromatography or headspace gas chromatography can be used.

2. **高效液相色谱法** 如果挥发性成分具有紫外吸收，如桂皮醛、丹皮酚、丁香酚等芳香族化合物，可用高效液相色谱法进行测定。

**(2) High Performance Liquid Chromatography** Volatile components with UV absorption, such as cinnamaldehyde, paeonol, eugenol, and other aromatic compounds, can be determined by HPLC.

## 第六节 多糖类成分分析
## 7.6 Analysis of Polysaccharide Components

PPT

### 一、概述
### 7.6.1 Overview

多糖是由 10 个以上单糖分子通过苷键聚合而成的高分子化合物，一般由几百个甚至几千个单糖分子组成。多糖经酸水解后能生成多分子单糖。组成多糖的单糖主要有 D- 葡萄糖、D- 半乳糖、L- 阿拉伯糖、L- 鼠李糖、D- 半乳糖醛酸和 D- 葡萄糖醛酸等。中药中常见的多糖有淀粉、菊糖、黏液质、果胶、树胶、纤维素和甲壳素等。近年研究发现一些中药中的多糖具有较强的生物活性，如香菇多糖、灵芝多糖、猪苓多糖具有抗肿瘤作用，昆布多糖具有抗动脉粥样硬化作用，人参多糖具有抗突变作用和免疫调节作用，茶叶多糖具有抗凝血和降血脂作用等。

多糖在浓酸的作用下可水解成单糖，继而脱水生成具有呋喃环结构的糠醛及其衍生物。糠醛衍生物可以和许多芳胺、酚类及具有活性次甲基基团的化合物缩合生成有色化合物，可利用糠醛形成反应区别不同类型的糖。

The polysaccharide is a high molecular compound which is polymerized by more than 10 monosaccharide molecules through the glycoside bond, generally composed of hundreds or even thousands of monosaccharide molecules. The main monosaccharides that makeup polysaccharide are D-glucose, D-galactose, L-arabinose, L-rhamnose, D-galacturonic acid and D-glucuronic acid. The common polysaccharides in traditional Chinese medicine are starch, inulin, mucilage, pectin, gum, cellulose, chitin, etc. In recent years, it has been found that some polysaccharides in traditional Chinese medicine have strong biological activity, for instance, lentinan, ganoderma lucidum polysaccharide and polyporus polysaccharide have an anti-tumor effect, laminarin has an anti-atherosclerotic effect, ginseng polysaccharide has antimutagenic and immunomodulatory effects, tea polysaccharide has anti-coagulation and hypolipidemic effect.

Polysaccharides can be hydrolyzed to monosaccharides under the action of concentrated acid and then dehydrated to produce furfural and its derivatives with a furan ring structure. Furfural derivatives can condense with several aromatic amines, phenols, and compounds with active methylene to produce colored compounds. Different types of saccharides can be distinguished by furfural formation reaction.

### 二、定性分析
### 7.6.2　Qualitative Analysis

#### （一）薄层色谱法
#### 1. Thin Layer Chromatography

常用的吸附剂或载体有硅胶、氧化铝、纤维素、硅藻土等。糖的极性大易吸附，在硅胶薄层上进行色谱时，点样量不宜过多（一般少于 5μg）。也可用强碱与弱或中等强度的酸所成的盐，代替水制备硅胶薄层板，降低硅胶吸附能力，增加样品承载量，使斑点集中，改善分离效果。常用的有 0.3mol/L 磷酸氢二钠溶液或磷酸二氢钠溶液、0.02mol/L 醋酸钠溶液、0.02mol/L 硼酸盐缓冲液和 0.1mol/L 亚硫酸氢钠水溶液等。硅胶薄层色谱常用极性较大的含水溶剂系统为展开剂，如正丁醇 - 醋酸 - 水等。常用的显色剂有硫酸溶液、α - 萘酚 - 硫酸试剂等。

Silica gel, alumina, cellulose, and diatomite are often used as adsorbents or carriers. The polarity of saccharide is high and easy to adsorb when the silica gel is used for TLC, the sample amount should not be too much (generally less than 5μg). Instead of water, the salt consisting of a strong base and a weak or moderately strong acid can reduce the adsorption capacity of silica gel, increase the load capacity of the sample, make the spots concentrated and improve the separation efficiency. Commonly used are 0.3mol/L disodium hydrogen phosphate solution or sodium dihydrogen phosphate solution, 0.02mol/L sodium acetate solution, 0.02mol/L borate buffer, and 0.1mol/L sodium bisulfite aqueous solution.The aqueous solvent system with high polarity is often used as a developing agent in silica gel thin layer chromatography, such as *n*-butyl alcohol-acetic acid-water, etc. The common chromogenic agents for silica gel TLC are alcohol solution of sulfuric acid, and α-naphthol-sulfuric acid reagents.

#### （二）纸色谱法
#### 2. Paper Chromatography

糖的纸色谱常用水饱和的有机溶剂为展开剂，其中以正丁醇 - 乙酸 - 水应用最为普遍。为增大 $R_f$ 值，可加乙酸、吡啶、乙醇等。对于难区分的糖，还可采用由硼酸、硼砂缓冲液浸过的滤纸，以硼酸、硼砂缓冲液饱和的正丁醇 - 乙酸乙酯溶剂系统下行法展开。纸色谱常用的显色剂基本与硅胶薄层色谱相同，但不宜用含硫酸的显色试剂。

The water-saturated organic solvent is often used as the developing agent for the paper chromatography of saccharide. *n*-butanol-acetic acid-water is the most commonly used. To increase the value of $R_f$, acetic acid, pyridine, ethanol, etc. can be added. For saccharides that are difficult to distinguish, the filter paper soaked by boric acid and borax buffer can also be developed by using the descending development method of *n*-butanol-ethyl acetate solvent system saturated with boric acid and borax buffer. The common chromogenic reagent used in paper chromatography is the same as silica gel thin layer chromatography, but the reagent containing sulfuric acid should not be used.

此外，采用高效液相色谱法鉴别糖时，多选用氨基柱，以乙腈 - 水为流动相，示差折光检测器检出不同单糖组分。用气相色谱法鉴别多糖时，可通过制备成三甲基硅烷化衍生物来增加挥发性；也可通过将醛糖用四氢硼钠还原成多元醇，然后制成乙酰化物或三氟乙酰化物来测定。若联用 MS 检测，不仅可测出多糖的组成，并且可测得单糖之间的摩尔比。还可采用电泳法鉴别多糖。

In addition，Amino column is often used to identify saccharide by HPLC, acetonitrile-water is used as mobile phase, different monosaccharide components are detected by differential refractive index detector. When identifying polysaccharide by gas chromatography, the volatilization can be increased by preparing trimethyl-silane derivatives. It can also be determined by reducing aldose with sodium borohydride to polyol and then making acetylate or trifluoroacetate. If combined with MS, not only the composition of polysaccharide but also the molar ratio of monosaccharide can be measured. Polysaccharides can also be measured by electrophoresis.

### 三、定量分析
### 7.6.3 Quantitative Analysis

（一）比色法
### 1. Colorimetric method

多糖的含量测定多采用比色法，在样品中加入适当的试剂显色后在可见光区测定吸光度，计算含量。常用的显色试剂有苯酚 - 硫酸、蒽酮 - 硫酸、3,5- 二硝基水杨酸（DNS）等。

The content of polysaccharides is determined by colorimetry, after adding an appropriate reagent to the sample for color development, the absorbance is measured in the visible region and the content is calculated. The commonly used color reagent is phenol-sulfuric acid, anthranone-sulfuric acid, 3,5-dinitrosalicylic acid (DNS), etc.

1. **苯酚 - 硫酸比色法** 多糖经浓无机酸处理脱水生成的糠醛或糠醛衍生物，能与酚类化合物缩合生成有色物质。通常使用的无机酸为硫酸，常用的酚有苯酚、地衣酚等。其中苯酚 - 硫酸应用较多。苯酚 - 硫酸试剂可与游离的或多糖中的己糖、戊糖和糖醛酸起显色反应，己糖在 490nm、戊糖及糖醛酸在 480nm 有最大吸收。苯酚 - 硫酸比色法是测定多糖的经典方法之一，苯酚和硫酸的用量、显色时间、温度、放置时间等因素均会影响测定结果。制作标准曲线时宜用相应的标准多糖，如用葡萄糖作对照品绘制标准曲线，应乘以校正系数 0.9。对杂多糖，根据各单糖的组成比及主要组分单糖的标准曲线的校正系数加以校正计算。

**（1）Phenol-Sulfuric Acid Colorimetry** Polysaccharides are dehydrated by concentrated inorganic acid to produce furfural or furfural derivatives, which can condense with phenolic compounds to produce colored substances. The commonly used inorganic acid is sulfuric acid. The phenol-sulfuric acid reagent can produce a chromogenic reaction with hexose, pentose and glucuronic acid, the maximum absorption of hexose at 490nm and pentose glucuronic acid at 480nm. The amount of phenol and sulfuric acid, the time of color development, temperature and other factors will affect the determination results. When the standard curve is made, the corresponding standard polysaccharide should be used. If the standard curve is drawn with glucose as the reference, the correction coefficient should be multiplied by 0.9. For heteropolysaccharides, according to the composition ratio of each monosaccharide and the calibration coefficient of the standard curve of the main component monosaccharide, the calibration was calculated.

**2. 蒽酮 - 硫酸比色法** 多糖遇浓硫酸脱水生成糖醛或其衍生物，可与蒽酮试剂缩合产生蓝绿色物质，于 620nm 波长处有最大吸收。色氨酸含量较高的蛋白质对显色反应有一定干扰。蒽酮不仅能与单糖也能与双糖、糊精、淀粉等直接起作用，样品也可不必经过水解。

（2）**Anthrone-Sulfuric Acid Colorimetry** The polysaccharide dehydrates with concentrated sulfuric acid to form furfural or its derivatives, which can condense with anthrone reagent to produce a blue-green substance with maximum absorption at the wavelength of 620nm. It should be noted that proteins with high tryptophan content interfere with the color reaction. Anthracene can not only interact with monosaccharides but also disaccharides, dextrin and starch directly, and the sample does not need to be hydrolyzed.

**3. 3,5- 二硝基水杨酸（DNS）比色法** 在碱性溶液中，3,5- 二硝基水杨酸与还原糖发生氧化还原反应，生成 3- 氨基 -5- 硝基水杨酸，该产物在煮沸条件下显棕红色，且在一定浓度范围内颜色深浅与还原糖含量成比例关系。因其显色深浅只与糖类游离出还原基团的数量有关，而对还原糖的种类没有选择性，故 DNS 方法适用于多糖（如纤维素、半纤维素和淀粉等）水解产生的多种还原糖。

（3）**3, 5-dinitrosalicylic Acid (DNS) Colorimetric Method** 3,5-dinitrosalicylic acid reacts with reducing sugar to produce 3-amino-5-nitrosalicylic acid in an alkaline solution, which is brownish red in boiling condition, and the color is proportional to the content of reducing sugar in a certain concentration range.DNS method applies to many reducing sugar systems produced by hydrolysis of polysaccharides (such as cellulose, hemicellulose, starch,etc.), because its color depth is only related to the number of reductive groups dissociated from sugars, and there is no selectivity for the types of reducing sugars.

（二）高效液相色谱法

## 2. High Performance Liquid Chromatography

单体多糖多以凝胶或离子交换树脂为 HPLC 法的固定相，以已知分子量的多糖对照品作对照，确定其分子量。再将其酸水解后进行 HPLC 法测定，确定单糖的种类和比例，以单糖的量推算多糖的量。测定多糖时常用氨基键合硅胶柱分离，示差折光检测器检测，但其稳定性差，可在流动相中加入 0.01%TEPA（四乙酸胺）改善。

The polysaccharides is determined by gel or ion exchange resin as the stationary phase of HPLC, taking polysaccharide with known molecular mass as a reference substance. The polysaccharide is hydrolyzed by acid and determined by HPLC to determine the type and proportion of monosaccharide. The amount of polysaccharide was calculated by the amount of monosaccharide. The polysaccharide was separated by an amino bonded silica gel column and detected by the differential refractive detector, However, its stability is poor, which can be improved by adding 0.01% TEPA (tetraacetic acid amine) into the mobile phase.

## 第七节　其他类型成分分析

# 7.7　Analysis of Other Types of Components

### 一、木脂素类成分分析

### 7.7.1　Analysis of Lignans

（一）概述

### 1. Overview

木脂素类结构中常有酚羟基、亚甲二氧基、甲氧基、羧基等取代基和内酯环，可利用这些官能团的性质和颜色反应进行木脂素类成分的检识和含量测定。

There are phenolic hydroxyl, methylenedioxy, methoxy, carboxyl group and lactone ring in lignans structure, the properties and color reactions of these functional groups can be used to detect and determine the content of lignans.

（二）定性分析

### 2. Qualitative Analysis

木脂素类母核没有共同的化学反应，只能利用分子结构中的官能团如酚羟基、亚甲二氧基、内酯环等的特征显色反应，用化学反应法进行初步鉴别，但专属性差。具有荧光的木脂素类根据其荧光颜色可用荧光法鉴别。

There is no common chemical reaction of lignans, so the characteristic color reaction of functional groups such as phenolic hydroxyl group, methylenedioxy group and lactone ring in molecular structure can only be used for preliminary identification. The fluorescent color of lignans with fluorescence can be observed.

薄层色谱法常被用于鉴别木脂素类成分，常用的吸附剂为硅胶，展开剂一般选用三氯甲烷 - 甲醇、三氯甲烷 - 乙酸乙酯等。薄层色谱展开后，有颜色木脂素可在日光下观察；有荧光的木脂素在 UV 光下观察；无色又无荧光的木脂素用 10% 硫酸乙醇液、茴香醛浓硫酸试剂、5%~10% 磷钼酸乙醇液或碘蒸气熏蒸显色后检视。这些非特征性的试剂对不同的木脂素类化合物可显示不同的颜色，常用于木脂素类成分的薄层鉴别。

TLC is often used to identify lignans. The commonly used adsorbent is silica gel, and the developing agents generally are trichloromethane - methanol, trichloromethane - ethyl acetate, etc. After TLC development, colored lignans can be observed directly in sunlight, fluorescent lignans are observed under UV light, colorless and non-fluorescent lignans need to be sprayed with chromogenic reagent, the most commonly used chromogenic reagents are 10% sulfuric acid ethanol solution, anisaldehyde concentrated sulfuric acid reagent, 5%-10% phosphomolybdate ethanol solution or fumigation with iodine vapor. These non-characteristic reagents can show different colors to different lignans, which are often used for thin layer identification of lignans.

（三）定量分析

### 3. Quantitative Analysis

根据测定目的不同可分为总木脂素含量测定和单体木脂素成分的含量测定。常用的方法有分光光度法、薄层色谱扫描法和高效液相色谱法等。

It can be divided into total lignans content determination and monomer lignans content determination according to different purposes. The common methods are spectrophotometry, thin layer chromatography, and high performance liquid chromatography.

**1. 分光光度法** 总木脂素的含量测定多采用此法。该方法的原理是利用木脂素分子结构中取代基的特征反应使其生成有色物质，采用分光光度法测定总木脂素含量。如结构中含有亚甲二氧基的木脂素类成分，与变色酸 - 浓硫酸试剂反应生成的有色物质在 570nm 处有最大吸收，在此波长测定吸光度，计算含量。但应注意，本法干扰较多，要求供试液纯度较高，需要进行阴性试验，以证明方法的专属性。

（1）**Spectrophotometry** This method is often used for the determination of total lignans. The principle of this method is to use the characteristic reaction of the substituent groups in the molecular structure of lignans to make them produce colored substances. For example, lignans with methylenedioxy group in the structure react with Labat reagent to produce a colored substance, which has the maximum absorption at 570nm, the absorbance is measured at this wavelength and the content is calculated. However, it should be noted that this method has many interferences and requires a higher purity of the test liquid, so a negative test is needed to prove the specificity of the method.

**2. 薄层色谱扫描法** 在可见光或紫外光区有吸收的木脂素类成分，用薄层吸收扫描法测定含量；能发出荧光或有荧光淬灭特性的木脂素类成分，可用薄层荧光扫描法测定含量。

（2）**TLCS** Lignans that can absorb visible or ultraviolet light are determined by thin layer absorption scanning method, and those that can emit fluorescence or have fluorescence quenching properties can be determined by thin layer fluorescence scanning method.

**3. 高效液相色谱法** 高效液相色谱法是目前测定单体木脂素含量的主要方法。一般以十八烷基硅烷键合硅胶为固定相，乙腈 - 水或甲醇 - 水系统为流动相，多采用紫外检测器检测。

（3）**HPLC** HPLC is the main method to determine the content of monomer lignans. In general, octadecyl silane bonded silica gel is used as the stationary phase, acetonitrile-water or methanol-water system as mobile phase, and UV detector is usually used.

## 二、有机酸类成分分析
## 7.7.2　Analysis of Organic Acids

（一）概述
### 1. Overview
有机酸类是指一类具有羧基的酸性有机化合物，根据结构不同可以分为脂肪族有机酸（琥珀酸、柠檬酸、苹果酸、酒石酸等）、芳香族有机酸（咖啡酸、阿魏酸、桂皮酸、水杨酸等）和萜类有机酸（甘草酸、齐墩果酸、熊果酸、山楂酸等）。多数有机酸具有多方面生物活性，如齐墩果酸可防治脂肪肝、抗动脉粥样硬化，绿原酸可抗菌、油酸可抗癌等。但是存在于关木通、青木香、广防己等中药中的马兜铃酸具有较强的肾毒性。

Organic acids refer to a class of acid organic compounds with carboxyl groups, it can be divided into aliphatic organic acids (such as succinic acid, citrate, malic acid, tartaric acid, etc.), aromatic organic acids (such as ferulic acid, cinnamic acid, salicylic acid, etc.) and terpene organic acids (such as glycyrrhizic acid, oleanolic acid, ursolic acid, maslinic acid, etc.) according to different structures. Most organic acids have a variety of biological activities, such as oleanolic acid can prevent fatty liver and atherosclerosis, chlorogenic acid can be antibacterial, oleic acid can be anti-cancer. However, aristolochic acid, which exists in traditional Chinese medicines such as Caulis Aristolochiae Manshuriensis, Dutchmanspipe root, and Aristolochia Fangchi, has strong renal toxicity.

（二）定性分析

## 2. Qualitative Analysis

有机酸的鉴别多采用薄层色谱法，常用硅胶或聚酰胺做吸附剂，极性较大的溶剂系统为展开剂，常在展开剂中加入一定量的甲酸、乙酸等抑制解离，防止斑点拖尾。薄层色谱展开后，有荧光的有机酸如绿原酸、阿魏酸等，可在 UV 光下观察；既无颜色又无荧光的有机酸常用硫酸乙醇、碘蒸气等显色。

Organic acids are often identified by TLC, silica gel or polyamide are commonly used as adsorbents, and the solvent system with greater polarity is the developer. To prevent the dissociation of organic acids in the process of development and cause the tailing of chromatographic spots, a certain amount of formic acid and acetic acid are often added into the developing agent. After the development of TLC, organic acids with fluorescence such as chlorogenic acid and ferulic acid can be observed under UV light, colorless and non-fluorescent organic acid need spray color reagent. Such as sulfuric acid ethanol and iodine vapor, etc.

（三）定量分析

## 3. Quantitative Analysis

总有机酸的测定常用酸碱滴定法或电位滴定法、分光光度法；有机酸单体成分的测定常用薄层色谱扫描法、高效液相色谱法、高效毛细管电泳法、气相色谱法等。

Titration analysis and spectrophotometry are used in the content determination of of total organic acid. The content determination of monomer organic acid by thin layer scanning, high performance liquid chromatography, high performance capillary electrophoresis, gas chromatography and so on.

1. 总有机酸的含量测定

**(1) Determination of Total Organic Acid**

（1）滴定法　药材中总有机酸的含量高于 1% 时，一般采用酸碱滴定法，由于中药提取液的颜色往往比较深，应用电位法指示终点。有机酸类成分酸性较弱时，采用非水溶液滴定法。

*Titration analysis*　When the content of total organic acid in medicinal materials is higher than 1%, the acid-base titration method is generally used. However, the color of the extract of traditional Chinese medicine is often dark, potentiometric method is applied to indicate the endpoint. When the organic acid component is weak in acidity, the non-aqueous solution titration method is used.

（2）分光光度法　利用某些有机酸可与显色剂反应生成有色物质的性质，采用分光光度法测定总有机酸含量。如以咖啡酸为对照，用三氯化铁 - 铁氰化钾显色，在 763nm 处测定蒲公英中总有机酸的含量。

*Spectrophotometry*　The content of total organic acid is determined by spectrophotometry according to the properties of some organic acids reacting with a chromogenic reagent to form colored substances. For example, the content of total organic acid in Taraxaci Herba is determined at 763nm, using ferric trichloride and potassium ferricyanide to develop color, taking caffeic acid as a reference substance.

2. 单体有机酸类成分的含量测定

**(2) Determination of Monomer Organic Acids**

中药中的各种有机酸均可采用高效液相色谱法测定含量。有机酸在水中很容易发生电离，产生多峰或拖尾现象，通常在流动相中加入冰醋酸、磷酸、磷酸盐缓冲液等抑制有机酸的离解。咖啡酸、绿原酸、没食子酸、桂皮酸、阿魏酸等有较强的紫外吸收，可选择紫外检测器，齐墩果酸、灵芝酸、熊果酸、山楂酸等成分紫外吸收弱，则选择通用型的蒸发光散射检测器效果较好。

The contents of all kinds of organic acids in traditional Chinese medicine can be determined by HPLC. Organic acids are easily ionized in water, resulting in multiple peaks or tails, glacial acetic acid, phosphoric acid, phosphate buffer and other substances are usually added to the mobile phase to inhibit the dissociation of organic acids. Caffeic acid, chlorogenic acid, gallic acid, cinnamic acid, ferulic acid, and other components have strong UV absorption, UV detector can be selected, the UV absorption of oleanolic acid, ganoderma acid, ursolic acid, maslinic acid, and other components is weak, so the general type of evaporative light scattering detector is better.

薄层色谱扫描法、毛细管区带电泳（CZE）法和毛细管胶束电泳（MECC）法也可用于有机酸的测定。具有挥发性的有机酸可用气相色谱法测定。非挥发性的有机酸可用衍生化法生成具有挥发性的衍生物后用气相色谱法测定。如在碱性条件下，γ-亚麻酸与三氟化硼-甲醇试剂反应生成具有挥发性的 γ-亚麻酸甲酯后，用气相色谱法测定。

TLCS, Capillary zone electrophoresis (CZE) and micellar electrokinetic capillary chromatography (MECC) are used in assay of monomer organic acids. Gas chromatography can be used for the determination of volatile organic acids. The non-volatile organic acids can be generated into volatile derivatives by derivatization and then determined by gas chromatography. For example, under alkaline conditions, γ-linolenic acid reacts with boron trifluoride-methanol reagent to produce volatile γ-linolenic acid methyl ester, which is then measured by gas chromatography.

### 三、香豆素类成分分析
### 7.7.3  Analysis of Coumarins

（一）概述
#### 1. Overview
小分子游离香豆素有挥发性和升华性，亲脂性强。香豆素类化合物因具有内酯结构，在其苯环或吡喃酮环上常有羟基、甲氧基、异戊烯基等取代基存在，利用这些官能团的性质可进行香豆素的定性和定量分析。香豆素类化合物具有抗菌、抗炎、抗凝血、扩张冠状动脉等生理活性。

Small molecule free coumarin has volatility, sublimation and strong lipophilicity. As coumarins have lactone structure, substituent group such as hydroxy, methoxy and isopentenyl often exist in benzene ring or α-pyranone ring, the properties of these functional groups can be used for qualitative and quantitative analysis of coumarin. Coumarins have antibacterial, anti-inflammatory, anti-coagulation, dilating coronary artery and other physiological activities.

（二）定性分析
#### 2. Qualitative Analysis
1. 化学反应法　用异羟肟酸铁反应鉴别内酯环；三氯化铁或重氮化试剂鉴别酚羟基；Gibb 试剂和 Emerson 试剂鉴别香豆素 $C_6$ 位或酚羟基对位是否有取代基。

（1）Chemical Reaction Method　The lactone ring was identified by ferric isohydroxamic acid reaction, identification of phenolic hydroxyl group by ferric trichloride or diazotization reagent, Gibb's reagent and Emerson reagent are used to identify whether there are substituents at the $C_6$ position or para-position of phenol hydroxy of coumarin.

2. 荧光法　香豆素母核本身无荧光，其 $C_7$ 位羟基衍生物却呈强烈的蓝色荧光，在碱性溶液中荧光增强；但若在 $C_7$ 位的邻位即 $C_6$ 或 $C_8$ 位引入羟基，则荧光减弱或消失；呋喃香豆素多显较弱的蓝色或褐色荧光；多个烷氧基取代的呋喃香豆素显黄绿色或褐色荧光。如秦皮的乙醇提取液在日光下显碧蓝色荧光，在 365nm 显亮蓝紫色荧光。

（2）**Fluorescence**　The molecular structure of coumarin has no fluorescence, but its $C_7$ hydroxyl derivatives show strong blue fluorescence, and the fluorescence is enhanced in alkaline solution. However, if hydroxyl groups are introduced at the $C_6$ or $C_8$ position, the fluorescence will weaken or disappear. Furanocoumarin has weak blue or brown fluorescence. Several alkoxys substituted furanocoumarins show yellow-green or brown fluorescence. For example, the ethanol extract of Fraxini Cortex shows blue fluorescence under sunlight and bright blue-purple fluorescence at 365nm.

3. **薄层色谱法**　薄层色谱鉴别香豆素常用的吸附剂为硅胶。游离香豆素极性较小，可用正己烷 - 乙酸乙酯为展开剂，香豆素苷根据极性选择不同比例的三氯甲烷 - 甲醇展开。展开后可直接观察荧光或者喷少量稀 NaOH 或 KOH 溶液使其荧光加强；或用三氯化铁 - 铁氰化钾、异羟肟酸铁、重氮化氨基苯磺酸等试剂显色，在日光下观察斑点呈现的黄、橙、红、棕、紫等颜色。

（3）**Thin layer Chromatography**　Coumarin is identified by TLC with silica gel as adsorbent. The polarity of free coumarin is relatively small, which can be developed by *n*-hexane-ethyl acetate. Coumarin glycoside is developed according to polarity by selecting different proportions of trichloromethane-methanol. The fluorescence can be observed directly or enhanced by spraying a small amount of dilute NaOH or KOH solution after deployment. The thin layer plate can also be colored with ferric trichloride-potassium ferricyanide, ferric isohydroxamic acid, diazotized aminobenzene sulfonic acid and other reagents, and then the yellow, orange, red, brown, purple and other colors of the spots are observed under sunlight.

（三）定量分析

3. **Quantitative Analysis**

1. **紫外 - 可见分光光度法**　当样品较纯时，可直接在合适波长下用紫外分光光度法测定。如以欧前胡素为对照，300nm 为测定波长直接测定白芷中总香豆素的含量。也可选择恰当的显色试剂显色后，测定总香豆素的含量。

（1）**Uv-visible spectrophotometry**　When the sample is relatively pure, it can be directly determined by UV spectrophotometry at the appropriate wavelength. For example, the content of total coumarin in angelica dahurica is directly determined by taking imperatorin as the reference substance and 300nm as the measuring wavelength. The content of total coumarin can also be determined by selecting the appropriate reagent for coloration.

2. **荧光光度法**　此法测定具有荧光的羟基香豆素类成分的含量，具有较高的灵敏度及选择性。当干扰成分较多时，可先用色谱法分离纯化。

（2）**Fluorometry**　This method has high sensitivity and selectivity in the determination of hydroxy coumarins with fluorescence. When there are many interfering components, they can be separated and purified by chromatography.

3. **薄层色谱扫描法**　经薄层色谱分离后的香豆素类成分，根据其具有紫外吸收、可产生荧光、能与不同试剂显色的特性，直接进行扫描或荧光扫描测定含量。

（3）**Thin Layer Chromatography Scanning**　The coumarins separated by TLC can be directly scanned or determined by fluorescence scanning according to their characteristics of ultraviolet absorption, fluorescence generation and color development with different reagents.

4. **高效液相色谱法**　由于香豆素类成分具有芳香环及其他共轭结构，紫外吸收较强，用高效液相色谱法测定时常选用紫外检测器，具有较高的灵敏度。固定相多为 ODS，流动相为不同比例的甲醇 - 水或乙腈 - 水。如补骨脂素、异补骨脂素、欧前胡素、异欧前胡素、秦皮甲素、秦皮乙素、蛇床子素等的含量测定。

（4）**High Performance Liquid Chromatography**   Because coumarins have aromatic rings and other conjugated structures and have strong UV absorption, UV detector is often used to determine coumarins by HPLC, which has high sensitivity. Most of the stationary phase is ODS, and the mobile phase is methanol-water or acetonitrile-water in different proportions, such as psoralen, isopsoralen, imperatorin, isoimperatorin, aesculin and aesculetin, osthole, etc.

5. **气相色谱法**   某些分子量小、具有挥发性的游离香豆素类成分，可用气相色谱法测定。常用 SE-30 石英毛细管柱、FID 检测器。如花椒毒素、香橙内酯、蛇床子素、欧前胡素均可用气相色谱法测定含量。

（5）**Gas Chromatography**   Some free coumarins with small molecular weight and volatility can be determined by gas chromatography with the SE-30 quartz capillary column and FID detector. For example, the content of Xanthotoxin, Citrus lactone, Osthole and Imperatorin can be determined by gas chromatography.

### 四、动物药成分分析
### 7.7.4   Component Analysis of Animal Medicine

（一）概述
### 1. Overview
动物药是指含有动物的角、骨、肉、皮、血及脂肪等成分的药物。按含有活性成分的结构特征可分为以下几类：蛋白质（酶）、多肽及氨基酸类，如鹿茸中的多肽；生物碱类，如地龙中的次黄嘌呤；多糖类；甾体类化合物，如熊去氧胆酸；酚、酮、酸类成分，如麝香中的麝香酮、胆汁酸；萜类成分等。

Animal medicine refers to the medicine containing animal horn, bone, meat, skin, blood and fat, and other components. According to the structural characteristics of the active ingredients, they can be divided into the following categories: proteins (enzymes), polypeptides and amino acids etc. Such as polypeptides in cervi cornu pantotrichum; alkaloids: Such as hypoxanthine in pheretima; polysaccharides; steroids: such as ursodeoxycholic acid; phenols, ketones, acid components: such as musk muscone and bile acid in moschus; terpenoids, etc.

（二）定性分析
### 2. Qualitative Analysis
以化学反应法和薄层色谱法为主，其中以薄层色谱法最为常用。

Chemical identification and TLC identification are the main methods, in which TLC identification is the most commonly used.

1. **化学反应法**   取蟾酥粉末 0.1g，加甲醇 5ml，浸泡 1 小时，滤过，滤液加对二甲氨基苯甲醛固体少量，滴加硫酸数滴，即显蓝紫色（蟾毒色胺类化合物反应）。取蟾酥粉末 0.1g，加三氯甲烷 5ml，滤过，滤液蒸干，残渣加醋酐少量使溶解，滴加硫酸，初显蓝紫色，渐变为蓝绿色（蟾毒和蟾毒配基反应）。

（1）**Chemical Reaction Method**   Take 0.1g of toad venom powder, add 5ml of methanol, soak for 1 hour, filter, add a small amount of p-dimethylaminobenzaldehyde to the filtrate, add several drops of sulfuric acid to make the filtrate blue and purple (reaction of toad poison tryptamine). Take 0.1g of toad venom powder, add 5ml of trichloromethane, filter, evaporate the filtrate to dry, add a small amount of acetic anhydride to the residue to dissolve it, add sulfuric acid, it turns blue-purple at first and turns blue-green gradually (the reaction of toad venom).

2. 薄层色谱法　龟甲及其制剂中的活性成分可用薄层色谱法鉴别。将龟甲的甲醇超声提取液、龟甲对照药材甲醇提取液和胆固醇对照品制成的对照液分别点于同一硅胶 G 薄层板上，用甲苯 - 乙酸乙酯 - 甲醇 - 甲酸（15：2：1：0.6）展开，喷以硫酸无水乙醇溶液，加热，供试品色谱中，在与对照药材色谱和对照品色谱相应的位置上，显相同颜色的斑点。

(2) **Thin Layer Chromatography**　The active components in tortoiseshells and their preparations can be identified by TLC. The methanol ultrasonic extract of tortoiseshell, the methanol extract of tortoiseshell reference material and the cholesterol reference material are respectively spotted on the same silica gel G thin layer plate, developed with toluene-ethyl acetate-methanol-formic acid (15:2:1:0.6). After the deployment, spray anhydrous ethanol solution of sulfuric acid, heat it, the chromatogram of the test sample shows spots of the same color as the control herbs or contrast in the same position.

（三）定量分析

### 3. Quantitative Analysis

采用化学分析法、高效液相色谱法、薄层色谱扫描法、气相色谱法等，其中以高效液相色谱法最为常用。

Chemical analysis, high performance liquid chromatography, thin layer chromatography scanning method and gas chromatography can be used for quantitative analysis, among which high performance liquid chromatography is the most commonly used.

1. 化学分析法　化学分析法用于各类总成分的测定。样品提取纯化后，选择适当的方法进行滴定；或将样品溶液适当处理得到纯的沉淀，干燥至恒重，根据质量换算出样品含量。如应用配位滴定法测定石决明中碳酸钙的含量。

(1) **Chemical Analysis**　Chemical analysis is often used for the determination of all kinds of total components. After sample extraction and purification, the appropriate method is selected for titration. The sample solution can also be treated with appropriate methods to obtain pure precipitation, and the precipitation can be dried to constant weight, and the sample content can be converted according to the mass of precipitation. For example, the coordination titration method is used to determine the content of calcium carbonate in Concha Haliotidis.

2. 高效液相色谱法　高效液相色谱法广泛应用于动物药及其制剂的含量测定。如采用高效液相色谱法测定冬虫夏草中腺苷的含量，斑蝥中斑蝥素的含量，蟾蜍中脂蟾毒配基、华蟾酥毒基的含量，牙痛一粒丸，六应丸，麝香保心丸。

(2) **High Performance Liquid Chromatography**　It is widely used in the determination of animal medicine and their preparations, such as HPLC method is used to determine the content of adenosine in Cordyceps Sinensis, cantharidin in Mylabris, resibufogenin and cinobufagin in Bufonid, resibufogenin and cinobufagin in Yatong Yili Wan, Shexiang Baoxin Wan, etc.

3. 薄层色谱扫描法　该方法是动物药及其制剂的有效成分含量测定方法之一，特别是胆酸等结构中没有共轭结构，无紫外吸收，无法用紫外检测器或荧光检测器测定含量，更适宜于用此法。如体外培养牛黄中胆酸的含量测定，灵宝护心丹中牛黄胆酸的含量测定。

(3) **Thin Layer Chromatography Scanning**　It is one of the methods for the determination of the effective components in animal medicines and preparations. In particular, there is no conjugated

structure in cholic acid and no UV absorption, so the content cannot be determined by a UV detector or fluorescence detector, which is more suitable for this method. For example, it is used to determine the content of cholic acid in Calculus Bbovis Cultured in vitro and Lingbao Huxin Dan.

**4. 气相色谱法**  气相色谱法具有高灵敏度、高选择性、分析速度快、所需试样量少等优点，可用于动物药熊胆、麝香、蟾酥等及其制剂的含量测定，多用氢火焰离子化检测器检测。

**(4) Gas Chromatography**  Gas chromatography has the advantages of high sensitivity, high selectivity, fast analysis speed, and small sample quantity, etc. It can be used for the determination of animal medicines such as bear gall, musk, venenum bufonis, and their preparations, and it is mostly detected by hydrogen flame ionization detector.

### 五、矿物药成分分析
### 7.7.5  Component Analysis of Mineral Medicine

（一）概述
#### 1. Overview

矿物药主要成分为无机化合物。涉及的无机元素主要包括存在于雄黄、砒霜中的砷；朱砂、轻粉中的汞；红丹、密陀僧中的铅；胆矾、铜绿中的铜；赭石、磁石中的铁；石膏、钟乳石中的钙；滑石、白石英中的硅；芒硝、玄明粉中的硫；大青盐、秋石中的氯等。

The main components of mineral medicine are inorganic compounds. The inorganic elements involved mainly include arsenic in realgar and arsenic trioxide; Mercury in cinnabar and calomel; Lead in red lead and lithargite; Copper in bluestone and verdigris; Iron in ochre and lodestone; Calcium in gypsum and stalactites; Silicon in soapstone and crystobalite; Sulfur in mirabilite and compound of glauber-salt; Chlorine in halite and prepared salt.

（二）定性分析
#### 2. Qualitative analysis

矿物药的鉴别多用离子反应、火焰反应、沉淀反应和气体反应等化学反应法和热分析法。

Chemical reaction methods such as ion reaction, flame reaction, precipitation reaction and gas reaction and thermal analysis are used in the identification of mineral medicines.

**1. 化学反应法**  根据中药所含的无机元素，采用化学反应进行鉴别。如鉴别胆矾时利用硫酸盐加氯化钡生成白色沉淀的性质；鉴别明矾时钾盐的焰色反应显紫色；利用燃烧时易熔融，火焰为蓝色，并有二氧化硫刺激性气味鉴别硫黄。

**(1) Chemical Reaction Method**  According to the inorganic elements contained in traditional Chinese medicine, the chemical reaction is used for identification. For example, the properties of white precipitate formed by sulfate and barium chloride can be used to identify bluestone; the flame reaction of potassium salt in alum is purple; Sulfur can be identified by the characteristics of easy melting, blue flame, and sulfur dioxide irritating smell.

**2. 热分析法**  热分析法是在程序控制温度下，记录物质的理化性质随温度变化的关系，研究其在受热过程中所发生的晶形转化、熔融、蒸发、脱水等物理变化或热分解、氧化等化学变化以及伴随发生的温度、能量或质量改变的仪器分析方法。用以对该物质进行物理常数、熔点和沸点的确定以及作为鉴别和纯度检查的方法。根据矿物药性质和检测目的不同，常用的热分析法有热重法、差热分析法、差示扫描量热法等。

**(2) Thermal Analysis**  Thermal analysis is an instrumental analysis method that records the relationship between physical and chemical properties of a substance and temperature changes under programmed temperature control, and studies the physical changes such as crystal transformation, melting, evaporation, and dehydration, or chemical changes such as thermal decomposition and oxidation, as well as the accompanying changes in temperature, energy or mass during the heating process. It is used to determine the physical constants, melting and boiling points, and as a method for identification and purity inspection. According to the different properties and detection purposes of mineral medicines, the commonly used thermal analysis methods include thermogravimetry, differential thermal analysis, differential scanning calorimetry, etc.

（三）定量分析

### 3. Quantitative analysis

矿物药的含量测定方法通常选择容量分析法和重量分析法，对含量较低的药物可选择可见分光光度法、原子吸收光谱法和电感耦合等离子体质谱法等。

Volumetric analysis and gravimetric analysis are usually used for the determination of mineral medicine, while visible spectrophotometry, atomic absorption spectrometry and inductively coupled plasma mass spectrometry can be selected for mineral medicine with lower content.

1. **化学分析法** 将矿物药样品分解制备成溶液，选择配位滴定、酸碱滴定和氧化还原滴定进行测定，如有干扰物质存在，应采用分离法或掩蔽法消除干扰。或将样品分解液通过适当处理后得到较纯的沉淀，干燥至恒重，根据重量换算出样品含量。

**(1) Chemical Analysis Method** The sample of mineral medicine is decomposed into solution, and complexometric titration, acid-base titration, and redox titration are selected for determination. If there are interfering substances, the separation method or masking method shall be adopted to eliminate the interference. The sample decomposition solution can also be properly treated to obtain pure precipitation, dried to constant weight, and the sample content can be converted according to the weight.

2. **可见分光光度法** 利用一些无机金属元素可与某些化合物形成有色配合物的性质，采用分光光度法进行测定。如可利用砷化氢与二乙基二硫代氨基甲酸银（Ag-DDC）三乙胺的氯仿溶液作用，产生新生态的银在510nm有吸收，以测定砷的含量；高价汞与双硫腙作用生成橙色化合物测定含汞的矿物药等。

**(2) Visible Spectrophotometry** The content of mineral medicine is determined by spectrophotometry by using the property that some inorganic metal elements can form colored complexes with some compounds. For example, the reaction of arsenide hydrogen and the chloroform solution of silver diethyldithiocarbamate (Ag-DDC) triethylamine can be used to produce newly formed silver with absorption at 510nm to determine the content of arsenic. Determination of mineral medicines containing mercury by the properties of orange compounds formed by the interaction of high valence mercury with dithizone.

3. **原子吸收光谱法** 该法能测定几乎全部金属元素，灵敏度高，选择性好，抗干扰能力强，适用范围广。近年来已广泛应用于矿物药及其制剂中各种微量元素的分析。

**(3) Atomic Absorption Spectrometry** Atomic absorption spectrometry can be used to determine almost all metal elements with high sensitivity, good selectivity, strong anti-interference ability, and wide application range. In recent years, it has been widely used in the analysis of various microelements in mineral medicines and their preparations.

4. **电感耦合等离子体光谱法** 根据测定原理不同分为电感耦合发射光谱法和电感耦合质谱法。测定时样品均由载气带入雾化后，以气溶胶形式进入等离子体的轴向通道，在高温和惰性气体中被充分蒸发、原子化、电离和激发。两种方法不同之处在于电感耦合发射光谱法发射出所含元素的特征谱线，经分光系统进入光谱检测器，依据元素特征谱线上的响应值与其浓度成正比的性质进行定量分析；而电感耦合质谱法则是样品气溶胶被蒸发、原子化、电离和激发后，转化成带正电荷的离子进入质谱仪采集系统，根据离子的质荷比进行定量分析。

**(4) Inductively Coupled Plasma Spectrometry** Inductively coupled plasma spectrometry can be divided into inductively coupled emission spectrometry and inductively coupled mass spectrometry according to different measurement principles. During the determination, the samples are carried into the axial channel of the plasma in the form of aerosols after being atomized by the carrier gas. They are fully evaporated, atomized, ionized and excited in the high temperature and inert gas. The difference between the two methods is that the characteristic spectral lines of the elements are emitted by inductively coupled emission spectrometry, and then enter the spectral detector through the spectroscopic system. Quantitative analysis is carried out according to the property that the response value of the characteristic spectral lines of the elements is directly proportional to their concentration. However, inductively coupled mass spectrometry is a process in which the sample aerosol is evaporated, atomized, ionized and excited, and then converted into positively charged ions, which are then collected in the mass spectrometer collection system and quantitatively analyzed according to the mass to charge ratio of the ions.

该技术具有多谱线同时检测、检测速度快、动态线性范围宽、灵敏度高等优点，可应用于矿物药及其制剂中各种微量元素的分析。

This technique has the advantages of simultaneous detection of multi-spectral lines, fast detection speed, wide dynamic linear range, and high sensitivity, and can be applied to the analysis of various microelements in mineral medicines and their preparations.

# 岗 位 对 接
# Post Docking

本章为中药学、中药制药、中药资源专业学生必须掌握的内容，为成为合格的中药质量评价与控制人员奠定坚实的基础。

This task is the content that students of traditional Chinese medicine major must master and lays a solid foundation for becoming qualified personnel of quality evaluation and control of traditional Chinese medicine.

本章内容对应岗位包括中药药师、中药购销员、中药调剂员、中药材种植员、中药材生产管理员的相关工种。

The corresponding positions of this task include TCM pharmacist, TCM buyer and seller, TCM dispensing staff, TCM material planting staff and TCM production manager.

上述从事中药服务、中药购销和中药材生产种植相关所有岗位的从业人员均需要掌握中药各类化学成分分析方法的内容，能熟记各类化学成分的结构特点和理化性质，学会应用中药各类成分提取、纯化、鉴别和含量测定的方法开展中药学服务工作。

The above practitioners engaged in TCM service, TCM purchase, and sale, and TCM production and planting need to master the contents of various chemical composition analysis methods of TCM, be familiar with the structural characteristics and physical and chemical properties of various chemical ingredients, and learn to apply the methods of extraction, purification, identification and content determination of various components of TCM to carry out pharmaceutical service.

# 重 点 小 结
# Summary of Key Points

中药所含的生物碱类、黄酮类、萜类、醌类、挥发性成分、甾体类、多糖类、木脂素类、有机酸类、香豆素类等化学物质群是其防病治病的物质基础，由于化学结构和理化性质的不同，其提取纯化、定性鉴别和含量测定等原理和方法存在很大差异。

Alkaloids, flavonoids, terpenoids, quinones, volatile components, steroids, polysaccharides, lignans, organic acids, coumarins and other chemical groups in traditional Chinese medicine are the material basis for disease prevention and treatment. Due to the different chemical structure and physical and chemical properties, the principles and methods of extraction, purification, qualitative identification, and content determination are quite different.

中药各类化学成分的分析包括定性分析和定量分析。常用的定性分析方法有化学反应法、重量法、薄层色谱法、纸色谱法、气相色谱法、电泳法、离子交换色谱法、荧光法等，矿物药还可应用热分析法定性鉴别，其中以薄层色谱法应用最为广泛。常用的定量分析方法有分光光度法、薄层色谱扫描法、高效液相色谱法、气相色谱法、滴定法等，矿物药还可应用原子吸收光谱法和电感耦合等离子体光谱法定量分析，其中以高效液相色谱法应用最为普遍。因此，需要重点注意薄层色谱法和高效液相色谱法的原理和应用。

The analysis of various chemical components of traditional Chinese medicine includes qualitative analysis and quantitative analysis. The commonly used qualitative analysis methods include chemical reaction method, weight method, thin layer chromatography, paper chromatography, gas chromatography, electrophoresis, ion exchange chromatography, fluorescence method, etc. Mineral drugs can also be identified by thermal analysis, among which thin layer chromatography is the most widely used. The commonly used quantitative analysis methods include spectrophotometry, TLC scanning, HPLC, gas chromatography, titration, etc. Mineral drugs can also be quantitatively analyzed by atomic absorption spectrometry and inductively coupled plasma spectrometry, among which HPLC is the most commonly used. Therefore, we should pay more attention to the principle and application of TLC and HPLC.

# 目 标 检 测

题库

**一、选择题**

**（一）单项选择题**

1. 采用 $C_{18}$ 色谱柱对中药中生物碱类成分进行 HPLC 分析时，常采用的离子对试剂是

    A. 十二烷基磺酸钠                 B. 乙二胺

    C. 溴化四甲基胺                 D. 磷酸盐缓冲液

2. 从中药水提液中萃取三萜皂苷的常用有机溶剂是

    A. 苯                              B. 乙酸乙酯

    C. 三氯甲烷                      D. 正丁醇

3. 采用酸性染料比色法测定中药中生物碱类成分时，影响生物碱及酸性染料存在状态的因素是

    A. 反应时间　　　　　B. 反应温度　　　　　C. 溶液 pH　　　　　D. 溶剂极性

4. 采用比色法测定中药中蒽醌类成分时，用三氯甲烷或乙醚提取，提取液蒸干后，再加甲醇溶解定容，作为供试品溶液。该方法测定的是

    A. 总蒽醌　　　　　B. 游离蒽醌　　　　　C. 结合蒽醌　　　　　D. 以上三者

5. 可以通过观察升华物的显色反应或晶型来进行鉴别的中药是

    A. 人参　　　　　B. 乌头　　　　　C. 大黄　　　　　D. 黄芩

6. 由于中药中多数三萜皂苷类成分具有末端吸收，因此 HPLC 法测定三萜皂苷含量时常用的检测器是

    A. 蒸发光散射检测器　　　　　　　　B. 紫外检测器

    C. 荧光检测器　　　　　　　　　　　D. 电化学检测器

7. 与 $Al^{3+}$ 反应用来鉴别中药中黄酮类成分，会出现阴性结果的基团是

    A. 3-OH　　　　　B. 5-OH　　　　　C. 7-OH　　　　　D. 邻二酚羟基

8. 关于中药中黄酮类成分的溶解性，以下说法错误的是

    A. 黄酮苷一般易溶于水、甲醇等强极性溶剂

    B. 黄酮苷糖链越长，则水溶性越大

    C. 苷元中羟基数越多，脂溶性越大

    D. 黄酮苷元易溶于甲醇、乙酸乙酯等有机溶剂

9. 有关多糖的纸色谱法鉴别，下列说法正确的是

    A. 常用 BAW 系统为展开剂

    B. 为减小 $R_f$ 值，可在展开剂中加入乙酸、吡啶、乙醇等

    C. 显色剂常用硫酸乙醇溶液、α - 萘酚 - 浓硫酸或茴香醛 - 浓硫酸试剂

    D. 喷显色剂后一般不需要加热，斑点即刻出现

10. 测定甾体总皂苷一般用

    A. 薄层色谱扫描法　　　　　　　　　B. 高效液相色谱法

    C. 气相色谱法　　　　　　　　　　　D. 重量法

11. 应用荧光法鉴别香豆素类成分时，下列说法错误的是

    A. 香豆素母核本身无荧光，其 $C_7$ 位羟基衍生物却呈强烈的蓝色荧光

    B. 碱性溶液中荧光减弱

    C. $C_7$ 位的邻位即 $C_6$ 或 $C_8$ 位引入羟基，则荧光减弱或消失

    D. 呋喃香豆素多显较弱的蓝色或褐色荧光

**（二）多项选择题**

1. 采用比色法测定中药中总黄酮类时，常用的显色系统是

    A. 氢氧化钠　　　　　　B. 亚硝酸钠　　　　　　C. 香草醛

    D. 硝酸铝　　　　　　　E. 茚三酮

2. 常用于中药中蒽醌类成分化学反应鉴别的试剂是

    A. 盐酸 - 镁粉　　　　　B. 碱溶液　　　　　　　C. 磷钼酸试液

    D. 醋酸镁甲醇试液　　　E. 茚三酮

3. 易溶于水的生物碱是

    A. 季铵碱　　　　　　　B. 大多数游离生物碱　　C. 含氮氧配位键的生物碱

    D. 仲胺碱　　　　　　　E. 麻黄碱

4. 采用比色法测定中药中三萜皂苷类成分时，常用显色剂的是

    A. 香草醛 - 硫酸           B. 碘化铋钾           C. 香草醛 - 高氯酸

    D. 醋酐 - 硫酸           E. 盐酸 - 镁粉

5. 有关中药挥发性成分的薄层色谱法鉴别，下列说法正确的是

    A. 吸附剂常用硅胶 G 或中性氧化铝

    B. 组成复杂的挥发油，双向展开或二次展开效果较好

    C. 含氧烃类常以正己烷（或石油醚）作展开剂

    D. 可根据挥发油成分中双键数目和位置不同，用硝酸银薄层分离，硝酸银在吸附剂中的
含量以大于 50% 为宜

    E. 含氧烃类用正己烷（或石油醚）- 醋酸乙酯展开

6. 中药所含总有机酸的含量测定，可用以下哪种方法

    A. 分光光度法           B. 高效液相色谱法           C. 酸碱滴定法

    D. 薄层色谱扫描法           E. 气相色谱法

# 第八章 不同类型中药的质量分析特点

# Chapter 8 Characteristics of Quality Analysis of Different Types of Traditional Chinese Medicine Samples

 学习目标 | Learning Goal

**知识要求：**

1. 掌握 固体和液体中药样品的质量分析特点。

2. 熟悉 半固体中药样品的质量分析特点。

3. 了解 外用膏剂的质量分析特点。

**能力要求：**

学会应用不同类型中药样品质量分析的特点去解决中药材（饮片）、提取物和中药制剂的质量分析。

**Knowledge Requirements**

**1. Master** The quality analysis characteristics of solid and liquid Chinese medicine samples.

**2. Familiar** The characteristics of quality analysis of semi-solid traditional Chinese medicine samples.

**3. Understand** The Characteristics of quality analysis of external ointment.

**Ability Requirements**

Learn to apply the characteristics of quality analysis of different types of Chinese medicine samples to solve the quality analysis of Chinese herbal medicines (pieces), extracts and Chinese medicine preparations.

中药按其物态可分为固体、半固体、液体、外用膏剂和其他类型，其质量分析的特点也各有不同。

Chinese medicine can be divided into liquid, semi-solid, solid, topical ointment and other types according to its physical state, and the characteristics of its quality analysis are also different.

## 第一节 液体中药的质量分析特点

## 8.1 Analysis of Liquid Chinese Medicine

PPT

液体中药样品包括挥发油、油脂以及合剂、酒剂、酊剂、注射剂等制剂。液体制剂的取样要有代表性，应摇匀后取样，还需要注意液体制剂中防腐剂、矫味剂对分析的影响。

Liquid traditional Chinese medicine samples include volatile oils, oils and fats, mixtures, medicinal wines, tinctures, injections and so on. Sampling of liquid preparations should be representative. Samples should be taken after shaking well, and attention should be paid to the influence of preservatives and flavoring agents on the analysis.

### 一、中药挥发油和油脂
### 8.1.1 Chinese Medicine Volatile Oil and Grease

挥发油是与水不相混的油状液体，多为单萜、倍半萜及其含氧衍生物。一般用一定浓度的乙醇，或用有机溶剂（如乙酸乙酯、石油醚）提取后分析。植物油脂可直接用有机溶剂溶解后进行分析，或衍生化后用 GC 进行分析。

Volatile oil is an oily liquid immiscible with water, mostly monoterpenes, sesquiterpenes and their oxygenated derivatives. Generally, ethanol with a certain concentration or organic solvents (such as ethyl acetate and petroleum ether) are used for extraction and analysis. Vegetable oils and fats can be directly dissolved in organic solvents for analysis or derivatized and analyzed by GC.

### 二、液体中药制剂
### 8.1.2 Analysis of Chinese Medicine Liquid Preparations

液体中药制剂包括合剂、酒剂、酊剂等。液体中药制剂中的溶剂大多为水或乙醇，根据目标成分的理化性质、溶剂种类及杂质情况，可采用液 - 液萃取法等进行样品前处理，以达到富集纯化目的。液体中药制剂常含有防腐剂、矫味剂等辅料，需要消除该类辅料成分对样品分析的干扰。此外还应注意样品取样的均匀性、代表性，一般应摇匀后再取样。

Chinese medicine liquid preparations include mixtures, medicinal wines, tinctures, etc. Generally, the solvent in Chinese medicine liquid preparations is water or ethanol. The appropriate separation and purification methods, such as liquid-liquid extraction can be selected, according to the physicochemical properties of the targeted components, the type of solvent, and the amount of impurities. Chinese medicine liquid preparations often contain auxiliary materials including preservatives and flavoring agents, thus, it is necessary to eliminate the interference of such auxiliary materials for sample analysis. In addition, liquid samples should be collected after shaking to get a uniform solution for further analysis.

（一）合剂与口服液
1. Mixtures and Oral Solution

合剂是传统汤剂的改进，溶剂多为水，杂质含量较大，特别是水溶性杂质，有一定的黏度，很难直接分析，大多情况下需纯化后进行分析。合剂常用纯化前处理方法有液 - 液萃取法和固相萃取法，可结合定性定量方法选择使用。在液 - 液萃取法中还可利用待测成分的酸、碱性，先将提取液酸化或碱化，再用有机溶剂进行萃取。口服液因其制剂制备工艺中多已含有纯化步骤，杂质含量相对较少，有的可稀释后或直接进行分析。但当药味较多、成分复杂时，分析前需纯化处理，方法与一般合剂相似。

The Chinese medicine mixture is an improve dose form of the traditional decoction. The solvent is mostly water, the impurity content is large, especially the water-soluble impurities, have a certain viscosity, it is difficult to directly analyze, in most cases it needs to be analyzed after purification. Commonly used purification pretreatment methods for mixtures include liquid-liquid extraction and solid-phase extraction, which can be used in combination with qualitative and quantitative methods. In the liquid-liquid extraction method, the acid and alkalinity of the components to be tested can also be used, and the extraction liquid is first acidified or alkalized, then extracted with an organic solvent. Oral liquids already contain purification steps in the preparation process of their preparations, and the content of impurities is relatively small, and some can be diluted or directly analyzed. However, when the medicine has more Chinese crude drug and complex components, it needs to be purified before analysis. The method is similar to the general mixtures.

### （二）酒剂、酊剂
### 2. Medicinal Wines and Tinctures

酒剂和酊剂因含醇量较高，因此蛋白质、多糖、黏液质、鞣质等水溶性大分子杂质较少，澄明度也好，样品的前处理相对简单，大多可直接进行分析。但对于一些成分复杂的酒剂、酊剂，仍需纯化处理后方可进行分析，常用的纯化方法是通过加热除去样品中的乙醇，然后再用适当的有机溶剂对待测成分进行萃取。当待测成分为生物碱类或酸性成分时，可先蒸去样品中的乙醇，碱化或酸化后，再用有机溶剂萃取。也可用柱层析法对除乙醇后的样品进行纯化处理。

There are few water-soluble macromolecular impurities such as protein, polysaccharides, mucus and gums in medicinal wines and tinctures of Chinese medicine with high ethanol and clarity. The sample pretreatment is relatively simple, and most of them can be analyzed directly. However, some medicinal wines and tinctures with complex components still need to be purified before analysis. The common purification method is to remove ethanol from the sample by heating, and then extract the components to be tested with an appropriate organic solvent. When the component to be tested is an alkaloid or acidic component, the ethanol in the sample can be distilled off first, then alkalized or acidified, and then extracted with an organic solvent. Column chromatography can also be used to purify the sample after removing ethanol.

### 三、中药注射剂
### 8.1.3 Chinese Medicinal Injection

中药注射剂一般以中药饮片或提取物为原料进行制备，其原料药物均有相应的质量控制，并严格按各品种规定的方法进行提取和纯化，在制备过程中除去了大量的杂质，同时在一定程度上保留了中药多成分的特点。因此，中药注射剂前处理方法较简便，通常可直接分析或经溶解、稀释后进行分析。对于药味较多，成分间干扰较大的注射剂，可根据成分的理化性质选择适宜的净化方法，其处理方法与合剂、口服液相似。

Traditional Chinese medicinal injection is generally prepared with decoction pieces or extractives as crude drugs, which are extracted and purified strictly according to the related specified requirements. During the preparation process, most of the impurities are removed, while the multi-component characteristics of TCM are retained to some extent. Therefore, the pretreatment method of CMI is relatively simple, and the injections can be analyzed directly or after dissolved and diluted. For CMI containing several Chinese medical materials, the interferences between components can be eliminated by choosing suitable purification methods, according to the physicochemical properties of the components. The method of purification is similar to the mixtures and oral solutions.

由于中药注射剂给药途径的特殊性，其质量要求较口服制剂更为严格。比如中药注射剂要进行指纹图谱研究，有关物质和相关物质的检查，以及安全性检查。

The requirements for quality analysis of CMI are more stringent than those of oral formulations. For example, traditional Chinese medicine injections are asked for fingerprint study, related substance and related substance inspection, and safety inspection.

### 四、实例
### 8.1.4　Examples

例 8-1　清开灵注射液

Example 8-1　The Quality Analysis of Qingkailing Zhusheye (Qingkailing Injection)

【指纹图谱】照高效液相色谱法测定。

**Fingerprint**　Carry out the method for high performance liquid chromatography.

**色谱条件与系统适用性试验**　以十八烷基硅烷键合硅胶为填充剂（色谱柱 Phenomenex Luna C18 250mm×4.6mm，5μm）；以乙腈为流动相 A，以 0.1% 甲酸溶液为流动相 B，梯度洗脱（略）；流速为 0.5ml/min；检测波长为 254nm，柱温为 25℃。理论板数按栀子苷峰计算，应不低于 100000。

*Chromatographic system and system suitability*　Use octadecylsilane bonded silica gel as the stationary phase (column, Phenomenex Luna C18，250mm×4.6mm，5μm), acetonitrile and 0.1% formic acid solution as the mobile phases, elute in gradient. Flow rate set at 0.5ml per minute. As detector a spectrophotometer set at 254nm, maintain the column temperature at 25℃. The number of theoretical plates for the column is not less than 100000, calculated with the reference to the peak of geniposide.

**参照物溶液的制备**　取栀子苷对照品适量，精密称定，加甲醇制成每 1ml 含 0.2mg 的溶液，即得。

*Reference solution*　Dissolve a quantity of geniposide CRS, accurately weighted, in methanol to produce a mixture containing 0.2mg per ml.

**供试品溶液的制备**　取本品，滤过，取续滤液，即得。

*Test solution*　Filter the injection and use the successive filtrate as the test solution.

**测定法**　分别精密吸取参照物溶液和供试品溶液各 10μl，注入液相色谱仪，测定，记录 85 分钟内的色谱图，即得。

*Procedure*　Inject accurately 10μl of the reference solution and the test solution separately into the column, record chromatogram within 85 minutes.

本品指纹图谱中应呈现与栀子苷对照品色谱峰保留时间一致的色谱峰，并应出现 10 个共有峰，以 1、3、5、6、7、8、9、10（S）号峰为标记，经中药色谱指纹图谱相似度评价系统软件计算，与对照指纹图谱相比较，相似度不得低于 0.80（图 8-1）。

The peak retention time in the chromatogram obtained with the test solution correspond to that in the chromatogram obtained with geniposide reference solution. Among 10 peaks, according to the similarity evaluation system for chromatographic fingerprint of TCM, calculate the similarity between the test solution fingerprint and the reference fingerprint. Not less than 0.80 marked with peak 1, 3, 5, 6, 7, 8, 9, 10 (S) (Fig.8-1).

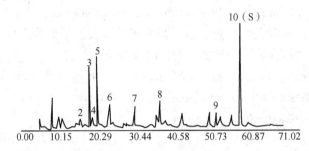

图 8-1　清开灵注射液对照指纹图谱

Fig. 8-1　Control fingerprint of Qingkailing injection

峰 10（S）：栀子苷

Peak 10 (S): Gardenoside

【检查】山银花　取本品 20ml，加盐酸 3 滴，边加边搅拌，滤过，滤液加氢氧化钠试液调节 pH 值至 7，用水饱和的正丁醇振摇提取 2 次，每次 30ml，合并正丁醇液，用氨试液洗涤两次，每次 30ml，分取正丁醇液，蒸干，残渣加甲醇 2ml 使溶解，作为供试品溶液。另取灰毡毛忍冬皂苷对照品，加甲醇制成每 1ml 含 1mg 的溶液，作为对照品溶液。照薄层色谱法（《中国药典》通则 0502）试验，吸取上述两种溶液各 2μl，分别点于同一硅胶 G 薄层板上，以三氯甲烷 - 甲醇 - 水（6：4：1）为展开剂，展开，取出，晾干，喷以 10% 硫酸乙醇溶液，在 105℃加热至斑点显色清晰。供试品色谱中，在与对照品色谱相应的位置上，不得显相同颜色的斑点。

**Inspections**　*Lonicerae flos*　To 20ml of the injection, add 3 drops of hydrochloric acid by stirring. Filter and adjust the pH value of filtrate to 7 with sodium hydroxide TS. Extract the filtrate with two 30ml quantities of *n*-butanol saturated with water, combine the *n*-butanol extracts, wash with two 30ml quantities of ammonia TS, and evaporate the *n*-butanol to dryness. Dissolve the residue in 2ml of methanol as the lest solution. Dissolve dipsacaceae saponin B CRS in methanol to produce a solution containing 1mg per ml as the reference solution. Carry out the method for thin layer chromatography (*Chinese Pharmacopoeia*, general chapters 0502), using silica gel as the coating substance and a mixture of chloroform, methanol and water (6：4：1) as the mobile phase. Apply separately 2μl of each of the above two solutions to the plate. After developing and removal of the plate, dry in air. Spray with a 10% solution of sulfuric acid in ethanol, heat at 105℃ to the spots clear. The spot in the chromatogram obtained with the test solution should not appear spot which corresponds in position and colour to the spot in chromatogram obtained with the reference solution.

**溶液的颜色**　精密量取本品 1ml，置 50ml 量瓶中，加水稀释至刻度，摇匀，与黄色 10 号标准比色液比较，应不得更深。

*Color of solution*　Measure accurately 1ml injection to a 50ml volumetric flask, dilute with water to volume and mix well. The color of the test solution should not intense than the yellow reference solution No 10.

**pH 值**　应为 6.8~7.5。

*pH value*　6.8-7.5.

**炽灼残渣**　精密量取本品 5ml，按照炽灼残渣检查法测定，每 1ml 应为 3.0~8.5mg。

*Residue on ignition*　Measure accurately 5ml of the injection, carry out the method of residue on ignition. It should not less than 3.0 and not more than 8.5mg per ml.

**总固体**　精密量取本品 2ml，置 105℃ 干燥至恒重的蒸发皿中，蒸干，在 105℃ 干燥 2 小时，移至干燥器中，冷却 30 分钟，迅速精密称定重量，每 1ml 遗留残渣应为 30~60mg。

*Total solid*　Measure accurately 2ml of the injection to a 105℃ tared evaporating dish. Evaporate to dryness, dry at 105℃ for 2 hours. Transfer to a desiccator and cool for 30 minutes. Weigh quickly and accurately. The residue should not less than 30mg and not more than 60mg per ml.

**有关物质**　除蛋白质、树脂、草酸盐外，应符合规定。

*Materials about injection*　Complies with the general requirement for determination of materials about injection, except protein, oxalate and potassium.

**蛋白质**　取本品 1ml，加鞣酸试液 1~3 滴，不得出现浑浊。

*Protein*　To 1ml of the injection, add 1-3 drops of tannic acid TS, opalescence should not be observed.

**树脂**　取本品 5ml，加三氯甲烷 10ml，振摇提取，分取三氯甲烷液，置水浴上蒸干，残渣加冰醋酸 2ml 使溶解，置具塞试管中，加水 3ml，混匀，放置 30 分钟，可有轻微浑浊，不得出现絮状物或沉淀。

*Resin*　Measure the injection 5ml, add 10ml of chloroform, extract by shaking, and evaporate the chloroform to dryness. Dissolve the residue in 2ml of glacial acetic acid and transfer to a stoppered tube, add 3ml of water, mix well and stand for 30 minutes. Opalescence slightly, and flocculus should not be observed.

**草酸盐**　取本品 5ml，置离心管中，滴加 6mol/L 盐酸溶液 5 滴，搅匀，离心，吸取上清液，滤过，取滤液 2ml，调节 pH 值至 5~6，加 3% 氯化钙溶液 2~3 滴，放置 10 分钟，不得出现沉淀。

*Oxalate*　Measure 5ml in a centrifugal tube, add 5 drops of 6mol/L hydrochloric acid, mix well, centrifuge. Filter the supernatant, measure 2ml of the filtrate, adjust the pH value to 5-6, add 2-3 drops of 3% solution of calcium chloride and allow to set for 10 minutes. No precipitate should be observed.

**重金属**　精密量取本品 1ml，置坩埚中，蒸干，再缓缓炽灼至完全灰化，放冷，照重金属检查法（《中国药典》通则 0821）第一法检查，含重金属不得过 10mg/kg。

*Heavy metals*　Measure accurately 1ml of the injection in a crucible, evaporate to dryness. Ignite slowly to complete charred, allow to cool, carry out the limit lest for heavy metals (*Chinese Pharmacopoeia*, general chapters 0821). Not more than 10mg per kg.

**异常毒性**　取本品，依法检查（《中国药典》通则 1141），静脉注射给药，剂量按每只小鼠注射 0.5ml，应符合规定。

*Abnormal toxicity*　Complies with requirement in the test for abnormal toxicity (*Chinese Pharmacopoeia*, general chapters 1141), using 0.5ml per mice by intravenous administration.

**过敏反应**　取本品，依法检查（《中国药典》通则 1147），应符合规定。

*Allergen*　Complies with requirement in the limit test for allergen (*Chinese Pharmacopoeia*, general chapters 1147).

**热原** 取本品，依法检查（《中国药典》1142），剂量按家兔体重每1kg注射5ml，应符合规定。

*Pyrogens* Complies with requirement in the test for pyrogens (*Chinese Pharmacopoeia*, general chapters 1142), using 5ml per kilogram of the rabbit's weight.

**溶血与凝聚** 取本品，依法检查（《中国药典》通则1148），应符合规定。

*Haemolysis and agglomertion* Complies with requirement in the limit test for hamolysis and agglomertion (*Chinese Pharmacopoeia*, general chapters 1148).

**其他** 应符合注射剂项下有关的各项规定（《中国药典》通则0102）。

*Other requirements* Complies with the general requirements for injection (*Chinese Pharmacopoeia*, general chapters 0102).

PPT

## 第二节 半固体中药的质量分析特点
## 8.2 Analysis of Semi-Solid Chinese Medicine

半固体中药样品包括流浸膏剂、浸膏剂、糖浆剂、煎膏剂（膏滋）和凝胶剂等。

Chinese medicine semi-solid preparations include liquid extracts, extracts, syrups and concentrated decoctions, etc.

### 一、流浸膏剂和浸膏剂
### 8.2.1　Extracts and Liquid Extracts

流浸膏剂和浸膏剂若杂质较多，则可用萃取法及柱色谱分离法等进行纯化处理。处理时，将样品稀释后，再采用液-液萃取法，根据待测成分的性质选取适宜溶剂萃取；也可将样品稀释后调节pH值，再用适宜的溶剂提取，以利于酸性、碱性成分的分离。当待测成分具有挥发性时，可采用蒸馏法提取。对于单味药材制成的流浸膏或浸膏，杂质相对较少，可以稀释后直接分析。

If there are many impurities in the flow extract and extract, they can be purified by extraction and column chromatography. Due to extracts and liquid extracts are relatively sticky, and the sample can be diluted, and then the liquid-liquid extraction method is applied. Meanwhile, the sample can also be diluted and adjusted to different pH value, and then extracted with a suitable solvent. When the targeted components are volatile, distillation can be used. For the liquid extracts or extracts of single herb with fewer impurities, the sample can be directly analyzed after dilution.

### 二、煎膏剂和糖浆剂
### 8.2.2　The Concentrated Decoctions and Syrups

煎膏剂、糖浆剂含有较多的糖或者蜜，溶液较黏稠，可在样品中加入适量的惰性材料（如硅藻土、纤维素等），经低温烘干后，按固体样品处理。亦或将样品先加水或稀醇稀释，按液体样品处理。若待测成分为酸性、碱性成分，可采用pH梯度萃取；也可采用固相萃取法将制剂中的大量糖分去除后进行质量分析；当待测成分为挥发性成分时，可采用水蒸气蒸馏。

Decoctions and syrups contain more sugar or honey, and the solution is more viscous. You can add an appropriate amount of inert materials (such as diatomite, cellulose, etc.) to the sample. After drying at low temperature, treat it as a solid sample. Alternatively, dilute the sample with water or dilute alcohol, and treat it as a liquid sample. If the component to be tested is acid or alkaline, pH gradient extraction can be used; solid phase extraction can also be used to remove a large amount of sugar in the preparation for quality analysis; when the component to be tested is volatile, distillation of water vapor can be used.

### 三、凝胶剂
### 8.2.3　Gel

单相分散系统基质的凝胶剂可分为水性凝胶剂与油性凝胶剂。水性凝胶基质一般由水、保湿剂（甘油或丙二醇）与水溶性高分子材料（卡波姆、海藻酸盐、西黄蓍胶、明胶等）构成；油性凝胶基质由液状石蜡与聚氧乙烯或脂肪油与胶体硅或铝皂、锌皂构成。两相分散系统基质的凝胶剂有乳状液型凝胶剂、混悬型凝胶剂等。凝胶剂需根据基质性质的不同。参考栓剂进行处理。

The gel of the single-phase dispersion system matrix can be divided into aqueous gel agents and oil gel agents. The water-based gel matrix is generally composed of water, humectants (glycerin or propylene glycol) and water-soluble polymer materials (carbomer, alginate, tragacanth, gelatin, etc.); the oily gel matrix is composed of liquid paraffin and polyoxygen ethylene or fatty oil and colloidal silicon or aluminum soap, zinc soap. The gel agents of the two-phase dispersion system matrix include emulsified gels agents, suspension gel agents, and so on. The gel should be based on the nature of the matrix. Refer to suppositories for treatment.

### 四、实例
### 8.2.4　Examples

例 8-2　小儿止咳糖浆

Example 8-2　Xiao'er Zhike Syrup

【鉴别】取本品 2ml，加水 6ml，摇匀，滤过，取滤液 1ml，加稀盐酸数滴，生成沉淀，再加氨试液适量，沉淀可溶解。

**Identification**　To 2ml, add 6ml of water, mix well filter. To 1ml of the filtrate, add several drops of dilute hydrochloric acid, a precipitate is produced, then add a quantity of ammonia TS, the precipitate can be dissolved.

## 第三节　固体中药的质量分析特点

## 8.3　Analysis of Solid Chinese Medicine

固体中药样品包括中药材、饮片、中药提取物及丸剂、散剂、栓剂、颗粒剂、片剂、胶囊剂等中药制剂。中药材、饮片以及全部或部分使用中药饮片细粉入药的制剂，因待测成分仍存在于植物组织、细胞中，因此，应注意提取溶剂、提取方法和提取时间的选择。而中药提取物，选用合适的溶剂溶解即可。此外，在中药制剂中还要注意辅料对分析的干扰，例如蜜丸中的糖和蜂蜜。

Solid Chinese medicine samples include Chinese medicinal materials, decoction pieces, Chinese medicine extracts and pills, powders, suppositories, granules, tablets, capsules and other Chinese medicine preparations. Traditional Chinese medicinal materials, decoction pieces, and all or part of the preparations using fine powders of traditional Chinese medicine decoctions, because the components to be tested are still present in plant tissues and cells, so attention should be paid to the choice of extraction solvent, extraction method, and extraction time. The Chinese medicine extracts can be dissolved in a suitable solvent. In addition, attention should be paid to the interference of excipients in the analysis of traditional Chinese medicine preparations, such as sugar and honey in honey pills.

## 一、中药材和饮片
### 8.3.1　Chinese Herbal Medicines (Pieces)

中药材（饮片）有完整性状特征可采用性状鉴别；无完整形状或特征不明显的可采用显微鉴别。在饮片的理化分析中，植物药其待测成分存在于植物组织、细胞中，不易溶出。因此，需要根据其质地粉碎成不同的粒度，然后采用适宜的方法进行提取。矿物药样品粉碎后，用适当的方法进行溶解或熔融后再进行测定。

Most of the decoction pieces remain the characteristics of surface, cutting specifications, colour and odour of Chinese Materia Medica. The description and microscopical identification are of great importance in judging the authenticity of decoction pieces. In physicochemical analysis, the components of the botanical drug to be tested are present in plant tissues and cells and are not easily dissolved. Therefore, it needs to be pulverized into different particle sizes according to its texture, and then extracted by an appropriate method. After crushing the mineral medicine sample, dissolve or melt it by an appropriate method and then measure.

注意炮制对饮片质量分析的影响，一些加入甘草、黑豆等辅料炮制的品种，辅料中的成分可作为饮片的指标成分，如法半夏可通过薄层检识甘草次酸，鉴别真伪。一些药材中的化学成分在加工过程中，有可能发生变化，如生地黄中的梓醇遇热不稳定，炮制后含量降低，不再作为熟地黄的指标成分。

The effect of processing on the chemical compositions should be noticed. Some decoction pieces are processed with licorice, black beans and other excipients, the ingredients from the excipients can be used as its maker compounds. For example, Pinellia Praeparatum Rhizoma (Fabanxia) can be identified by detecting glycyrrhetinic acid with TLC method. On the other hand, some components in decoction pieces may be changed in the processing such as catalpol, the marker compound of Rehmannia Radix. It can be destroyed by heating and the content in Rehmannia Radix Praeparata is too low to detect.

饮片在保存过程中，易生虫、发霉，产生微生物毒素，为便于保存和改善饮片外观，在饮片中非法添加色素、杀虫剂等有害物质及使用硫黄熏蒸等现象时有发生，因此，在中药饮片的质量分析中应注意对外源性有害物质进行检查，保证用药安全。

In addition, some decoction pieces are fumigated with sulfur or added illegal additions, such as pigments, pesticides and other harmful substances, to prevent insects, mildew or facilitate the preservation and improve the appearance. Therefore, in the quality analysis of decoction pieces, the inspection of exogenous harmful substances should be inspected to ensure the safety in clinical practice.

### 二、固体中药制剂
### 8.3.2 Solid Chinese Medicine Preparations

固体中药制剂包括丸剂、片剂、颗粒剂、散剂、栓剂等。

There are many kinds of solid preparations of traditional Chinese medicines (TCM), including pills, tablets, granules, powders, suppositories, etc.

#### （一）丸剂
#### 1. Pills

水蜜丸、水丸、浓缩丸、糊丸、蜡丸等可以直接研细或粉碎后进行提取。滴丸含有大量的聚乙二醇（6000、4000）等水溶性基质和硬脂酸、氢化植物油等水不溶性基质。基质对其分析的影响较大，因此，须将基质与待测成分分离。对一些酸性或碱性待测成分，可以通过酸化或碱化处理，使其游离或成盐后，用有机溶剂或水提取，从而使待测成分与基质分离。蜜丸中由于含有大量的炼蜜，不能直接研细或粉碎，可将其剪碎或用小刀将其切成小块后，加溶剂进行提取；如果测定蜜丸中待测成分有较强的脂溶性，也可用水将蜜丸溶解，离心后取药渣，再用合适的溶剂对药渣进行提取；也可直接加甲醇、乙醇等亲水性有机溶剂对切成小块的蜜丸直接提取；或者采用硅藻土（0.5~2倍）等惰性材料与蜜丸研磨，使蜜丸分散均匀，再用合适的溶剂提取。另外还应注意，有些成分能被硅藻土吸附，造成回收率偏低。

Most pills can be ground or pulverized directly for extraction except honeyed pills, which contain a large amount of honey and need special handling. Dropping pills contain a large amount of water-soluble bases such as polyethylene glycol (6000, 4000) and water-insoluble bases such as stearic acid and hydrogenated vegetable oil. The matrix has a great influence on its analysis. Therefore, the matrix must be separated from the components to be tested. For some acidic or alkaline components to be tested, they can be freed or salted by acidification or alkalization, and then extracted with organic solvents or water to separate the components to be tested from the matrix. For extracting fat-soluble component, the honeyed pills can be dispersed with water, centrifuged to obtain the residue, then extracted the residue with organic solvent. Another method is to extract the honeyed pills directly with hydrophilic organic solvents after cut into small pieces. In addition, the honeyed pill can be dispersed with kieselguhr (0.5-2 times) and then extracted with solvent. It should be noted that some components might be adsorbed on the kieselguhr tightly, and resulting in a low recovery rate.

#### （二）片剂
#### 2. Tablets

中药片剂一般用提取物制备，也有部分片剂含药材原粉。片剂在制备过程中常加有一定量的赋形剂，如淀粉、糊精、糖粉、硫酸钙等，赋形剂可能会影响片剂的分析，但由于这些赋形剂多数是水溶性的，可以选择有机溶剂进行提取，排除其干扰。有的片剂还加入中药饮片细粉，一些成分仍存留在植物组织、细胞中，需要选择合适的溶剂和提取方法进行提取。常用片剂的处理方法为将片剂研碎（糖衣片要先去除糖衣）、过筛后提取。

Chinese medicinal tablets are generally prepared with extracts, and some tablets contain crude powder of materials. Excipients such as starch, dextrin, sugar powder, microcrystalline cellulose, and calcium sulfate are often used during the preparation process, which may affect on the quality analysis of the tablet. It is important to note that the excipients of tablets are generally water-soluble, and their interference can be removed when the tablets is extracted with a suitable organic solvent. Some also add fine powder of Chinese herbal medicine, ingredients still remain in plant tissues and cells, and need to choose appropriate solvent and extraction method for extraction. The commonly used tablet processing method is to crush the tablets (the sugar-coated tablets must be removed from the sugar-coated tablets), sieve and extract.

片剂的含量常以每片中所含被测成分的重量来表示。若有效成分明确、结构已知、规格具体，则常按标示量计算的百分含量来表示每片中有效成分测得的实际含量与标示量的符合程度。但在实际生产中，不可能做到每个药片的重量完全一致，因此，常用平均片重作为每片重量进行含量测定的计算。为了使取样具有代表性，一般取 10~20 个药片，精密称定，计算平均片重，然后研细、混匀后，从中精密称取适量，作为每次分析用的样品。按标示量计算百分含量的算式如下：

Tablet content is expressed in terms of the weight of the marker component contained in each piece. If the active ingredient and the specification of the tablet are clear, its percentage content, calculated by the labeled amount, is often used to indicate the degree of conformity between the measured content and the labeled amount per tablet. However, the weight of each tablet can not be completely consistent. And the average tablet weight is usually used as the tablet weight to calculate the content. The method is as follows: Weigh accurately 10-20 tablets and calculate the average weight, pulverize to fine powder and mix well, then weigh an appropriate amount accurately to analysis. The formula for calculating the percentage content is as follows:

$$标示量（\%）= \frac{样品中被测成分测得的实际含量 \times 平均片重}{标示量} \times 100\% \qquad (8\text{-}1)$$

$$\text{Labeled amount}（\%）= \frac{\text{the measured content} \times \text{the average tablet weight}}{\text{labeled amount}} \times 100\% \qquad (8\text{-}1)$$

含量均匀度是保证治疗量与极量接近、剂量小而作用强的药物的安全性和有效性，以及提高含辅料较多、主药与辅料分散性差、不易混合均匀的片剂质量的重要指标。《中国药典》规定，片剂、硬胶囊剂、颗粒剂或散剂等，每一个单剂标示量小于25mg 或主药含量小于每一个单剂重量 25% 者，应根据《中国药典》通则 0941 对其进行含量均匀度检查。

Content uniformity could influence the safety and efficacy of the narrow therapeutic range drugs, especially those which have low dose and high excipient/API (active pharmaceutical ingredient) ratio. It also reflect the quality of the drugs that the raw materials is difficult to mixed evenly in the preparation process due to poor drug dispersity. For tablets, hard capsules, granules or powders containing less than 25mg or active pharmaceutical ingredient comprising less than 25% of a single-dose unit by weight, the test for content uniformity should be carry out and comply with the requirements specified in *Chinese Pharmacopoeia* (general chapters 0941).

除另有规定外，取供试品 10 个，照各品种项下规定的方法，分别测定每一个单剂以标示量为 100 的相对含量 $X_i$，求其均值 $\overline{X}$ 和标准差 $S$（$S = \sqrt{S = \dfrac{\sum_{i=1}^{n}/(X_i - \overline{X})^2}{n-1}}$）以及标示量与均值之差的绝对值 $A$（$A = |100 - \overline{X}|$）。

Unless otherwise specified, take 10 dosage units of the substance being examined, carry out the method as specified in the monograph and determine separately the relative content $x_i$, of each dosage unit which is expressed 100 as the labelled amount. Calculate the mean value $\overline{X}$, the standard deviation

$S$ ( $S=\sqrt{\dfrac{\sum_{i=1}^{n}/(X_i-\overline{X})^2}{n-1}}$ ) and the absolute value $A$ ( $A=|100-\overline{X}|$ ) which is the difference between the labelled amount and the mean value.

若 $A+2.2S \leqslant L$，则供试品的含量均匀度符合规定；

If $A+2.2S \leqslant L$, the substance being examined complies with the requirements for content uniformity；

若 $A+S>L$，则不符合规定；

If $A+S>L$, the substance being examined fails to comply with the requirements for content uniformity；

若 $A+2.2S>L$，且 $A+S<L$，则应另取供试品 20 个复试。

If $A+2.2S>L$, and $A+S<L$, then repeat the test using another 20 dosage units.

根据初、复试结果，计算 30 个单剂的均值 $\overline{X}$、标准差 S 和标示量与均值之差的绝对值 $A$。再按下述公式计算并判定。

According to the results of the first and the repeated tests of 30 dosage units, calculate the mean values $\overline{X}$, the standard deviation $S$ and the absolute value $A$ which is the difference between the labelled amount and the mean value. Then calculate and judge as follows.

当 $A \leqslant 0.25L$ 时，若 $A^2+S^2 \leqslant 0.25L^2$，则供试品的含量均匀度符合规定；若 $A^2+S^2 > 0.25L^2$，则不符合规定。

When $A \leqslant 0.25L$, if $A^2+S^2 \leqslant 0.25L^2$, the substance being examined complies with the requirements for content uniformity; If $A^2+S^2 \leqslant 0.25L^2$, the substance being examined fails to comply with the requirements for content uniformity.

当 $A>0.25L$ 时，若 $A+1.7S \leqslant L$，则供试品的含量均匀度符合规定；若 $A+1.7S>L$，则不符合规定。

When $A>0.25L$, if $A+1.7S \leqslant L$, the substance being examined complies with the requirements for content uniformity; $A+1.7S>L$, the substance being examined fails to comply with the requirements for content uniformity.

上述公式中 $L$ 为规定值。除另有规定外，$L=15.0$；单剂量包装的口服混悬液、内充非均相溶液的软胶囊、胶囊型或泡囊型粉雾剂、单剂量包装的眼用、耳用、鼻用混悬剂、固体或半固体制剂 $L=20.0$；透皮贴剂、栓剂 $L=25.0$。

$L$ in the above formulas is specified. Unless otherwise specified, $L=15.0$. Single-dose oral suspension, soft capsule filled with heterogeneous solution, capsule or blister powder, single-dose ophthalmic, otic, nasal suspension, solid or semi-solid preparation, $L=20.0$. Transdermal patches, suppositories, $L=25.0$.

（三）颗粒剂

### 3. Granules

中药颗粒剂在制备时大多采用醇沉法除去了大部分水溶性杂质，且制剂呈颗粒状态，待测成分易溶出，因此在分析时，可根据待测成分和干扰成分的性质选择适宜的溶剂直接进行提取，提取方法常用超声法或回流法。对于含药材细粉的颗粒剂，应注意考察提取时间和温度，使待测成分充分溶出。

颗粒剂大多含有乳糖、糊精、淀粉等辅料，用水或低浓度乙醇提取时，所得提取液黏稠，而用有机溶剂提取时，容易形成不溶性块状板结物，包裹和吸附待测成分，影响提取效率。因此，应根据所加辅料的特点选择合适的方法和溶剂进行提取和纯化，以免干扰待测成分的分析。此外，对于一些成分较复杂的中药颗粒剂，需要进一步采用萃取法、沉淀法或柱色谱法等方法排除干扰。

Most of the traditional Chinese medicinal granules are prepared by alcohol precipitation to remove most of the water-soluble foreign matter. The components are easily dissolved out from the granule. Therefore, it can be extracted directly with the suitable solvent, which is selected based on the chemical properties of the marker compound and the interference components. Ultrasonic method and reflux method are often used in the extraction of granule. For granules containing fine powder of crude drug, attention should be paid to select extraction time and extraction temperature. Granules usually contain excipients such as lactose, dextrin, starch, etc. When the granule is extracted with water or low concentration ethanol, the extract solution may be thick. For organic organic solvent extraction, the granule is easy to form insoluble bulk plate and affects the extraction efficiency. In addition, for some granules with complex components, precipitation or column chromatography can be used to purify the extract. Therefore, extraction and purification methods should be optimized for analysis of granules, according to the characteristics of the excipients and the target compound.

### （四）散剂
### 4. Powders

中药散剂多为药材粉末混合而成，因此，组织碎片的显微特征是判断散剂真伪的重要依据。一些含毒性药物、液体药物的散剂，在制备中常添加一定比例的辅料进行分散和吸收（液体药物），如磷酸钙、淀粉、糊精、蔗糖、乳糖、葡萄糖等；还有一些散剂中会加入食用色素如胭脂红、靛蓝等着色以保证药粉混合的均匀性。因此，散剂分析时，应注意选择适宜的提取分离方法，排除辅料和色素的干扰，同时应注意对毒性及贵重药材进行分析。

Most traditional Chinese medicinal powders of TCM contain fine powder of crude drugs. It is important to identify the powders using the microscopic identification method. For the powders containing toxic drug and/or liquid drug, some precipitations such as calcium phosphate, starch, dextrin, sucrose, lactose, glucose, etc. are used to disperse or absorb the drugs. In addition, to ensure the uniformity of the mixture, some pigments such as carmine and indigo are added. Therefore, in the quality analysis of powders, it is necessary to select the appropriate extraction and isolation method to exclude interference from the precipitations and the pigments.

### （五）栓剂
### 5. Suppositories

栓剂中的基质主要有油脂性基质和水溶性基质，油脂性基质包括天然油脂类如可可脂、香果脂、半合成或全合成脂肪酸甘油酯类和氢化植物油等；水溶性基质主要有甘油明胶、聚乙二醇类、泊洛沙姆等。此外，栓剂中还含有表面活性剂、抗氧剂、增塑剂等添加剂。这些辅料对栓剂的分析带来一定困难。目前，除去栓剂中基质的主要方法有：①将栓剂用硅藻土等惰性材料分散，再选择适宜的溶剂加热提取，如基质为亲水性的，一般用有机溶剂提取，基质为油脂性的，一般用水或稀醇提取。②对于油脂性基质的栓剂，若待测成分亲水性强，可将栓剂切成小块，加适量水，于温水浴上加热使其融化，搅拌一定时间，取出于冰浴中再使基质凝固，将水溶液滤出，如此反复2~3次，可将亲水性成分提出；若制剂原料为药材粉末，亦可用石油醚等低极性的有机溶剂回流、脱脂后再进行提取。③对于水溶性基质的栓剂，可根据待测成分的性质用不同浓度的乙醇、甲醇或亲水性有机溶剂直接提取。此外，若栓剂中待测成分为有机酸、生物碱等酸碱性化合物，可结合酸碱萃取的方法，更好的去除基质的干扰。

Suppository bases may be conveniently classified as oleaginous (fatty) bases and water-soluble bases. The oleaginous bases mainly include cocoa butter, oleum linderae, semi-synthetic and fully synthetic fatty acid glycerides and hydrogenated vegetable oil, etc.; while the water-soluble bases include glycerin-gelatin, polyethylene glycol, poloxamer, etc. In the quality analysis of suppositories, particular attention must be given to excluding the interferences of excipients. The generally pretreatment methods of the suppositories are as follows: ① The suppository is dispersed with inert materials such as kieselguhr, then extracted with solvent. If the bases is hydrophilic, the suppository may be extracted with organic solvent; if the bases is fatty, water or dilute alcohol may be used. ② For the suppository with fatty bases, when the marker compounds is hydrophilic, cut the suppository into small pieces, add some water, melt the mixture with warm water bath and stir for a while, then solidify the bases with ice bath, filter out the aqueous solution, repeat the above procedure 2-3 times to ensue the extraction rate. Moreover, if the suppository contains medicinal powder, the fatty bases can be removed by refluxing with a low-polarity organic solvent such as petroleum ether. ③ For the suppository with water-soluble bases, it can be extracted directly with different concentrations of ethanol, methanol, or hydrophilic organic solvents, according to the properties of its mark compound. In addition, if the marker compound in suppository are acid-base compounds such as organic acids and alkaloids, it may be better to use acid-base extraction method to exclude the interference of excipients.

（六）胶囊剂

## 6. Capsules

中药软胶囊制剂中的内容物除挥发油或油类物质外，多为中药提取物与植物油等辅料组成的黏稠状液体，在样品预处理时应注意排除辅料对检测的干扰。当软胶囊内容物为挥发油或油类组分时，可考虑做旋光度或折光率检查，由于其内容物为均一性良好的液体，质量分析可以参照液体制剂，如可直接将内容物用乙醚、乙醇等溶剂溶解稀释后进行分析。当软胶囊内容物为提取物与植物油等组成的黏稠状液体时，质量分析可以参照半固体制剂，如可在内容物中加入适量硅藻土等惰性材料，低温烘干后，按固体样品处理；如待测成分为极性较大的成分，可用乙醚、石油醚等溶剂先去除基质干扰。软胶囊取样时应剪破囊材，再挤出内容物，如内容物黏附在囊壳内壁，则可用有机溶剂洗涤囊壳，洗涤液与样品一同后处理。

Except for volatile oils or oils, the contents of Chinese medicine soft capsule preparations are mostly viscous liquids composed of crude extracts and excipients such as vegetable oils. The pretreatment method should be rationally designed to eliminate the interference of such excipients. When the content of soft capsule is volatile oil or oil component, the optical rotation or refractive index can be checked. Since the content is a liquid with good uniformity, quality analysis can refer to the methods of liquid preparations. For example, the content can be directly dissolved and diluted with solvents such as ether and ethanol for analysis. When the content of soft capsule is a viscous liquid composed of crude extract and vegetable oil, quality analysis can refer to the method of semi-solid preparations. For example, an appropriate amount of diatomite can be added, and the sample in solid form will be yielded after drying. For the sample pretreatment, the capsule shells should be cut and the contents squeeze out. If the sticky contents adhere to the inner wall of the capsule shell, the capsule shell can be washed with an appropriate solvent.

硬胶囊剂进行分析时，应将内容物从胶囊中全部倾出，然后按颗粒剂或散剂的处理方法进行分析。

For the quality analysis of hard capsules, the contents should be poured out of the capsules, and then the pretreatment method of the granules or powders can be rationally designed according to the physicochemical properties of the targeted compounds.

### 三、实例
### 8.3.3　Examples

例 8-3　元胡止痛软胶囊

Example 8-3　Yuanhu Zhitong Soft Capsule

【鉴别】取本品内容物 0.5g，加甲醇 50ml，超声处理 30 分钟，滤过，滤液蒸干，残渣加水 10ml 使溶解，用浓氨试液调节 pH 值至 9~10，用乙醚振摇提取 3 次，每次 10ml，合并乙醚液，挥干，残渣加甲醇 1ml 使溶解，作为供试品溶液。另取延胡索对照药材 1g，同法制成对照药材溶液。照薄层色谱法（《中国药典》通则 0502）试验，吸取上述两种溶液各 5μl，分别点于同一硅胶 G 薄层板上，以正己烷 - 二氯甲烷 - 甲醇（7.5 : 4 : 1）为展开剂，置氨蒸气预饱和的展开缸内，展开，取出，晾干，置碘蒸气 10 秒钟后，置紫外光灯（365nm）下检视。供试品色谱中，在与对照药材色谱相应的位置上，显相同颜色的斑点。

**Identification**　To 0.5g of the contents, add 50ml of methanol, ultrasonicate for 30 minutes, filter, evaporate the filtrate to dryness, dissolve the residue in 10ml of water, alkalify with concentrated ammonia TS to adjust to pH 9-10, and then extract with three 10ml quantities of ether with shaking. Combine the ether extracts and evaporate the filtrate to dryness, dissolve the residue in 1ml of methanol as the test solution. Prepare a solution of 1g of Corydalis Rhizoma reference drug in the same manner as the reference drug solution. Carry out the method for thin layer chromatography, using silica gel G as the coating substance and a mixture of *n*-hexane, dichloromethane and methanol (7.5 : 4 : 1) as the mobile phase. Apply separately 5μl of each of the two solutions to the plate. After developing in a chamber pre-equilibrated with ammonia vapor and removal of the plate, dry it in air, expose the plate to iodine vapour for 10 seconds, examine under ultraviolet light at 365nm. The spots in the chromatogram obtained with the test solution correspond in position and color to the spots in the chromatogram obtained with the reference drug solution.

## 第四节　外用膏剂的质量分析特点
## 8.4　Analysis of Chinese Medicine Topical Ointment

### 一、乳膏剂、软膏剂
### 8.4.1　Ointments and Creams

对于乳膏剂，可先采用一些方法破乳化，如加热、加电解质、加相反类型乳化剂等，再用适当溶剂将待测成分提取出来，进行分析。软膏剂通常可采用以下方法处理：

For the quality analysis of ointments and creams, the pretreatment method should be rationally designed to eliminate the interference of excipients. For the creams, the emulsion can be broken by heating, adding electrolyte or the opposite type of emulsifier, and then the appropriate solvent is used to extract the targeted components. The following pretreatment methods can be considered for ointments and creams:

**滤除基质法**　取适宜溶剂添加至适量软膏中，加热熔化软膏，然后自然冷却使基质凝固与上清液分层，过滤或离心去除基质，滤液或上清液作为供试液进行分析。

*Filtration method*　Weigh a certain amount of ointment, add appropriate solvent, and heat the ointment to make it liquefied, then cool it. After the matrix is solidified, separate the supernatant from the matrix for further analysis.

**离心法** 取样品直接加适宜的溶剂混匀，再进行离心、滤过，滤液可作为供试液进行分析。

*Centrifugation method* The sample is mixed with suitable solvent, then centrifuged and filtered, and the filtrate can be used for further analysis.

**提取分离法** 先用不混溶的有机溶剂将基质提取后除去，再进行分析。也可用有机溶剂将样品溶解，再用酸性或碱性水溶液进行萃取分离后分析。

*Extraction and separation method* The sample is extracted with immiscible organic solvent and removed, and then determined. The sample can also be dissolved with organic solvent and be extracted and separated with acid or alkaline aqueous solution.

**灼烧法** 若软膏的待测成分为无机物，可通过灼烧软膏以除去基质，再用适宜溶剂溶解残渣作为供试液进行分析。

*Burning method* For inorganic substances as the targeted components in ointment, the sample is burned to remove the matrix for further analysis.

### 二、膏剂
### 8.4.2　Plasters

膏剂处方中多含有细料药的细粉这一类主要药物组分，一般在工艺中的下丹成膏后将其兑入和混匀，是膏剂质量分析的主要对象。膏剂样品前处理的难点和重点主要是去除其基质的干扰，由于膏剂基质具有易溶于三氯甲烷的特点，如果目标待测成分难溶于三氯甲烷，则可用三氯甲烷去除基质后再进行质量分析；也可根据目标待测成分的理化性质选取合适的溶剂直接提取后再进行质量分析。

For the plasters preparations, most of the fine materials are main drugs and thus are the main targeted components for quality analysis of pastes. The plaster preparations always contain various complex matrix, so the pretreatment method should be rationally designed to eliminate the interference of such excipients. When the targeted component is insoluble in chloroform, chloroform can be used to remove the plaster matrix. In addition, the plasters can also be extracted with a suitable solvent according to the physicochemical properties of the targeted components.

### 三、贴膏剂
### 8.4.3　Cataplasms

橡胶贴膏剂处方复杂，主药成分少，质量分析时容易受基质的干扰。分析时，可直接在橡胶贴膏剂表面测定待测成分，也可以根据待测成分的理化性质，采用合适的方法提取橡胶贴膏剂中的待测成分后进行分析。若橡胶贴膏剂中的待测成分在一定条件下能形成特定性状的结晶，则可以对待测成分进行显微鉴别。若含有樟脑、薄荷脑、冰片等挥发性成分，可采用升华法等将待测组分与基质分离后进行质量分析。

*Adhesive plasters* Adhesive plasters have the characteristics of complex components and low content, so the pretreatment method should be rationally designed to eliminate the interference of the complex matrix. For example, it can be determined the targeted components directly on the surface of the adhesive plasters by using a specific chemical reaction or with the help of an instrument. Meanwhile, the adhesive plasters can also be extracted with proper solvent for further quality analysis. When the targeted components on the adhesive paste can form crystals with specific properties under certain conditions, the identification can be done by microscope. When the adhesive plasters contain volatile components such as camphor, menthol or borneol, the sublimation method can be used to separate the targeted component from the matrix.

凝胶贴膏剂的基质具有亲水性，可先用极性溶剂将含药基质与盖衬分离后，再根据待测成分的理化性质采用适宜溶剂提取后分析。

*Hydrogel plasters* Because the hydrogel plasters contain hydrophilic matrix, the matrix with targeted components can be separated from the backing with a polar solvent and then extracted with a suitable solvent according to the physicochemical properties of the targeted components.

### 四、实例
### 8.4.4 Examples

例 8-4　麝香镇痛膏
Example 8-4　Shexiang Zhentong Plaster

【鉴别】取本品 10 片，除去盖衬，剪成小块，置 250ml 烧瓶中，加乙醇 100ml，加热回流 1 小时，取乙醇液，浓缩至约 2ml，加 5% 硫酸溶液 20ml，搅拌，滤过，滤液置分液漏斗中，加氨试液使成碱性，用二氯甲烷振摇提取 2 次（30ml、20ml），合并二氯甲烷液，蒸干，残渣加无水乙醇 1ml 使溶解，作为供试品溶液。另取硫酸阿托品对照品，加无水乙醇制成每 1ml 含 2mg 的溶液，作为对照品溶液。照薄层色谱法（通则 0502）试验，吸取供试品溶液 20μl、对照品溶液 5μl，分别点于同一硅胶 G 薄层板上，以乙酸乙酯 - 甲醇 - 浓氨试液（17∶2∶1）为展开剂，展开，取出，晾干，喷以稀碘化铋钾试液。供试品色谱中，在与对照品色谱相应的位置上，显相同颜色的斑点。

**Identification** To 10 pieces, Remove off the cover lining and cut into small pieces; place in a 250ml flask, add 100ml of ethanol, heat under reflux for 1 hour; separate the ethanol liquid, concentrate to about 2ml and add 20ml of 5% sulfuric solution; stir and filter; transfer the filtrate to a separating funnel and adjust the filtrate to base with ammonium TS, extract by shaking with dimethylmethane for 2 times (30ml, 20ml); combine the dimethylmethane liquid, evaporate to dryness and dissolve the residue in 1ml of anhydrous ethanol as the test solution. Dissolve a quantity of atropine sulfate CRS in anhydrous ethanol to produce a solution containing 2mg per ml as the reference solution. Carry out the method for thin layer chromatography, using silica gel G as coating substance and a mixture of ethyl acetate, methanol and concentrated ammonia TS (17: 2: 1) as mobile phase. Apply separately 20μl of the test solution and 5μl of the reference solution to the plate. After developing and removal of the plate, dry in air, spray with dilute potassium iodobismuthate TS. The spot in chromatogram obtained with the test solution corresponds in position and color to the spot in chromatogram obtained with the reference solution.

## 岗 位 对 接
## Post Docking

本章为中药学、中药制药、中药资源与开发等相关专业学生必须掌握的内容，为成为合格的中药质量分析人员奠定坚实的基础。

This task is the content of students majoring in Chinese medicines, Chinese medicines pharmacy, Chinese medicines resources and development, and lays a solid foundation for becoming a qualified Chinese medicines analyzer.

本章内容对应岗位包括中药质量检验、制剂生产、新药研发等相关工种。

The corresponding positions of this task include quality inspection of Chinese medicines, medicine preparations production, and new drug research and development.

上述从事中药质量分析相关所有岗位的从业人员均需要掌握各类中药质量分析特点，学会应用本章所学内容开展各类中药质量分析工作。

The above-mentioned practitioners should master the characteristics of all kinds of Chinese medicine quality analysis to carry out pharmaceutical service.

# 重 点 小 结
# Summary of Key Points

中药按其物态可分为液体、半固体、固体、外用膏剂和其他类型，其质量分析的特点也各有不同。中药材、饮片以及全部或部分使用中药饮片细粉入药的制剂，因待测成分仍存在于植物组织、细胞中，因此，应注意提取溶剂、提取方法和提取时间的选择。而中药提取物，选用合适的溶剂溶解即可。此外，在中药制剂中还要注意辅料对分析的干扰，例如蜜丸中的糖和蜂蜜。液体制剂的取样要有代表性，应摇匀后取样，还需要注意液体制剂中防腐剂、矫味剂对分析的影响。

Chinese medicine can be divided into liquid, semi−solid, solid, topical ointment and other types according to its physical state, and the characteristics of its quality analysis are also different. Chinese medicinal materials, decoction pieces, and all or part of the preparations using fine powder of decoction pieces of Chinese medicine, because the components to be tested still exist in plant tissues and cells, therefore, attention should be paid to the choice of extraction solvent, extraction method and extraction time. The Chinese medicine extract can be dissolved in a suitable solvent. In addition, attention should be paid to the interference of excipients in the analysis of traditional Chinese medicine preparations, such as sugar and honey in honey pills. Sampling of liquid preparations should be representative. Samples should be taken after shaking. It is also necessary to pay attention to the influence of preservatives and flavoring agents in liquid preparations on analysis.

# 目 标 检 测

题库

## 一、选择题

（一）单项选择题

1. 需进行甲醇量检查的剂型是
   A. 酒剂和酊剂　　　　B. 酒剂和口服液　　　　C. 合剂和口服液　　　　D. 合剂和酒剂

2. 合剂与口服液最常用的净化方法为
   A. 液 – 固萃取　　　　B. 液 – 液萃取　　　　C. 蒸馏法　　　　D. 沉淀法

3. 进行总固体量检查的剂型是

    A. 糖浆剂         B. 酒剂         C. 酊剂         D. 口服液

4. 《中国药典》规定，要检查不溶物的剂型是

    A. 流浸膏剂         B. 浸膏剂         C. 糖浆剂         D. 煎膏剂

5. 硬胶囊剂的内容物，照《中国药典》水分测定法，除另有规定外，水分不得超过

    A. 9.0%         B. 10.0%         C. 12.0%         D. 6.0%

6. 膏药质量分析可利用其基质易溶于（     ）溶剂的特点，将基质除去。

    A. 甲酸         B. 甲醇         C. 三氯甲烷         D. 乙醇

7. 橡胶膏剂特有的质量要求是

    A. 酸碱度         B. 含膏量         C. 黏着力试验         D. 耐热试验

8. 颗粒剂均匀度检查时，不能通过一号筛和能通过五号筛的颗粒和粉末总和不得过

    A. 10%         B. 20%         C. 15%         D. 30%

9. 一般中药注射液树脂检查，可取注射液 5ml，加（     ）溶液 1 滴，放置 30 分钟，应无树脂状物析出。

    A. 30% 磺基水杨酸                       B. 硫代乙酰胺溶液

    C. 盐酸                                  D. 鞣酸

10. 片剂中所含成分含量较高，结构明确，为保证单剂量的准确性，还应进行

    A. 崩解时限检查                       B. 溶出度检查

    C. 溶散时限检查                       D. 含量均匀度检查

11. 中药注射剂含量限度指标（生产用）的制定，至少需要（     ）批样品的实测数据。

    A. 3 批         B. 10 批         C. 20 批         D. 5 批

12. 下列选项中，属于栓剂的一般检查项目的是

    A. 融变时限检查                       B. 溶出度检查

    C. 溶散时限检查                       D. 溶化性检查

13. 下列处理方法中，最适于提取脂肪栓中的亲脂性成分的是

    A. 加入硅藻土分散后再进行提取         B. 用亲脂性有机溶剂直接提取

    C. 用石油醚回流脱脂后，再进行提取     D. 用熔融冰浴凝固法除去基质后再提取

14. 下列选项中，需要检查乙醇含量的是

    A. 片剂         B. 流浸膏         C. 浸膏         D. 注射剂

15. 有效成分制成的注射剂，主药成分含量应不少于

    A. 60%         B. 70%         C. 80%         D. 90%

（二）多项选择题

1. 口服液质量检查的项目为

    A. 相对密度             B. pH 值             C. 装量差异

    D. 重量差异             E. 性状

2. 在贮存时间内允许有微量轻摇易散的沉淀的剂型包括

    A. 合剂     B. 口服液     C. 酒剂     D. 酊剂     E. 注射剂

3. 半固体制剂的质量要求包括

    A. 性状             B. 装量差异             C. 微生物限度

    D. 甲醇量             E. 重量差异

4. 对于乳剂型软膏，可采用以下（     ）方法使乳剂破裂，再使用适当溶剂将药物提取出来。

    A. 超声             B. 加热             C. 振摇

D. 加电解质       E. 加相反类型乳化剂

5. 橡胶膏剂的质量分析特点有
  A. 离心测定法      B. 直接测定法      C. 提取测定法
  D. 镜检测定法      E. 色谱测定法

6. 去除大蜜丸中蜂蜜干扰的方法有
  A. 硅藻土吸附法      B. 冰浴凝固法      C. 酸碱萃取法
  D. 有机溶剂提取法      E. 水洗法

7. 颗粒剂应检查
  A. 粒度    B. 溶化性    C. 水分    D. 溶散时限    E. 均匀度

8. 下列哪些试剂可用于中药注射剂中鞣质的检查
  A. 鸡蛋清      B. 铁氰化钾      C. 四苯硼酸钠
  D. 二乙基二硫代氨基甲酸银    E. 磺基水杨酸

9. 水丸的一般质量检查项目包括
  A. 相对密度      B. 水分      C. 装量差异
  D. 重量差异      E. 性状

10. 中药注射剂的检查项目包括
  A. pH 值      B. 异常毒性      C. 澄明度
  D. 鞣质      E. 草酸盐

11. 需进行溶散时限检查的剂型是
  A. 大蜜丸      B. 水丸      C. 片剂
  D. 蜡丸      E. 浓缩丸

12. 下列关于中药注射剂指纹图谱叙述正确的是
  A. 中药注射剂的指纹图谱应全面反映注射剂所含成分的信息
  B. 中药注射剂中含有的大类成分，一般都应在指纹图谱中得到体现
  C. 同一注射剂可建立多张指纹图谱
  D. 指纹图谱的评价可采用相似度等进行评价
  E. 中药注射剂应分别建立原料、中间体和制剂的指纹图谱

## 二、思考题

三九胃泰胶囊处方为三叉苦、九里香、两面针、木香、黄芩、茯苓、地黄、白芍，以下为其鉴别检查项之一，请解释下划线标注步骤的目的和意义。

取本品内容物 0.4g，①加乙醇 30ml，加热回流 1 小时，放冷，滤过，滤液蒸干，残渣加水20ml，加热使溶解，放冷，②用盐酸调节 pH 值至 1~2，用乙酸乙酯 30ml 振摇提取，分取乙酸乙酯液，蒸干，残渣加乙醇 1ml 使溶解，作为供试品溶液。③另取黄芩对照药材 0.2g，加乙醇20ml，同法制成对照药材溶液。再取黄芩苷对照品，加甲醇制成每 1ml 含 1mg 的溶液，作为对照品溶液。照薄层色谱法（通则 0502）试验，吸取上述三种溶液各 2μl，分别点于同一聚酰胺薄膜上，④以乙酸乙酯 - 甲醇 - 醋酸（4∶1∶10）为展开剂，展开，取出，晾干，⑤喷以 2% 三氯化铁乙醇溶液。供试品色谱中，在与对照药材色谱和对照品色谱相应的位置上，显相同颜色的斑点。

# 第九章　生物样品内中药成分分析

## Chapter 9　Analysis of Ingredients of Chinese Medicine in Biological Samples

 学习目标 | Learning Goal

**知识要求：**

**1. 熟悉** 生物样品的制备方法，生物样品分析方法的建立与验证。

**2. 了解** 生物样品内中药成分分析的目的、意义和特点。

**能力要求：**

学会应用生物样品内中药成分分析解决中药化学成分的吸收、分布、排泄和代谢。

### Knowledge Requirements

**1. Familiar** The method for preparing biological samples, establishment and verification of biological sample analysis method.

**2. Understand** The purpose, significance and characteristics of the analysis of traditional Chinese medicine components in biological samples.

### Ability Requirements

Learn to apply Chinese medicine composition analysis in biological samples to solve the absorption, distribution, excretion and metabolism of Chinese medicine composition.

---

生物样品内中药化学成分分析是中药分析的重要分支，主要研究生物体内中药化学成分及其代谢物质与量变化规律。中药成分复杂，其药效是多种化学成分共同作用的结果。通过分析中药中化学成分在生物样本中的质变和／或量变规律，可阐明其药效物质及其变化规律，为中药的研制、质量控制指标和剂型的改进、临床合理用药及其作用机理探讨等提供科学依据，保证临床用药安全、有效、合理，推进中药现代化的进程。

The analysis of the chemical composition of traditional Chinese medicine in biological samples is an important branch of traditional Chinese medicine analysis. It mainly studies the changes of the chemical composition of Chinese traditional medicine and its metabolic substances and quantities *in vivo*. The composition of traditional Chinese medicine is complex, and its efficacy is the result of a combination of various chemical ingredients. By analyzing the qualitative and/or quantitative changes of the chemical constituents in traditional Chinese medicines in biological samples, they can clarify their medicinal substances and their changing rules. They are for the development of traditional Chinese medicines, the improvement of quality control indicators and dosage forms, the rational use

医药大学堂
WWW.YIYAODXT.COM

226

of medicines and their mechanism of action. Provide scientific basis to ensure the safety, effectiveness, and rationality of clinical medicine and promote the process of modernization of traditional Chinese medicine.

## 第一节 概述
## 9.1 Overview

### 一、生物样品内中药成分分析的意义和任务
### 9.1.1 Significance and Task of Analysis of Chinese Medicine Components in Biological Samples

以往中药质量的控制和评价，主要着眼于在体外对其进行鉴别、检查和含量测定。随着临床中药学、临床药理学和现代分析技术的发展，以及人们对中药在机体内的吸收、分布、代谢和排泄过程与疗效关系的进一步认识，发现药理作用强度有时因个体差异而显著不同，即"化学等价而生物学不等效"，因此，中药分析不但要进行体外研究，更需要研究中药化学成分在生物体内的表现形式及变化规律，以便获得体内代谢过程的信息，从而有助于科学评价中药的生产、研发、临床疗效和质量评价。

In the past, with regard to the control and evaluation of the quality of traditional Chinese medicine, the main focus has been on identification, inspection, and content determination in vitro. With the development of clinical Chinese pharmacy, clinical pharmacology and modern analytical techniques, as well as people's further understanding of the relationship between the absorption, distribution, metabolism and excretion process of traditional Chinese medicine in the body and the therapeutic effect, it is found that the intensity of pharmacological effects sometimes varies significantly due to individual differences, That is, "chemically equivalent and biologically not equivalent", therefore, Chinese medicine analysis not only requires in vitro research, but also needs to study the manifestations and changes of the chemical composition of traditional Chinese medicine in the organism in order to obtain information about the metabolic process in the body, so that It helps to scientifically evaluate the production, research and development, clinical efficacy and quality evaluation of traditional Chinese medicine.

生物样品内中药成分分析的任务：建立生物样品内中药成分的分析方法，以解决生物样品内待测成分浓度低、基质组成复杂、干扰大的问题。分析生物样品内中药成分及其代谢产物的存在状态及动态变化规律。

The tasks of analyzing the composition of traditional Chinese medicine in biological samples are as follows: The establishment of an analytical method for the composition of traditional Chinese medicine in biological samples to solve the problems of low concentration of components to be tested in biological samples, complex matrix composition, and large interference. The analysis of the existence state and dynamic changes of traditional Chinese medicine components and their metabolites in biological samples.

### 二、生物样品内中药成分分析的特点
### 9.1.2 Characteristics of the Analysis of Traditional Chinese Medicine Components in Biological Samples

**干扰因素多** 生物样品内含有大量内源性物质，如蛋白质、脂肪等有机物和 Na⁺、K⁺ 等无机物，同时，进入体内的其他化学成分也会影响或干扰测定。

*Many interference factors* Biological samples contain a large amount of endogenous substances, such as organic substances such as protein and fat, and inorganic substances such as $Na^+$ and $K^+$. At the same time, other chemical components entering the body will also affect or interfere with the measurement.

**样品量少** 生物样品的取样，总量往往受限，且不易重复获得。

*Small sample size* The total amount of biological samples collected is often limited, and it is not easy to obtain repeatedly.

**待测成分浓度低** 一般血药浓度在 ng/ml，因此，对分析方法的灵敏度要求较高。

*The concentration of the component to be tested is low* The general blood drug concentration is ng/ml. Therefore, the sensitivity of the analytical method is high.

**样品稳定性差** 生物样品中有多种酶，取样后仍可作用于被测物，使被测物不稳定。

*Poor sample stability* There are many enzymes in biological samples, which can still act on the test object after sampling, making the test object unstable.

**待测成分存在形式多样** 中药化学成分在生物体内经过代谢可产生一种或多种代谢产物，母体药物和代谢物又能与内源性生物大分子结合，使得待测成分在生物体内以原型、结合型、缀合物、代谢物等多种形式存在。

*There are various forms of the tested component* The chemical components of the traditional Chinese medicine can be metabolized in the organism to produce one or more metabolites, prototype drugs and metabolites can also be combined with endogenous biological macromolecules, so that the components to be tested exist multiple forms, such as prototypes, conjugates, glycoconjugates, metabolites and so on.

## 第二节 生物样品的制备
## 9.2 Preparation of Biological Samples

生物样品是指来自生物机体的各种体液、器官、组织及排泄物等，包括血液、尿液、唾液、头发、胆汁、脑脊液、胃液、胰液、淋巴液、脏器及组织、乳汁、精液等，其中常用的生物样品是血液（血清、血浆、全血）、尿液、唾液及胆汁。

Biological samples refer to various body fluids, organs, tissues and excretions from biological organisms, etc., such as blood, urine, saliva, hair, bile, cerebrospinal fluid, gastric juice, pancreatic juice, lymphatic fluid, organs and tissues, milk, semen, etc. Among them, blood (serum, plasma, whole blood), urine, saliva and bile are the commonly used biological samples.

### 一、常用的生物样品
## 9.2.1　Common Biological Samples

（一）血样
### 1.　Blood Sample

血液样品包括血浆、血清、全血，主要用于血清化学、药物代谢动力学、临床治疗药物浓度检测，以及代谢组学等的研究。血药浓度通常指血浆或血清中药物浓度。药物在体内达到稳态血药浓度时，血浆中药物浓度通常可以反映药物在体内作用部位的状况，故血浆是进行体内药物分析最常用的样品。

Blood samples include blood plasma, blood serum, and whole blood, which are mainly used for the study of serum chemistry, pharmacokinetics, clinical therapeutic drug concentration detection, and metabolomics. Blood drug concentration usually refers to the drug concentration in plasma or serum, not the whole blood drug concentration. When drug reaches steady-state blood concentration *in vivo*, the drug concentration in plasma usually reflects the status of the drug at the site of action *in vivo*, so plasma is the most commonly used sample for drug analysis *in vivo*.

1. **血样的采集**　动物实验时，可从心脏、动脉或静脉取血；人体取血时通常从静脉取血。采血量取决于临床或动物实验要求、血药物浓度及分析方法的灵敏度等。常用注射器、负压管、毛细管或特殊的微量采血管采集血样。

**(1) The collection of blood samples**　In animal experiments, blood should be taken directly from the heart, arteries or veins. Blood is usually taken from vein in human body. The amount of blood can be collected according to the requirements of clinical or animal experiments, the drug concentration in the blood and the sensitivity of analytical methods, etc. Syringes, negative pressure tubes, capillaries or special micro-sampling vessels are usually used to collect blood.

2. **血样的处理**
**(2) Treatment of blood samples**

**血浆的制备**　将采集的血液置于含有抗凝剂的试管中，混合后以 2500~3000rpm/min 离心 5~15 分钟，使之与血细胞分离，淡黄色上清液即为血浆。抗凝剂常用肝素的钠盐、钾盐。另外，还有 EDTA、枸橼酸盐、氟化钠、草酸盐等。

*Plasma preparation*　The collected blood is placed in a test tube containing anticoagulant, and then centrifuged at 2500-3000r/min for 5-15 minutes after mixing to separate it from the blood cells. The yellow supernatant is plasma. Heparin is a common anticoagulant, commonly used its sodium salt, sylvite salt. In addition, there are EDTA, citrate salt, fluoride sodium, oxalate salt.

**血清的制备**　将采集的血液置于试管中，静置 0.5~1 小时。再以 2500~3000r/min 离心 5~10 分钟，上层的澄清淡黄色液体即为血清。

*Serum preparation*　The collected blood is placed in a test tube and left to rest for 0.5-1 hour. The clarified yellowish liquid on the upper layer is the serum after centrifugation at 2500-3000r/min for 5-10 minutes.

（二）尿样
### 2.　Urine Sample

体内药物清除，主要是通过尿液，将药物以原型（母体药物）或代谢物及缀合物等形式排出。尿液的特点有：药物浓度较高，收集量大，收集简单。目前代谢组学的研究多以尿液为研究样品。由于尿液浓度变化较大，所以通常测定一定时间内尿液中的药物总量，如8小时、12小时、24小时内累积量，需要同时记录下尿液体积。动物实验，如采集24小时尿液，一般8点给药，之后排出的尿液全部储存于干净的容器中，直到次日上午8时。常用的容器有涂蜡的一次性纸杯、玻璃杯等，准确量好体积后贮存。常用代谢笼（配有刻度储尿瓶）。

The drugs in the body are mainly eliminated through urine excretion in prototype, metabolite and conjugate. Urine is characterized by high drug concentration, large collection volume, simple collection. Now, most studies on metabolomics take urine as the research sample.

Because urine concentration changes greatly, it is necessary to measure the total amount of drugs in urine within a certain period of time, such as the cumulative amount within 8 hours, 12 hours and 24 hours. Urine volume should be recorded at the same time. In animal experiments, if the urine is collected for 24 hours, the drug is usually administrated at 8 o′clock, after which all the urine is stored in a clean container until 8 o′clock the next morning. Commonly used containers are disposable paper cups coated with wax and glasses, which can be stored after accurately measuring the volume. Metabolic cages (with graduated urine storage bottles) used in animal metabolomics.

（三）唾液样品

### 3. Saliva Sample

由于一些药物的唾液药物浓度与血浆游离药物浓度密切相关，这种情况下，可通过测定唾液药物浓度代替血浆药物浓度，并可用于药物代动力学研究。唾液的采集，应尽量在刺激少的安全状态下进行，一般是漱口后15分钟。用插有漏斗的试管接收口腔内自然流出或经舌在口内搅动后流出的混合唾液。另外也可采用物理（嚼石蜡片、小块聚四氟乙烯、橡胶或纱布球等）或化学（酒石酸、硝酸毛果云香碱等）等方法刺激，以其在短时间内得到大量的唾液。唾液采集后，应立即测量其除去泡沫部分的体积，以2000~3000r/min离心10~15分钟，取上清液作为待测样品。

Since some drugs concentration in saliva are closely related to free drug concentration in plasma, in this case, salivary drug concentration can be measured in place of plasma drug concentration and can be used in pharmacokinetic studies. Saliva collection should be carried out in a safe state without stimulation, usually 15 minutes after gargling, received in a tube with a funnel that flows naturally from the mouth or discharges after agitation by the tongue. In addition, the mixture collection can also be stimulated by physical methods (chewing paraffin slices, small pieces of polytetrafluoroethylene, rubber or gauze balls, etc.) or chemical methods (tartaric acid, nitric acid, etc.) to obtain a large amount of saliva in a short time. After collection, the saliva volume removing foam part should be measured immediately, then, following centrifugation for 10-15 minutes at 2000-3000r/min, take the supernatant as the sample to be tested.

（四）组织

### 4. Tissue Sample

研究药物体内吸收、分布及药物中毒死亡时，常采用动物组织。常用的脏器组织有心、肝、肺、肾、脑等。实验动物处死后、迅速取出组织样品（脑、心、肝、脾、肺、肾），生理盐水洗去组织的血液，滤纸吸干水分，精密称重。分析前需匀浆，制成均匀化的水性基质溶液，然后采用以下方法制备样品：

Animal tissues are often used in animal experiments to study drug absorption, distribution and death from drug poisoning. Commonly used organs and tissues are heart, liver, lung, kidney, brain, etc. After the experimental animals were sacrificed, the tissue samples (brain, heart, liver, spleen, lung, kidney) were quickly removed, the physiological waves were used to wash away the blood wave of the tissue, the filter paper was used to absorb water and weighed accurately. Prior to analysis, all samples need to be homogenized to make a homogenized aqueous matrix solution, and then samples are prepared by the following methods:

1. **蛋白沉淀法** 向组织匀浆液中加入甲醇、乙腈、高氯酸、三氯醋酸等沉淀剂，蛋白质沉淀后，离心取上清液直接分析或处理后再分析。

**(1) Protein precipitation** Methanol, acetonitrile, perchloric acid, trichloroacetic acid and other precipitants were added to the tissue homogenate. After protein precipitation, the supernatant centrifugated is for analysis or extraction before analysis.

2. **酸水解或碱水解法** 向组织匀浆中加入一定量的酸或碱，水浴中加热，待组织液化后，过滤或离心，取上清液备用。

**(2) Acid hydrolysis or alkaline hydrolysis** A certain amount of acid or alkali is added to the tissue homogenate and then heats in a water bath until the tissue is liquefied, filter or centrifuge and take the supernatant for use.

3. **酶水解法** 向组织匀浆中加入一定量 Tris 缓冲液，水浴上水解一定时间，待组织液化后过滤或离心，取上清液备用。

**(3) Enzyme hydrolysis** Add a certain amount of Tris buffer to the tissue homogenate, hydrolyze on a water bath for a certain time, filter or centrifuge after the tissue is liquefied, and take the supernatant for use.

### 二、生物样品的前处理
### 9.2.2 Pretreatment of Biological Samples

生物样品的前处理，是生物样品分析中极其重要的一个环节，由于生物样品的复杂性，其前处理过程也很难规定固定的模式和程序，需结合实验要求，采取适当的处理手段，从而保证生物样品内中药化学成分的准确分析。

The pretreatment of biological samples is an extremely important step in the analysis of biological samples. Due to the complexity of biological samples, it is difficult to set a fixed model and procedure for the pretreatment process. It is necessary to adopt appropriate pretreatment methods in combination with the experimental requirements to ensure the accurate analysis of the chemical components of Chinese medicines in biological samples.

#### （一）沉淀蛋白
#### 1. Precipitated Protein

血样或组织匀浆样品分析时，应先去除样品中的蛋白质，以便测定药物的总浓度；同时还可以通过提高样品的洁净度，达到保护仪器性能，延长使用寿命的作用。目前，可采用的除蛋白方法有以下几种：

When analyzing a blood sample or a tissue homogenate sample, the protein in the sample should be removed to determine the total concentration of the drug; at the same time, the cleanliness of the sample can be improved to protect the performance of the instrument and extend the service life. Currently, the following protein removal methods are available:

1. **加入与水相混溶的有机溶剂** 水溶性的有机溶剂可使蛋白质分子内及分子间的氢键发生变化，使蛋白质凝聚，释放出与蛋白质结合的化学成分。通常加入有机溶剂的体积为血浆或血清的 1~3 倍，超速离心，可除去 90% 以上的蛋白质。加入有机溶剂的种类不同，析出蛋白质沉淀形状、pH 值不同。用甲醇或乙腈时，上清液 pH 值 8.5~9.5；用乙醇或丙酮时，上清液 pH 值 9~10。甲醇或乙腈是反向 HPLC 中常用的有机相，且均有较高的沉淀蛋白的效率，是常用的蛋白质沉淀剂，其中乙腈的沉淀效率比甲醇更高。

**(1) Add an Organic Solvent Miscible with Water** The water-soluble organic solvent can change the hydrogen bonds within and between the molecules of the protein, cause the protein to aggregate, and release the chemical components bound to the protein. Usually the volume of organic solvent added is 1-3 of plasma or serum. Ultracentrifugation can remove more than 90% of the protein. Different types of organic solvents are added, the precipitated protein precipitate shape and pH value are different. When using methanol or acetonitrile, the pH value of the supernatant is 8.5-9.5; when using ethanol or acetone, the pH value of the supernatant is 9-10. Methanol or acetonitrile is a commonly used organic phase in reverse HPLC and has a high efficiency of protein precipitation. It is a commonly used protein precipitating agent, in which acetonitrile has a higher precipitation efficiency than methanol.

**2. 加入中性盐** 中性盐能将与蛋白质结合的水置换出来，从而使蛋白质脱水沉淀。常用的中性盐，有饱和硫酸盐、镁盐、磷酸盐及枸橼酸盐等。加入量为血浆或血清的 2 倍，超速离心，便可除去 90% 以上的蛋白质，所得上清液的 pH 值为 7.0~7.7。

**(2) Add Neutral Salt** A neutral salt replaces the water that binds to the protein, which dehydrates and precipitates the protein. Commonly used neutral salt are saturated sulfate, magnesium salt, phosphate and citrate salt, ect. Adding twice the amount of plasma or serum, ultracentrifugation can remove more than 90% of the protein, and the supernatant has a pH of 7.0-7.7.

**3. 加入强酸** 加入强酸使溶液的 pH 低于蛋白质的等电点，蛋白质的阳离子与酸形成不溶性盐而沉淀。常用的强酸有 10% 三氯醋酸、6% 高氯酸、硫酸–钨酸混合液及 5% 偏磷酸等。加入量为血浆或血清的 0.6 倍，超速离心，可去除 90% 以上的蛋白质，所得上清液的 pH 值为 0~4。

**(3) Add Strong Acid** When the pH is lower than the isoelectric point of the protein, the protein exists as a cation. After the addition of strong acid, it can form insoluble salt with protein cation and precipitate. Commonly used strong acid are 10% trichloroacetic acid, 6% perchloric acid, sulfuric acid-tungstate mixed solution and 5% partial phosphoric acid, ect. The added amount is 0.6 times of plasma or serum. Ultracentrifugation can remove more than 90% of the protein. The pH value of the supernatant is 0-4.

**4. 加入含锌盐及铜盐的沉淀剂** 当溶液的 pH 值大于蛋白质的等电点时，蛋白质以阴离子形式存在，可与金属阳离子形成不溶性盐而沉淀。常用的金属沉淀剂有 $CuSO_4$-$Na_2WO_4$、$ZnSO_4$-NaOH 等。加入量为血浆或血清的 1~3 倍，超速离心，可去除 90% 以上的蛋白质，所得上清液的 pH 值为 5.7~7.3（$CuSO_4$-$Na_2WO_4$）或 6.5~7.5（$ZnSO_4$-NaO）。

**(4) Add Metal Precipitant Containing Zinc Salt and Copper Salt** When the pH of the solution is greater than the isoelectric point of the protein, the protein is present as an anion, so metal cation that form an insoluble salt with the negatively charged carboxyl group of a protein to precipitate. Commonly used metal precipitators are $CuSO_4$-$Na_2WO_4$, $ZnSO_4$-NaOH, etc. Adding 1-3 the amount of plasma or serum, over 90% of the protein can be removed by ultracentrifugation. The pH value of the supernatant is 5.7-7.3 ($CuSO_4$-$Na_2WO_4$) or 6.5-7.5 ($ZnSO_4$-NaOH) .

**5. 超滤法** 本法是以多孔性半透膜（超滤膜）作为分离介质的一种膜分离技术。通过选用不同孔径的不对称性微孔膜，按照截留分子量的大小，可分离 300~1000kDa 的可溶性生物大分子物质。血样中游离药物的测定，用相对分子量截留值在 5 万左右的超滤膜，采用加压（$2kg/cm^2$）过滤法或高速离心法即可。

**(5) Ultrafiltration**　This method is a membrane separation technique with porous semi-permeable membrane (ultrafiltration membrane) as the separation medium. By selecting asymmetric microporous membranes with different pore sizes, soluble biomolecules of 300-1000kDa can be separated according to the size of interception molecular weight. The determination of free drugs in blood can use the ultrafiltration membrane with interception molecular weight around 50000, with 2kg/cm$^2$ pressure filtration or high speed centrifugation.

6. **酶水解法**　对于一些酸不稳定及与蛋白结合牢固的成分，可用酶解法。最常用的酶是枯草菌溶素，可使组织溶解，释放出化学成分。在 pH 值 7.9~11.0 的范围内蛋白质肽键降解，温度 50~60℃，具有最大活力。

**(6) Enzyme Hydrolysis**　Enzymatic hydrolysis can be used for some components that are unstable and bind to protein firmly. The most commonly used enzyme is subtilisin, which dissolves tissues and releases chemical components. Within the range of pH value 7.9-11.0, the protein peptide bond is degraded, the temperature is 50-60℃, and it has the maximum vitality.

（二）净化和富集

## 2. Purification and Enrichment

1. **液 - 液萃取法**　液 - 液萃取法是一种经典的分离纯化方法。有机试剂的种类、有机相和水相的体积比、水相的 pH 值等是该方法应用的关键。液－液萃取法，有时会发生乳化现象，造成被测物质的损失。可提取前在水相中加入适量的 NaCl，减轻乳化程度。当发生轻微乳化时，可通过离心，使水相和有机相完全分开。若发生严重乳化时，可置于低温冰箱使水相快速冻凝，破坏乳化层，融化后离心。

**(1) Liquid-Liquid Extraction**　Liquid-liquid extraction is a classic separation and purification method. The type of organic reagent, the volume ratio of the organic phase and the aqueous phase, the pH value of the aqueous phase, etc. are the key to the application of this method. In the liquid-liquid extraction method, emulsification sometimes occurs, resulting in the loss of the measured substance. Appropriate amount of NaCl can be added to the water phase before extraction to reduce the degree of emulsification. When a slight emulsification occurs, the water phase and the organic phase can be completely separated by centrifugation. If severe emulsification occurs, it can be placed in a low-temperature refrigerator to quickly freeze and freeze the aqueous phase, destroy the emulsified layer, and centrifuge after melting.

2. **固相萃取法**　固相萃取法是基于液相色谱的分离原理建立起来的分离纯化方法，具有无乳化现象、提取回收率高、样品用量少、方法的重现性好等特点，能满足 GC、HPLC、MS 等多种分析方法的需求，是一种更适合生物样品纯化的技术方法。

**(2) Solid-Phase Extraction**　The solid phase extraction method is a separation and purification method based on the separation principle of liquid chromatography. It has the characteristics of no emulsification, high extraction recovery rate, small sample consumption, and good method reproducibility. It can meet need for multiple analytical methods (GC, HPLC, MS, etc.), is a technical method that is more suitable for the purification of biological samples.

3. **固相微萃取法**　是在固相萃取的基础上，发展起来的一种新型样品预处理方法。固相微萃取法是基于待测成分在萃取涂层与样品之间的吸附或溶解－解析平衡而建立起来的集萃取、浓缩、进样等功能于一体的技术。该方法装置便携、易于操作、重现性好、灵敏度高、回收率高、样品用量少、无需溶剂或极少量溶剂，已成为目前生物样品前处理技术中应用最广泛的方法之一。目前，已实现了与液相色谱和气相色谱的联用。

**(3) Solid Phase Microextraction**  The method is a new type of sample pretreatment method developed on the basis of solid phase extraction. This method of solid-phase microextraction is based on the adsorption or dissolution-analysis equilibrium of the components to be tested between the extraction coating and the sample. The method is portable, easy to operate, has good reproducibility, high sensitivity, good recovery rate, small sample consumption, no solvent or very small amount of solvent, and has become one of the most widely used methods in biological sample pretreatment technology. At present, the combination with liquid chromatography and gas chromatography has been realized.

（三）缀合物的水解

## 3. Hydrolysis of the Conjugate

缀合物是中药中的化学成分或其代谢物与机体的内源性物质结合生成的产物。形成缀合物的内源性物质有葡萄糖醛酸、硫酸、甘氨酸、谷胱甘肽和醋酸等，其中葡萄糖醛酸、硫酸是形成缀合物最重要内源性物质。含有羟基、羧基、氨基和巯基的待测成分与葡萄糖醛酸形成葡萄糖醛酸苷缀合物，含有酚羟基、芳胺及醇类的待测成分与硫酸形成硫酸酯缀合物。尿中待测成分多数呈缀合状态，其极性较原型药物大，不宜被有机溶剂提取。为了测定尿液中待测成分总量，无论是直接测定或萃取分离，均需要进行水解，释放出待测成分。

A conjugate is a product produced by the combination of chemical components or metabolites in traditional Chinese medicine with endogenous substances in the body. Endogenous substances that form conjugates include glucuronic acid, sulfuric acid, glycine, glutathione, and acetic acid, among which glucuronic acid and sulfuric acid are the most important endogenous substances that form conjugates. The test component containing hydroxyl, carboxyl, amino and mercapto groups forms glucuronide conjugate with glucuronic acid, and the test component containing phenolic hydroxyl group, aromatic amine and alcohol forms sulfuric acid ester conjugate. Most of the components to be tested in urine are in a conjugated state, and its polarity is greater than that of the prototype drug, so it should not be extracted by organic solvents. In order to determine the total amount of components to be tested in urine, whether it is direct determination or extraction and separation, it is necessary to carry out hydrolysis to release the components to be tested.

1. **酸水解**  通常使用无机酸，如盐酸。酸的用量、浓度、反应时间和温度等条件，基于待测成分的理化性质，通过实验而定。该方法简便、快速，但专一性较酶水解差。

**(1) Acid Hydrolysis**  Usually inorganic acids such as hydrochloric acid are used. Conditions such as the amount, concentration, reaction time and temperature of the acid are determined by experiments based on the physical and chemical properties of the measured ingredients. This method is simple and fast, but the specificity is worse than enzymatic hydrolysis.

2. **酶水解**  适用于与酸及受热不稳定的待测成分。常用葡萄糖醛酸糖苷酶或硫酸酯酶，可分别水解待测成分的葡萄糖醛酸苷缀合物和硫酸酯缀合物。实际常使用葡萄糖醛酸苷酶 – 硫酸酯酶的混合酶，在 pH 4.5~7.0，37℃厌氧条件下培育数小时进行水解。

**(2) Enzymatic Hydrolysis**  Applicable to acid and thermally unstable components to be tested. Commonly used glucuronidase or sulfatase, can hydrolyze the glucuronide conjugate and sulfate conjugate of the component to be tested respectively. In practice, a mixed enzyme of glucuronidase-sulfatase is often used, which is incubated for several hours at pH 4.5-7.0 and 37℃ under anaerobic conditions for hydrolysis.

3. **溶剂解**  通过加入溶剂，使缀合物（主要是硫酸酯）在萃取过程中发生分解，称为溶剂解。例如，尿中的甾体硫酸酯在 pH 为 1 时，加乙酸乙酯提取，产生溶剂解。

**(3) Solvolysis**　By adding a solvent, the conjugate (mainly sulfate) is decomposed during the extraction process, which is called solvolysis. For example, urinary steroid sulfate is extracted with ethyl acetate at a pH of 1, resulting in solvolysis.

目前，对缀合物的分析逐渐趋向于直接测定缀合物的含量，以获得体内以缀合物形式存在的药物量，以及体外排出药物中缀合物的比率，为了解药物代谢情况提供更多信息。

At present, the analysis of conjugates has gradually tended to directly determine the content of conjugates in order to obtain the amount of drugs present in the form of conjugates in the body and the ratio of conjugates excreted in vitro, which provides more insights into drug metabolism much information.

---

## 第三节　生物样品分析方法的建立与验证

## 9.3　Establishment and Verification of Biological Sample Analysis Methods

PPT

### 一、生物样品分析方法的建立
### 9.3.1　Establishment of Biological Sample Analysis Methods

#### （一）检测条件的优化
#### 1. Optimization of Testing Conditions

取待测成分和内标物（必要时）的标准物质，按拟定的分析方法（不包含样品的预处理）测定，根据结果，确定最佳分析检测条件、最适宜的测定浓度和检测灵敏度。采用色谱分析法时，可通过调整色谱柱、流动相组成比例及流量、检测波长、柱温、进样量、内标物的浓度及其加入量等条件，从而获得良好的色谱参数、适当的峰面积比值（待测成分与内标物）及保留时间和足够的方法灵敏度。

The amount of pure product to be tested and internal standard (necessary) is determined according to the proposed analysis method (excluding the pretreatment part of biological samples). According to the analytical results, the optimal concentration, sensitivity and optimal detection conditions. Good chromatographic parameters in chromatographic separation method can be obtained by changing chromatographic column, mobile phase and its flow rate, detection wavelength, column temperature, the injection volume, the concentration of the internal standard and its added amount and so on. In this way, good chromatographic parameters, appropriate peak area ratio (component to be tested and internal standard), retention time and the good sensitivity of method are obtained.

#### （二）分离条件的优化
#### 2. Optimization of Separation Conditions

1. **空白溶剂试验**　取待测成分的非生物基质溶液，按拟定的分析方法进行预处理，并测定空白值的响应信号。空白响应信号将影响方法的灵敏度和专属性。可通过改变实验条件，降低空白试剂的信号，使其不干扰药物的测定。

**(1) Blank Solvent Experiments**　An abiotic matrix solution of the component to be tested is pretreated according to the proposed analytical method, and the response signals for the blank value

医药大学堂
WWW.YIYAODXT.COM

are determined. Blank value chromatographic information will affect the sensitivity and specificity of the method. Therefore, by changing the experimental conditions, the signal of the blank reagent can be reduced so that it will not interfere with the determination of the drug.

2. **空白生物基质试验**　主要用来考察生物基质中内源性物质对待测成分的干扰，在测定药物、特定的活性代谢物、内标物质等的"信号窗"内，不应出现内源性物质信号。即取空白生物基质，如空白血浆，按拟定的分析方法，进行处理并分析，不应对待测成分有干扰。

(2) **Blank Biological Matrix Experiments**　It is mainly used to investigate the interference of endogenous compounds in the biological matrix with the measured components. Endogenous substances should not be detected in the "signal window" for the drugs, specific active metabolites and internal standard substances, etc. Blank biological matrix is taken and treated and analyzed according to the proposed analysis method, and no interference with the measured components.

3. **模拟生物样品试验**　取空白生物基质，加入待测成分标准物质，制成模拟生物样品，按照"空白生物基质试验"相同的方法处理分析，考察方法的线性、范围、精密度、准确度和灵敏度等指标，检验生物基质中内源性物质以及可能共同存在的其他成分对测定的干扰程度。若采用色谱法进行测定，多数情况下需考虑用内标法定量，同时还应考察待测成分、内标物质与内源性代谢物或其他成分的分离情况。

(3) **Simulated Biological Sample Experiments**　The simulated biological sample is made by adding the purity of the components to be tested into the blank biological matrix. After the same treatment and analysis of the blank biological matrix, investigate the linearity, range, precision, accuracy and sensitivity of the method, and examine the degree of interference of the endogenous substances in the biological matrix and other components that may coexist with the determination. If the chromatographic method is adopted for determination, the internal standard method should be considered for quantification in most cases, investigate the separation of the components to be tested and internal standard substances or endogenous metabolites or other components.

4. **实际生物样品的测定**　经过"空白生物基质"和"模拟生物样品试验"，所确定的分析方法及其条件还不能完全确定是否适合于实样测定，还需进行实际生物样品的测定，考察代谢物对药物、内标物的干扰，从而选择避免干扰并适合样品实际情况的分析方法，验证方法的可行性。

(4) **Actual Biological Sample Determination**　After "blank biological matrix" and "simulated biological sample" tests, the analytical methods and conditions can′t be fully determined whether they are suitable for real sample determination, and needs to determine the actual biological samples, inspects the metabolite to the drug and internal standard interference after analyzing method determinated, thus avoiding interference and suiting actual condition to further validate the feasibility of method.

（三）质控样品及意义

### 3. Quality Control Aamples and Significance

未知生物样品的测定，应在分析方法建立并完成验证之后进行。在实际生物样品的测定过程中，应对分析数据的质量进行必要的监控。质控样品（quality control，QC），系指将一定量待测成分加入空白生物基质中，配制模拟生物样品，用于分析全程的质量控制，包括分析方法的精密度、准确度、提取回收率及样品稳定性等评价。一般配成低（LQC）、中（MQC）、高（HQC）3个质量浓度的质控样品。

The measurement of unknown biological samples should be carried out after the analytical method is established and the verification is completed. During the measurement of actual biological samples, the quality of the analysis data should be necessarily monitored. Quality control (QC) refers to adding a certain amount of components to be tested into a blank biological matrix to prepare a simulated biological sample for quality control of the entire process, including the precision, accuracy and extraction recovery rate of the analytical method and sample stability evaluation. It is generally formulated into three samples of quality concentration, which is low quality concentration (LQC), medium quality concentration (MQC) and high quality concentration (HQC).

每个未知样品一般只测定 1 次，必要时（有充分理由证实该测定结果异常时）可重复测定。每批样品测定的同时应建立相应的标准曲线，并随行间隔测定高、中、低至少 3 个质量浓度的质控样品（QC）。QC 样品应由浓度低至高或高至低的顺序以一定间隔，均匀穿插于整个分析批，与生物样品同时测定，根据质控样品的测定结果，评判该分析批的数据是否可被接受或拒绝。

Each unknown sample is generally measured only once, if necessary (when there are sufficient reasons to prove that the measurement result is abnormal), the measurement can be repeated. The corresponding standard curve should be established at the same time of the determination of each batch of samples, at the same time, the quality control samples (QC) of at least 3 concentrations (high, medium, and low) should be determined at intervals. QC samples should be evenly interspersed throughout the analysis batch at a certain interval in the order of low to high or high to low, and measured simultaneously with the biological sample. According to the measurement results of the quality control sample, judge whether the data of the analysis batch can be accepted or rejected.

每一个分析批内，应随机穿插分析至少 6 个 QC 样品，若未知样品数目较多时，应增加浓度质控样品数，使其数目大于未知样品总数的 5%。指控样品的测定结果的偏差一般应小于 15%，RSD≤15%，最多允许 1/3 同一浓度质控样品结果超限。若质控样品的测定结果不符合上述要求，则该分析批样测试结果作废。

In each analysis batch, at least 6 QC samples should be randomly interspersed. If there are a large number of unknown samples, the number of concentration of quality control samples should be increased so that the number is greater than 5% of the total number of unknown samples. The deviation of the measurement results of the QC sample should generally be less than 15%, RSD ≤ 15%, and at most 1/3 results of the QC samples in the same concentration of quality control are allowed to exceed the limit. If the measurement result of the quality control sample does not meet the above requirements, the test result of the analysis batch sample is invalid.

### 二、生物样品分析方法的验证
### 9.3.2　Verification of Biological Sample Analysis Methods

（一）专属性
#### 1. Selectivity
专属性系指生物样品中所含内源性和外源性物质及相应的代谢物质存在的情况下，所用的方法能准确测定待测物质的能力，通常表示所检测的相应信号应属于待测成分所特有。如果有多个分析物，应保证每个分析物都不被干扰。

Specificity refers to the ability of the method used to accurately determine the substance to be tested in the presence of endogenous and exogenous substances and corresponding metabolites contained in the biological sample, usually indicating that the corresponding signal detected should belong to the substance to be tested specific to the ingredients. If there are several analytes, ensure that each analyte is not disturbed.

对于质谱法，则应考虑分析过程中的基质效应，对于结构一致的化合物，必要时可通过二极管阵列检测器（HPLC-DAD）和质谱检测器（LC-MS）确证被测定色谱峰的单纯性和同一性；结构未知代谢物的测定，可采用 LC-NMR 进行结构的初步推测后，考察其干扰情况。

For mass spectrometry, the matrix effect in the analysis process should be considered. And for compounds with the same structure, the simplicity and identity of the chromatographic peaks determined can be confirmed through the diode array detector and mass spectrometry detector, while for metabolites with unknown structure, LC-NMR can be used for the preliminary prediction of the structure firstly, and then interference situation can be investigated.

（二）标准曲线与线性范围

## 2. Standard Curve and Linearity Range

标准曲线系指生物样品中所测定成分的浓度与响应值的相关性，通常用回归分析方法获得，并以相关系数评价标准曲线的线性程度。标准曲线的最高与最低浓度的区间为线性范围。待测成分模拟生物样品的浓度应在线性范围内，并应达到试验要求的精密度和准确度。

A standard curve is the relationship between instrument response and known concentrations of the analyte, usually obtained by regression analysis, and its linearity is evaluated by correlation coefficient. The interval between the highest and lowest concentrations of the standard curve is a linearity range. The concentration of the component to be tested in the simulated biological sample should be in the range and reach the precision and accuracy required by the test.

标准曲线的建立，一般要求 5~7 个浓度的标准模拟生物样品（不包括空白生物样品），其线性范围，应能覆盖全部待测生物样品中的药物浓度，不能使用线性范围外推的方法，计算未知生物样品中的药物浓度。建立标准曲线所使用的模拟生物样品的基质应与待测含药生物样品的基质相同。

The establishment of the standard curve generally requires standard simulated biological samples with 5-7 concentrations, whose linearity range should cover drug concentration in all biological samples to be tested, and the method of linearity range extrapolation cannot be used to calculate the drug concentration in biological samples. The simulated biological sample used to establish the standard curve should be prepared with the same biological matrix as the biological sample to be tested.

（三）精密度与准确度

## 3. Precision and Accuracy

精密度是指在确定的分析条件下相同生物介质中相同浓度样品的一系列测量值的分散程度。常用模拟生物样品的相对标准偏差表示。生物样品数量较大，往往在 1 个分析批内难以完成全部样品的分析，因此，为了评价不同分析批之间由于实验条件的微小改变对分析结果可能产生的影响，精密度除需评价批内精密度外，尚需评价批间精密度。

Precision refers to the degree of dispersion of a series of measured values of samples of the same concentration in the same biological medium under certain analytical conditions. Relative standard deviation of commonly used simulated biological samples. The number of biological samples is large, and it is often difficult to complete the analysis of all samples in one analysis batch. Therefore, in order to evaluate the possible impact of small changes in experimental conditions on the analysis results between different analysis batches, the precision needs to be evaluated in the batch. In addition to precision, batch precision needs to be evaluated.

准确度系指在确定的分析条件下测得的生物样品中待测成分的浓度与其真实浓度的接近程度。通常用模拟生物样品的实测浓度与标示浓度的相对回收率或者相对误差表示。相对回收率或相对误差的计算如下：

Accuracy refers to how close the concentration of the component to be measured in the biological sample measured under the determined analysis conditions is to its true concentration. Usually expressed by the relative recovery or relative error of the measured concentration of the simulated biological sample and the labeled concentration:

$$相对回收率（Relative\ Recovery）= \frac{M}{A} \times 100\% \qquad （9\text{-}1）$$

$$相对误差（Relative\ Error）= \frac{M-A}{M} \times 100\% \qquad （9\text{-}2）$$

式中，$M$ 为模拟生物样本中待测成分的实测浓度；$A$ 为加入的待测成分的标示浓度。

Where: $M$ is the measured concentration of the tested component in the simulated biological sample; $A$ is the labeled concentration of the added tested component.

精密度和准确度考察通常选择模拟生物样品的低、中、高 3 个质量浓度，各浓度至少 5 个样品。低浓度一般选择在标准曲线最低浓度的 3 倍以内；高浓度在标准曲线最高浓度的 70%~85% 附近；中间浓度在高、低浓度的几何浓度附近。测定批间精密度时，应在不同天（每天 1 个分析批）连续制备并测定，至少有连续 3 个分析批，即不少于 45 个样品的分析结果。各样品与随行的标准曲线同法操作，分别测定 1 次。精密度的 RSD 一般应小于 15%，在标准曲线最低浓度附近，精密度的 RSD 应小于 20%。准确度的相对回收率通常在 85%~115% 范围内（相对误差不超过 ±15%），在标准曲线最低浓度附近，准确度的相对回收率应在 80%~120%（相对误差不超过 ±20%）。

Precision and accuracy surveys usually choose low, medium, and high quality concentrations of simulated biological samples, with at least 5 samples of each concentration. The low concentration is generally selected within 3 times the lowest concentration of the standard curve; the high concentration is around 70%-85% of the highest concentration of the standard curve; the intermediate concentration is near the geometric concentration of the high and low concentrations. When measuring the precision between batches, it should be continuously prepared and measured on different days (1 analytical batch per day), and there should be at least 3 consecutive analytical batches, that is, the analysis results of not less than 45 samples. Each sample and the accompanying standard curve were operated in the same way, and were measured once. The precision RSD should generally be less than 15%, and the precision RSD should be less than 20% around the lowest concentration of the standard curve. The relative recovery rate of accuracy is usually in the range of 85%-115% (relative error does not exceed ± 15%), the relative recovery rate of accuracy should be 80%-120% (the relative error does not exceed ± 20%).

（四）定量限与检测限

## 4. Limit of Quantification and Limit of Detection

定量限是指分析方法在符合准确度和精密度要求的前提下，待测成分能够被定量测定的最低浓度，通常以标准曲线上的最低浓度点表示。检测限是指试样中被测成分能被检测出的最低浓度，一般以信噪比 S/N=3（或 2）时的相应浓度表示。

The limit of quantification refers to the lowest concentration at which the component to be measured can be quantitatively determined under the premise that the analysis method meets the requirements of accuracy and precision, usually expressed as the lowest concentration point on the standard curve. The detection limit refers to the lowest concentration at which the measured component in the sample can be detected.

（五）样品稳定性

## 5. Sample Stability

生物样品数量大，采集后，通常在1个工作日内难以完成全部样品的分析；且随着自动进样系统的广泛应用，多个制备样品会同时置于进样盘中等待分析；同时，虽然一般情况下，每个未知生物样品测定1次，但有时亦需进行复测。因此，为了确保分析结果的可重复与可靠性，分析过程中样品的稳定性显得尤为重要。样品稳定性验证内容包括长期贮存、室温、冷冻、冻融条件下的稳定性，以确定生物样品的存放条件和时间；另外还包括标准贮备液以及样品处理后的溶液（制备样品）中待测成分的稳定性。

The number of biological samples is large, and it is usually difficult to complete the analysis of all samples within 1 working day after collection; and with the wide application of automatic sampling systems, multiple prepared samples will be placed in the sample tray for analysis at the same time; Although under normal circumstances, each unknown biological sample is measured once, but sometimes it is necessary to retest. Therefore, in order to ensure the repeatability and reliability of the analysis results, the stability of the samples during the analysis process is particularly important. The sample stability verification content includes the stability under long-term storage, room temperature, freezing, and freeze-thaw conditions to determine the storage conditions and time of the biological sample; it also includes the standard stock solution and the solution (prepared sample) to be tested Ingredient stability.

1. **长期稳定性**　考察整个样品分析期间，含药生物样品长期储存条件（–20℃或–80℃）的稳定性，确定生物样品的存放条件和时间。考察的时间，应超过收集第一个样品至最后一个样品被分析所需的时间。

(1) **Long-term stability**　Check the stability of long-term storage conditions (–20°C or –80°C) of drug-containing biological samples during the entire sample analysis period to determine the storage conditions and time of biological samples. The inspection time should exceed the time required to collect the first sample until the last sample is analyzed.

2. **短期室温稳定性**　考察生物样品在室温等待处理、处理过程及制备完成等待进样过程中样品中待测成分的稳定性，以保证检测结果的重现性和准确性。根据实际操作在室温中需维持的时间，将样品于室温下放置相应时间，在不同时间点取样分析，与0小时的结果进行比较。

(2) **Short-term room temperature stability**　Examine the stability of the components to be tested in the samples waiting for processing, processing and sample preparation and waiting injection during room temperature, to ensure the reproducibility and accuracy of the test results. According to the time that the actual operation needs to be maintained at room temperature, the sample is placed at room temperature for a corresponding time, sampled and analyzed at different time points, and compared with the result of 0 hours.

3. **冻融稳定性**　待测成分的冻融稳定性考察应至少经历3次冻融循环测定。各样品于预期贮存温度（通常先设定为–20℃）贮存24小时后，置室温自然融化后取样分析。再将相应样品在相同条件下冷冻24小时，如此反复冻融循环2次以上，比较各次分析结果。若待测成分在预期储存温度（–20℃）下不稳定，则应置–80℃进行冻融稳定性考察。

(3) **Freeze-thaw stability**　The freeze-thaw stability of the components to be tested should be determined by at least 3 freeze-thaw cycles. Each sample is stored at the expected storage temperature (usually set to -20°C first) for 24 hours, and then left to melt at room temperature for sampling and analysis. Then freeze the corresponding samples for 24 hours under the same conditions, and repeat the freeze-thaw cycle more than 2 times, and compare the results of each analysis. If the component to be

tested is unstable at the expected storage temperature (-20°C), it should be placed at -80°C for freeze-thaw stability investigation.

稳定性试验中至少取高、低浓度的模拟生物样品，按照相应的条件下可能需要的存放时间确定考察时间点，每个样品重复 3 次，其平均值的偏差应在 0 时测定值的 ±5% 以内（需要衍生化处理的样品在 ±15% 以内）。

In the stability test, at least high and low concentrations of simulated biological samples are taken, and the investigation time point is determined according to the storage time that may be required under the corresponding conditions. Each sample is repeated 3 times, and the deviation of the average value should be within 5% the measured value (samples requiring derivatization treatment are within ± 15%) at 0h.

（六）提取回收率

## 6. Extraction Recovery

提取回收率又称为绝对回收率，是指从生物介质中回收得到待测成分的响应值与标准物质产生的响应值的比值，通常用 % 表示。要求考察高、中、低 3 个浓度的模拟生物样品，各浓度至少 5 个样品。另取等量的相应浓度的标准溶液，加入到空白生物介质中，制备相应的标准对照溶液，同法平行测定。将模拟生物样品的检测信号与未经处理的标准溶液的检测信号比较，计算提取回收率［式（9-3）］。

Extraction recovery rate, also called absolute recovery rate, refers to the ratio of the response value of the component to be tested recovered from the biological medium to the response value generated by the standard substance, usually expressed in %. It is required to investigate three simulated biological samples with high, medium and low concentrations, each with at least 5 samples. Take another equal amount of the corresponding standard solution of the corresponding concentration, add it to the blank biological medium, prepare the corresponding standard control solution, and measure in parallel with the same method. Compare the detection signal of the simulated biological sample with the detection signal of the untreated standard solution to calculate the extraction recovery rate.

$$R=A_{\mathrm{T}}/A_{\mathrm{S}}\times100\% \tag{9-3}$$

式中，$R$ 为提取回收率，$A_{\mathrm{T}}$ 为模拟生物样品制备处理后的检测信号；$A_{\mathrm{S}}$ 为未经处理的标准溶液的检测信号。

Where, $R$ is the extraction recovery rate, $A_{\mathrm{T}}$ is the detection signal after the preparation of the simulated biological sample; $A_{\mathrm{S}}$ is the detection signal of the untreated standard solution.

采用内标法时，应同时测定内标物的提取回收率，方法同待测成分，仅需要制备 1 个浓度 5 个模拟生物样品即可。

When using the internal standard method, the extraction recovery rate of the internal standard should be measured at the same time. The method is the same as that of the component to be tested, and only one concentration of 5 simulated biological samples needs to be prepared.

通常各浓度待测成分的提取回收率均应≥50%；且高、中浓度的 RSD 应≤15%，低浓度的 RSD 应≤20%。

Generally, the extraction recovery rate of each concentration of the component to be tested should be ≥50%; and the RSD of high and medium concentration should be ≤ 15%, and the RSD of low concentration should be ≤ 20%.

# 岗 位 对 接
# Post Docking

本章为中药学、中药制药、中药资源与开发等相关专业学生必须掌握的内容，为成为合格的中药分析人员奠定坚实的基础。

This task must be mastered by students majoring in traditional Chinese medicine, traditional Chinese medicine pharmacy and traditional Chinese medicine resources, and lay a solid foundation for becoming qualified Chinese medicine service personnel.

本章内容对应岗位包括中药新药研发等相关工种。

The corresponding positions of this task include research and development of new Chinese medicine and so on.

上述从事中药新药研发相关所有岗位的从业人员均需要熟悉制备方法，生物样品分析方法的建立与验证，学会应用本章所学内容开展中药分析工作。

The above-mentioned practitioners in all positions related to traditional Chinese medicine service need to familiar with preparation method, establishment and verification of biological sample analysis method, and learn to apply analysis of ingredients of Chinese medicine in biological samples to carry out traditional Chinese medicine analysis services.

# 重 点 小 结
# Summary of Key Points

生物样品是指来自生物机体的各种体液、器官、组织及排泄物等，常用的生物样品是血液（血清、血浆、全血）、尿液、唾液及胆汁。生物样品的前处理，是生物样品分析中极其重要的一环，由于生物样品的复杂性，其前处理过程也很难规定固定的模式和程序，需结合实验要求，采取适当的处理手段，建立适合生物样品中待测成分测定的分析方法，并通过严格的方法学验证，从而保证生物样品内中药化学成分测定结果的准确性。

Biological samples refer to various body fluids, organs, tissues and excretions from biological organisms. Commonly used biological samples are blood (serum, plasma, whole blood), urine, saliva and bile. The pre-processing of biological samples is an extremely important part in the analysis of biological samples. Due to the complexity of biological samples, it is difficult to specify a fixed model and procedure for the pre-processing process. It is suitable for the analysis method for the determination of the component to be tested in the biological sample, and through strict methodological verification, so as to ensure the accuracy of the determination result of the chemical composition of the traditional Chinese medicine in the biological sample.

题库

# 目　标　检　测

## 一、选择题

### （一）单项选择题

1. 代谢中药成分的主要脏器是
   A. 肺　　　　　　　B. 肾　　　　　　　C. 脾　　　　　　　D. 肝

2. 血样包括的种类有
   A. 血清、血浆、全血　　　　　　　B. 血浆、全血、血色素
   C. 血清、血色素、全血　　　　　　D. 全血、白蛋白、血清

3. 血浆制备过程中，最常用的抗凝剂是
   A. 枸橼酸　　　　　B. EDTA　　　　　C. 肝素　　　　　D. 氟化钠

4. 不属于均匀生物样本的是
   A. 血样　　　　　　B. 尿液　　　　　　C. 脏器组织　　　　D. 唾液

### （二）多项选择题

1. 代谢中药成分的脏器有
   A. 肺　　　　　B. 肝　　　　　C. 脾　　　　　D. 肾　　　　　E. 脑

2. 生物样品的稳定性试验包括
   A. 短期稳定性　　　　　B. 长期稳定性　　　　　C. 冻融稳定性
   D. 重复性　　　　　　　E. 中间精密度

3. 药物的药动学研究内容包括
   A. 吸收　　　　　B. 分布　　　　　C. 代谢　　　　　D. 排泄　　　　　E. 生物转化

4. 药物在生物体内存在的形式有
   A. 原型药　　　　B. 结合物　　　　C. 代谢物　　　　D. 缀合物　　　　E. 游离型

## 二、简单题

1. 简述生物样品内中药分析的特点。
2. 简述生物样品内去除蛋白质的方法。
3. 简述生物样品内中药定量分析方法学考察的内容。

# 第十章　中药质量标准的制定

# Chapter 10　Establishment of Quality Standards for Traditional Chinese Medicine

 学习目标｜Learning Goal

知识要求：

1. **掌握**　中药质量标准的主要内容和制定方法。
2. **熟悉**　中药质量标准制定的原则、前提和一般程序。
3. **了解**　中药的稳定性研究。

能力要求：

学会应用中药质量标准的主要内容和制定方法解决中药的质量控制与评价。

**Knowledge Requirements**

**1. Master**　The main contents and formulating method of Chinese medicine quality standard.

**2. Familiar**　The principles, prerequisites and general procedures for the formulating quality standards of TCM.

**3. Understand**　Study on the stability of traditional Chinese medicine.

**Ability Requirements**

Learn to apply the main content of Chinese medicine quality standards and formulating methods to solve the quality control and evaluation of Chinese medicine..

## 第一节　概述

## 10.1　Overview

PPT

### 一、制定质量标准的目的、意义

### 10.1.1　Purpose and Significance of Establishing Euality Standards

药品是一种特殊的商品，其质量的优劣直接关系到用药者的身心健康和用药安全，为保证人民群众身心健康与安全，必须制定药品质量标准。质量标准是中药新药研究中重要的组成部分，制定出符合中药特点、科学、先进、切实可行的质量标准对于保证中药的安全有效、质量稳定可控具有重要的意义，同时对指导药品生产、供应、使用、检验和管理，以及推动药品的国际交流与贸易具有重要意义。

Drug is a special commodity whose quality is directly related to the physical and mental health and medication safety of users. Quality standards are important parts in the study of new drug of TCM, and to develop standards which fit the characteristics of Chinese traditional medicine as well as being scientific, advanced and practical is of great importance to ensure the safety, effectiveness, stability and controllability of TCM, meanwhile, it is also of great value to the international communications and trade in pharmaceutical production, supply, use, inspection and management.

### 二、制定质量标准的原则和前提条件
### 10.1.2 Principles and Prerequisites for Establishing Quality Standard

（一）制定中药质量标准的原则

#### 1. Principles for the Establishment of Quality Standards for Traditional Chinese Medicine

中药质量标准的制定，要以中医药理论为指导思想，坚持质量第一，充分体现"安全有效、技术先进、经济合理、传承创新、科学、实用、规范"的原则。

The formulation of Chinese medicine quality standards must be guided by Chinese medicine theory, adhere to quality first, and fully embody the principles of safety and effectiveness, advanced technology, economical rationality, inheritance and innovation, science, practicality and standardization.

（二）制定中药质量标准必须满足的前提条件

#### 2. Preconditions for the Establishment of Quality Standards for Traditional Chinese Medicine

1. **处方组成固定** 中药制剂处方药味与份量是制定质量标准的依据，直接影响评价指标的选定和限度的制定。无论是成方还是临床验方，均需在制定质量标准前明确处方的组成。

**(1) The composition of prescription is fixed** The quality standard is based on the ingredients of traditional Chinese medicine preparation, which directly affects the selection of evaluation index and the formulation of limit, so both clinically experienced prescriptions and set prescriptions are all needed defining ingredients before establishing quality standards.

2. **原辅料稳定** 中药提取物、中药制剂质量标准制定之前，首先要制定中药材的质量标准，中药材同名异物、同物异名及多基源现象较常见，直接影响药材的质量，因此，必须明确中药材的基源。其次要制定饮片和辅料的质量标准。为保证药品质量和临床疗效稳定，最好从道地产区购进合格的药材。在新药临床研究、中试及后期生产时，均应严格按照质量标准的规定投料。

**(2) Stability of raw and auxiliary materials** Quality standards for Chinese medicinal extracts and preparations should be formulated after quality standards of Chinese medicinal materials are formulated , whereas the phenomenons that different Chinese medicinal materials have the same chinese name, the same Chinese medicinal materials have different chinese names and Chinese medicinal materials with polybasic sources are so common which affect the quality of medicinal materials directly, so the sources of Chinese medicinal materials must be clear. It is necessary to establish the quality standards for decoction pieces and pharmaceutical excipients. In order to ensure the quality and clinical efficacy of medicines, it is best to purchase qualified medicinal materials from genuine producing areas.

In the clinical study of new drugs, the pilot test or the later stage of production, the produce should be strictly in accordance with the prescript quality standard.

3. **工艺稳定**　在处方和原辅料都确定后，可结合临床给药方式确定剂型，再筛选生产工艺条件，制备工艺稳定后，再开展质量标准的实验设计。如果原辅料、处方相同，但工艺不同，可造成所含成分不同，会直接影响到鉴定、检查和含量测定等项目的建立和限度的规定。

**(3) Processing stability**　After the prescription and the pharmaceutical excipients are determined. The dosage form can be determined in combination with the clinical administration rote, and then the production process conditions can be screened. After the preparation process is stable, the experimental design of the quality standard can be carried out. If the prescription and pharmaceutical excipients, prescriptions are the same, but the process is different, it can cause different components, and will directly affect the establishment of identification, inspection, content determination, other items and limitations.

因此，处方组成固定，提取物、中药制剂处方和制备工艺固定，原辅料质量标准完备是制定中药质量标准的前提条件。

Therefore, that the prescription composition is fixed, that the extract, the traditional Chinese medicine preparation prescription and the preparation craft are fixed, and that the pharmaceutical excipients quality standard is complete, which are the prerequisite conditions to formulate the traditional Chinese medicine quality standards.

### 三、质量标准研究程序
### 10.1.3　Procedures of the Quality Standards

#### （一）依据法规制定总体方案
#### 1. Formulating the Overall Plan in Accordance with Laws and Regulations

中药质量标准研究的设计方案应根据《药品管理法》《中药新药质量标准研究的技术要求》《药品注册管理办法》等法律法规进行，质量标准拟定的各项内容参照现行版的《中国药典》。

The design plan for the study of quality standards of traditional Chinese medicine shall be carried out in accordance with *the Law on Drug Administration*, *the Technical Requirements for the Study on the Quality Standards of New Chinese Medicine*, and *the Measures for the Administration of Drug Registration*, The content of the draft quality standard refers to the current version the *Chinese Pharmacopoeia*.

#### （二）查阅文献资料
#### 2. Literature Review

查阅研究对象所涉及的各味中药的主要化学成分及理化性质、与功能主治有关的药效学及质量控制相关的国内外文献资料，为质量标准的制定提供参考依据。

The main chemical components, physical and chemical properties, pharmacodynamics and index of quality control related to the functions of various traditional Chinese medicines involved in the study are reviewed to provide reference for the formulation of quality standards.

#### （三）实验研究
#### 3. Experimental Research

根据质量标准研究方案和查阅文献的结果，对拟定的各项内容逐一进行研究，积累原始实验数据，为质量标准制定提供科学依据。

According to the research plan of quality standards and the results of literature review, the proposed contents are studied one by one, and the original experimental data is accumulated to provide scientific basis for the formulation of quality standards.

### （四）制定质量标准草案和编写起草说明
### 4. Formulating the Draft Quality Standards and Drafting Instructions

根据实验研究结果，参照现行版《中国药典》相对应的中药质量标准的内容和格式，整理数据和制定质量标准草案，选择准确、灵敏、简便和快速的检测方法纳入标准，其内容既要结合实际，又要与国际先进水平接轨，既要符合规范化的要求，又要结合临床应用。同时编写起草说明对制定的质量标准加以解释说明。

According to the experimental results, data is to be organized, quality standards shall be drafted, and accurate, sensitive, simple and rapid testing methods are to be included in the standards whose content should be connected with practice, matched with the international advanced technology, meet with the requirements of standardization, and combined with clinical application, referring to the contents and format of the quality standards of traditional Chinese medicine corresponding to the current edition of the *Chinese Pharmacopoeia*. Apart from that, a drafting note is also prepared to explain the quality standards settlement.

## 第二节　中药质量标准的主要内容
## 10.2　Main Contents of the Quality Standards for Traditional Chinese Medicine

### 一、中药材（饮片）
### 10.2.1　Chinese Medicinal Materials (Decoction Pieces)

中药材和饮片质量标准正文按名称、来源、性状、鉴别、检查、含量测定等顺序编写。未列饮片和炮制项的，其名称和药材名相同，则同为饮片和药材标准；列在药材项下的饮片，列出【炮制】项，与药材相同的内容只列出项目名称，内容用"同药材"表述，不同于药材的项目需逐项列出，并规定相应的指标。同时增加【性味与归经】【功能与主治】【用法与用量】【注意】【贮藏】等项目；单列饮片的标准内容，其来源简化为"本品为××的炮制加工品"，增加【制法】项，收载相应的炮制工艺。其余同上，具体见下文。

The texts of quality standards for Chinese medicinal medicines and decoction pieces are written in the order of name, sources, description, identification, test, and content determination. If the pieces and processed items are not listed, the name and the name of the medicinal materials are the same, and they are the same as the standard of pieces and medicinal materials; If the pieces are listed under the item of medicinal materials, the item of "Processing" should be listed, items are the same as the standard of pieces and medicinal materials, expressed with "same medicinal materials", items different from medicinal materials need to be listed item by item, and the corresponding indicators should be specified. At the same time, add items such as "Property and Flavor" "Meridian Tropism" "Action and Indications" "Administration and Dosage" "Precautions and Warnings" "Storage" and other items; the standard content of the single-piece decoction pieces, the source of which is simplified as "this product is ×× processing "Products" , add the item "processed" to include the corresponding processing technology. The rest is the same as above, see below for details

**名称** 名称包括中文名、汉语拼音名和拉丁名或英文名。

*Title* adopted Chinese names, Chinese phonetic alphabet and English name or Latin name.

**来源** 来源包括原植（动）物的科名、中文名、拉丁学名、药用部位、采收季节和产地加工等。矿物药包括该矿物的类、族、矿石名或岩石名、主要成分及产地加工等。

*Sources* The family names of the original plants (animals), Chinese names, Latin names, medicinal parts, harvesting seasons and post harvest processing are all included. To mineral medicines, the class, family, name of ore or rock, main ingredients and processing of origin of the mineral shall be contained.

**性状** 列出药材、饮片的形状、大小、表面（色泽、特征）、质地、断面及气味等。

*Description* The shape, color, size, surface characteristics, texture, section and flavor of medicinal materials, and decoction pieces

**鉴别** 列出鉴别药材、饮片真伪的方法，包括经验鉴别、显微鉴别（组织切片、粉末或表面制片、显微化学）、理化鉴别。

*Identification* Methods of identifying the authenticity of medicinal materials and decoction pieces including empirical identification, microscopic identification (tissue sections, powder or surface fabrication, microscopic chemistry), physical and chemical identification, which should be list.

**检查** 列出水分、纯净程度、重金属及有害元素、农药残留量、黄曲霉素、有关毒性成分等限量或者含量检查项目及限度。

*Test* List the limit or content inspection items and limits of moisture, ash, acid insoluble ash, heavy metals, arsenic salts, pesticide residues, aflatoxins related toxic components etc.

**浸出物** 列出所需的溶剂和测定方法，并规定限度。

*Extractives* List the required solvents and measurement methods, and formulate limits.

**特征图谱或指纹图谱** 列出相应的测定方法，采用色谱法建立的，需列出色谱条件和系统适用性实验，并附其对照图谱，指认色谱峰对应的成分。特征图谱需说明特征峰和相对保留时间，指纹图谱需按中药色谱指纹图谱相似度评价系统评价。并规定供试品指纹图谱与对照品指纹图谱的相似度。

*Characteristic Chromatography or Fingerprint* List the corresponding determination methods, established by chromatographic methods, the chromatographic system and system suitability experiments need to be listed, and their control chromatography are attached to identify the components corresponding to the chromatographic peaks. The characteristic chromatography should indicate the characteristic peak and relative retention time. The fingerprint should be evaluated according to the similarity evaluation system of chromatographic fingerprint of traditional Chinese medicine. It also specifies the similarity between the fingerprint of the test sample and the fingerprint of the reference product.

**含量测定** 列出含量测定的方法和相应的限度标准。

*Assay* List the content determination method and the corresponding limit standard.

**炮制** 药材项下饮片标准中均需列出炮制项，描述炮制方法。与药材性状不同的需要描述饮片性状。

*Processing* items should be listed in the decoction standard under the item of medicinal materials to describe the prepared method. Different from the traits of medicinal materials, the traits of decoction pieces need to be described.

**性味与归经** 按中医药理论与经验概括其四气五味和归经。

*Property and Flavor and Meridian Tropism* Four Qi five flavors and meridian tropism should be summed up according to the theory and experience of traditional Chinese medicine.

**功能与主治** 按中医药或民族医药学的理论和临床用药经验概述功能主治。

*Action and Indications* According to the theory of traditional Chinese medicine or ethnic medicine and clinical medication experience, action and indication are summarized.

**用法与用量** 如是常规水煎内服，只按成人一日剂量描述，必要时酌情增减，另有规定除外。

*Administration and Dosage* If it is taken orally, it is only described according to the adult's daily dose, and if necessary, increase or decrease as appropriate, unless otherwise specified.

**注意** 说明主要的禁忌和不良反应。

*Precautions and Warnings* Explain the main contraindications and adverse reactions.

**贮藏** 注明贮存与保存的基本要求。

*Storage* Specify the basic requirements for storage and preservation.

## 二、植物油脂和提取物
## 10.2.2 Herbal Oils, Fats and Extractives

**名称** 名称包括中文名、汉语拼音名及英文名。

*Title* adopted Chinese names, Chinese phonetic alphabet and English name.

**来源** 说明其以何种中药或药用植物加工制得。

*Sources* The source of the Chinese medicinal materials (decoction pieces) or medicinal plants should be described.

**制法** 除挥发油和油脂、有效成分不写制法外，其他粗提物、有效部位和组分提取物均需列出制法项，详细说明制备方法。

*Procedure* The details of preparations of crude extracts, effective parts and component extracts need to be described in the preparation methods except volatile oil, grease and active ingredients.

**性状** 挥发油和油脂需规定外观颜色、气味、溶解度、相对密度和折光率等；粗提物和有效部位提取物需规定外观颜色、气味等；有效成分提取物需规定外观颜色、溶解度、熔点、比旋度等。

*Description* The color, smell, solubility, relative density and refraction of volatile oils and fats need to be specified; The appearance, color and smell of the crude extracts and the extracts of the effective part need to be specified; The appearance color, solubility, melting point and optical rotation of the active ingredient extract need to be specified.

**鉴别** 描述鉴别真伪的方法，方法要求同中药材和饮片，但不做形态、显微鉴别。

*Identification* The method of describing the identification of authenticity is the same as the method of identifying Chinese medicinal materials and decoction pieces, but it does not need morphological and microscopic identification.

**检查** 植物油脂和提取物的检查项目应视具体情况而定，分别列出相应检查项目及限度。每个项目及限度为一个独立段落。

*Test* The examination items of herbal oils, fats and extractives should be depended on the actual situation and corresponding examination items and limits should be listed. Each item and its limits occupy a separated paragraph.

**特征图谱或指纹图谱** 同中药材（饮片）的方法和要求。

*Characteristic Chromatography or Fingerprint*    Same methods and requirements as that of Chinese medicinal materials (decoction pieces).

**含量测定**    列出含量测定方法，并规定其限度标准。

*Assay*    Methods for determination of content shall be listed and limits specified.

**贮藏**    注明其贮存与保管的基本要求。

*Storage*    The basic requirements for storage is indicated.

**制剂**    部分有明确制剂的植物油脂或提取物列出可制成的制剂。

*Preparations*    For some specific herbal oils, fats or extractives, what it can make should be listed.

### 三、中药制剂
### 10.2.3    Traditional Chinese Medicine Preparations

（一）名称
#### 1. Title

中药新制剂的命名，应避免混乱，力求明确、简短、科学，采用不易产生误解、混淆和夸大的名称；一般不另起商品名，以避免一药多名。属于国家标准收载而改变剂型的中药品种，除更新剂型名称外，原则上仍采用原来标准名称。

The naming of new preparations of traditional Chinese medicine should avoid confusion, and try to be clear, brief and scientific. Generally another trade name should not be given to avoid multiple names. The traditional Chinese medicine class which belongs to the national standard collection but change the form should still use the original standard name in principle, except the name of renewal form.

（二）处方
#### 2. Ingredients

处方中需要炮制的均用括号注明，未注明炮制的均为净制的生药材。需要保密的处方，应按保密品种申报。处方均应符合以下要求：

All the medicines in the ingredients needed to be processed should be indicated in parentheses, and the unspecified materials should be dealt as raw. Ingredients requiring confidentiality shall be declared in accordance with the type of confidentiality. Ingredients should meet the following requirements:

1. **处方组成**    列出处方中的不同药味和用量，辅料及附加剂一般不列入处方中，在制法中加以说明。

(1) **The Composition of the Ingredients**    The composition and the dosage of the ingredients should be listed, while the accessories and additives are generally not included in the ingredients and should be described in the method.

2. **处方中药味的名称**    国家标准收载的药材，应使用最新版规定的名称。地方标准收载的品种与国家药品标准名称相同而来源不同的，应另起名称。国家标准未收载的药材，应采用地方标准名称，并注明。

(2) **Title of Ingredients**    The title listed in the latest edition shall be used for the medicinal materials contained in the national standard. If the varieties contained in the local standard have different origin but same Chinese names as the national drug standards, a separate name shall be given. To medicinal materials not contained in the national standard, the local standard name shall be adopted and indicated.

3. **处方中药味的排列顺序**    根据中医理论，按君、臣、佐、使顺序排列，非传统处方可按药物作用主次（主药、辅药）排列。书写时从左到右，由上至下。

**(3) Order of Chinese Medicine in Ingredients** According to the theory of traditional Chinese medicine, Chinese medicine needs to be arranged according to the order of monarch, minister, assistant and guide, and non-traditional ingredients are arranged according to the primary and secondary action of drugs (main medicine, auxiliary medicine). Writing should follow the order of left to right, top to bottom.

4. **处方量** 处方中各药味用量一律使用法定剂量单位，重量以"g"、容量以"ml"表示。全处方量应以制成 1000 个剂型单位的成品量为准。

**(4) Prescription Quantity** The prescribed dosage of each drug is in the legal dose unit, and the weight is expressed as "g", capacity "ml". The whole prescription quantity shall be based on 1000 products unit.

（三）制法

## 3. Procedure

制法项下主要叙述处方中药物共多少味（包括药引、辅料），各味药处理的简单工艺。对质量有影响的关键工艺参数应列出，如时间、温度、相对密度、pH 等。中药材粉末的粉碎度用"粗粉""中粉""细粉""极细粉"等表示，不列筛号。一般一个品名收载一个剂型的制法。蜜丸可并列收载大蜜丸、小蜜丸和水蜜丸；制备蜜丸的炼蜜量要考虑地域气候、习惯差异，规定一定幅度，但不能影响用药剂量。如"100g 粉末加炼蜜 100~120g 制成大蜜丸"。常规或《中国药典》已经规定的炮制不需要叙述，特殊炮制加工在附注中叙述。

In the preparation of the method, the total number of drugs in the prescription (including guiding drug introduction, excipients), the simple process of each drug treatment is mainly described. Control conditions (e.g. time, temperature, relative density, pH value, etc.) for key processes that have an impact on quality need to be listed. The degree of crushing of Chinese medicinal materials is expressed as "coarse powder", "medium powder", "fine powder", "extreme fine powder" and so on, and the screen size needn't to be listed. Generally, a class should contain a preparation of one dosage form. Honey pill class can contain large honey pill, small honey pill and water honey pill. The difference of regional climate and habits should be considered in the quantity of refined honey in preparation of honey pills, and a certain range should be stipulated but can't affect the dosage of medicine.Loog powder plus 100-200g honey to make big honey pill. Processing products which are prescribed by the Convention or the *Chinese Pharmacopoeia* do not need to be described, and special processing is described in the notes.

（四）性状

## 4. Description

制剂的性状与原料的质量和工艺有关。中药制剂的性状主要包括成品的形状、形态、颜色及气味等。颜色、形态、性状后用"；"隔开。如为复合色，描写时主色调在后，如棕红色，以红色为主，色泽的描述避免使用各地理解不同的术语，如土黄色、肉黄色、咖啡色等。如有包糖衣的片剂、丸剂，应除去包衣后描述其性状；如果包衣为药物衣，则先描述包衣的颜色，再描述去包衣后的性状。硬胶囊应除去囊壳后，观察内容物的性状。剧毒药和外用药只描述气，不描述味。

The characters of preparation is related to the quality and process of the raw material. The character of TCM preparation refers to the shape, form, color odor and taste of product. semicolons are used after the color, shape and character. If the color of the preparation is compound color, the main one is later when it is described, to describe the color, terms that are different in various places should be avoided, such as yellow color like soil, skin yellow color, coffee color, etc. If there are sugar-coated tablets or pills, the characters should be described after removing the coating. If the coating is drug coating, the color of coating is described firstly, and then the characteristics of core are described. The hard capsule should be removed from the capsule, and the content of the property should be observed. Only the odor, not the taste of strongly toxic drugs and external use ones are described.

（五）鉴别

### 5. Identification

常用的鉴别方法有显微鉴别、一般理化鉴别及色谱鉴别等。

The commonly used identification methods include microscopic identification, general physical and chemical identification and chromatographic identification.

1. **显微鉴别**　应突出描述易观察到的特征。正文写"取本品，置显微镜下观察"，其后描述药材的鉴别特征，每味药材鉴别的特征都用句号分开。

**(1) Microscopic Identification**　Microscopic features that can be easily observed should be highlighted firstly. The text says "take this product and observe under microscope", and then describes the identification characteristics of the medicinal materials. The identification characteristics of each medicinal material are separated by a full stop.

2. **一般理化鉴别**　样品制成的供试品溶液，分别做两项鉴别试验，且二者的鉴别试验叙述较短，可写在一项鉴别中；如叙述较长，再无其他鉴别，则先写处理方法，再写"溶液（或滤液）照下述方法试验"；如鉴别不止两项，鉴别试验叙述较长，需分别做鉴别试验时，可分项叙述。

**(2) General Physical and Chemical Identification**　If the sample solution for two identification tests, and the description of the two identification experiments is short, it can be written in a single identification；If the description is long and there is no other identification, the treatment method is written firstly, then "solution (or filtrate) according to the following method test"comes next. If the identification is more than two, and the narrative is longer, where separated identifications are needed, itemization is possible.

3. **色谱鉴别**　一般先写供试溶液的制备，再写对照溶液的制备，最后写实验方法。如用上一鉴别项下的供试品溶液，不再重复写供试品溶液的制备，而是先写对照品（或对照药材）溶液的制备，再写吸取鉴别（×）项下的供试品溶液与上述对照品（或对照药材）溶液各"×"μl。如果用上一鉴别的溶液（滤液）或药渣，再处理才能制成供试品溶液的，应先写供试品溶液的制备，书写时的格式为，取鉴别（×）项下的（滤液）或药渣，再写（滤液）或药渣的处理方法。对于TLC展开条件苛刻的应注明展开条件，如展开的温度、相对湿度等。

**(3) Chromatographic Identification**　Generally write the preparation of the test solution first, then the preparation of the reference solution, and finally write the experimental method. If the test solution under the previous identification item is used, the preparation of the test solution is no longer repeated, but the preparation of the reference solution is written first, and then apply the test solution under the item of identification (×) and the above control solution "×" μl. If the solution (filtrate) of the previous identification is used, the preparation of the test solution should be written first. The format when writing is, take the solution (filtrate) of under identification (×), then write treatment method of solution (filtrate). For TLC deployment conditions that are harsh, the deployment conditions should be noted, such as the temperature and relative humidity of the deployment environment.

（六）检查

### 6. Test

先描述通则以外的项目，其他应符合该制剂项下的有关各项规定。通则规定的或通则以外检查项目，如果需要列出具体数据，其描述顺序为相对密度、pH 值、乙醇量、总固体、干燥失重、水中不溶物、酸不溶物、重金属、砷盐等。

Items other than general chapters are first described and other requirements comply with the general requirments for the corresponding preparation. For examination items specified in the general chapters or beyond the general chapters, if it is necessary to list specific data, the order of description shall be relative density, pH value, ethanol content, total solids, loss on drying, insoluble substances in water, acid insoluble substances, heavy metals, arsenic salt, etc.

### （七）浸出物测定
### 7. Extractives

列出所需的溶剂和测定方法，并规定限度。

List the required solvents and measurement methods, and specify limits.

### （八）含量测定
### 8. Content Determination

按照下列顺序独立成段，列出含量测定方法名称、测定方法的条件与要求、对照溶液制备方法、供试溶液制备方法、测定法、含量限度。

In the following order, the method name, the conditions and requirements of the method, the preparation method of the reference substance, the preparation method of the test substance, the determination method and the content limit are described in separate paragraphs.

### （九）功能与主治
### 9. Actions and Indications

功能的描述应使用中医术语，力求简明扼要。突出主要功能，使能指导主治，并应与主治衔接。书写时先功能、后主治，中间用句号隔开，以"用于"二字连接。如有明确的西医病名，一般可写在中医病名之后，如丹红注射液等。

The function should be described with TCM terminology concisely and simplicity. The main function should be highlighted, can guide the indications. In writing, function first, then the indications, separated by a full stop with the word "for" connection. If there is a clear western medicine disease name, generally it can be written after the disease name of traditional Chinese medicine, such as Danhong Injection.

### （十）用法与用量
### 10. Administration and Dosage

先描述用法，后描述一次用量及一日使用次数；同时可供外用的，则列在服法之后，并用句号隔开。如用温开水送服的内服药，则写"口服"；如需要用其他方法送服的应写明。除特殊需要明确者外，不需要写饭前或饭后服用。用量一般为成人有效剂量；儿童使用或以儿童使用为主的中药制剂，应注明儿童剂量或不同年龄儿童剂量。剧毒药物要注明最大剂量。不同的功能主治，用法用量也不同，须逐一写明。

The administration should be described firstly, then the dosage and times of daily; For both oral administration and topical administration, topical administration should be list after the dosage and times of daily for oral administration, and separated by a period. For example, drug for oral administration with warm water, write "For oral administration"; if drug for oral administration with other methods, method should be specified. It is not necessarily marked to take it before or after meals except for special needs. The dosage is generally the effective dose for adult; For use traditional Chinese medicine by children or mainly by children, the dosage for children or different ages should be indicated. The maximum dose for highly toxic drugs should be indicated. Different "Actions and Indications", "Administration and Dosage" are different, should by list item by item.

（十一）注意

## 11. Precautions and Warnings

包括各种禁忌，如孕妇及其他疾病和体质方面的禁忌、饮食的禁忌或注明该药为剧毒药等。

This part includes various contraindications, such as those of pregnant women and other diseases and physical contraindications, dietary contraindications or the designation of the drug as a highly toxic drug.

（十二）规格

## 12. Strength

规格的写法以重量计、以装量计、以标示量计等。以重量计的，如丸、片剂，注明每丸（或每片）的重量；以装量计的，如液体制剂、散剂、糖浆剂等，注明每包（或每瓶）的装量；以标示量计的，注明每片的含量。同一品种有多种规格时，量小的在前，依次排列，最后不列标点符号。规格在 0.1g 以下的，用"mg"，以上用"g"；液体制剂用"ml"。

The specification shall be written by weight, loading quantity, indicating quantity, etc. If it is calculated by weight, such as pill or tablet, it indicates the weight of per pill (or tablet); For liquid preparations, dispersions, syrups, etc., if measured by volume, the quantity of each package (or bottle) is indicated; In labeled quantities, the content of per tablet is indicated. When the same variety has a variety of specifications, the small quantity is in the front in order of arrangement, not listed at the end of the specification. If the specification is less than 0.1g, "mg" shall be used; more than 0.1, "g" shall be used; To liquid preparations, "ml" should be used.

（十三）贮藏

## 13. Storage

根据稳定性和影响因素的研究结果，结合制剂的特性，注明保存的条件与要求。除特殊要求外，一般品种可注明"密封"；需要在干燥处保存，又怕热的品种，加"置阴凉干燥处"；遇光易变质的品种要加"避光"等。

Storage refers to the basic requirements for the storage of traditional Chinese medicine preparations. The conditions and requirements for preservation need to be indicated according to the results of the study of stability and influencing factors, combined with the characteristics of the preparation. Except for special requirements, general varieties may be marked "preserve in tightly closed container"; For those which should be stored in a dry place and kept away of heat, "store in a cool and dry place" added. To varieties prone to spoilage when exposed to light, "protect from light" should be added.

## 第三节　中药质量标准起草说明

## 10.3　Drafting Instruction for Quality Standard of Traditional Chinese Medicines

PPT

中药质量标准起草说明是对制定的质量标准的详细注释，应按照质量标准项目逐条说明，充分反映标准制定的全过程。起草说明包括理论性解释和全部试验过程与数据的总结，即使部分内容未列入质量标准正文，也应编写在内，有助于判断制定标准的合理性及各种检测方法的可靠性。

Drafting instruction for quality standard of traditional Chinese medicines is the detailed explanation for the formulated quality standard. It explains all items in quality standard point by point, and fully represents the overall procedure of standard formulation. Drafting instruction contains theoretical explanation and summary of experience and data obtained from all practical work. Even though some contents are not listed in quality standard, they should be recorded in drafting instruction, which is useful to evaluate the rationality of standard formulation and dependability of various test methods.

### 一、中药材和饮片
### 10.3.1　Chinese Medicinal Material (Decoction Pieces)

（一）名称
#### 1. Title
阐明确定该名称理由和依据，植物的科名、拉丁学名主要参考 *Flora of China*、《中国植物志》等相关卷册的核定。炮制品的名称需与药材名相呼应，如制何首乌、清半夏、炙甘草。

Clarify the reason and basis for defining the name, The family names and Latin names of plants are mainly referred to the approval of related volumes such as *Flora of China*. The name of the processed product should be consistent with the name of the medicinal material, such as Polygoni multiflori Radix Praeparata, Pinelliae Rhizoma Praeparatum Cum Alumine and Glycyrrhizae Radix et Rhizoma Praeparata Cum Melle.

（二）来源
#### 2. Sources
简要说明历史沿革、目前使用和生产的药材品种和饮片情况。

Briefly describe the history, current usage and production of species and pieces of medicinal materials.

1. **基源**　记录该药材基源鉴定的详细资料。确定药材药用部位的理由及有关试验研究资料。引种或野生变家养的植物、动物药材，应有与原种、养的植物、动物对比的资料。如单列饮片需简化为"本品为×××的炮制加工品"，增加【制法】项，写明炮制工艺。

**(1) Origin**　Record the detailed information of the origin identification of the medicinal material. Reasons for conforming the medicinal part of medicinal material and the related experimental research data should be presented. Plant and animal medicinal materials that are introduced from elsewhere or changed to cultivation from wild should have the information of comparison with the original plants and animals. The decoction pieces listed as an independent unit need to be simplified as "this product is the processed product of ×××", and the "Preparation" item is also added to indicate the processing craft.

2. **生境**　详细说明原植（动）物的形态描述、生态环境、生长特性、产地及分布。主产的省、市、自治区名称，按产量大小次序排列。道地药材产地明确的可写明具体的产地。

**(2) Habitat**　Explain in detail the morphological description, ecological environment, growth characteristics, locality and distribution of the original plant (animal). The names of provinces, municipalities, and autonomous regions where are the main producing region are listed in order of output. The county name can be written if the origin of genuine regional drug is clear.

3. **采收时间**　采收时间应进行考察，并列出考察资料。写明最佳采收时间（季节）及其研究资料，采收时间须控制于某生长阶段的药材应明确规定，如"春季花未开放时采收""果实成熟时采收"；采收时间段不严格的药材应规定采收质量好的采收时间段，如"以枝叶茂盛时采收为佳"；采收时间对药材质量无影响的药材，规定"全年均可采收"。

**(3) Harvesting Time** The harvest time should be investigated and the obtained data should be listed. The optimal harvest time (season) and the related research data should be indicated. The medicinal material whose harvest time must be controlled at a certain growth stage should be clearly specified, such as "harvest when flowers are not open in spring", and "harvest when fruits are mature". For medicinal material with a non-strict harvesting time period, a harvesting time period with good quality should be specified, e.g. "better harvest when the foliage is flourishing". For the medicinal material which harvesting time has not effect on quality, it is stipulated that "they can be harvested throughout the year".

**4. 产地加工** 阐明产地加工的方法及研究资料。有的药材因地区习惯不同，加工方法有差别，尽量选择质量具有代表性的一种方法，必要时也可列两种。对药材质量及形状有影响的加工处理方法应重点说明，如"趁鲜切片后干燥"。若需在产地加工成片（段），应明确说明。

**(4) Origin Processing** Clarify the processing methods and the related research data. If the medicinal material has different processing methods due to different regional habits, a representative method (two methods, if necessary) tries to be selected. Processing methods that have an impact on the quality and shape of medicinal materials should be emphasized, such as "fresh material is sliced before dry". If it needs to be processed into pieces (sections) at the place of origin, it should be clearly stated.

**（三）性状**

**3. Description**

说明该药材标本的来源、性状描述的依据及其他需要说明的问题。对药材、饮片的实际形态进行描述，并附彩色照片。多基源的植（动）物药材，其性状无明显区别者，可合并描述；有明显区别者，应分开描述。应尽量多描述断面特征。列出曾发现过的伪品、类似品与本品性状的区别点。

Explain the source of the medicinal specimen, the basis for characterization, and other issues that need to be explained. Describe the actual form of medicinal materials and decoction pieces, and attach the color photos. If there are no obvious differences in the traits of plants (animals) from multi-sources, they can be described together; if there are obvious differences, they should be described separately. Describe as many cross-section features as possible. List the differences between this product and the found fakes and similar products.

**（四）鉴别**

**4. Identification**

应阐明选用各项鉴别的依据并提供全部研究资料。例如横切面或粉末显微特征应提供彩色照片，照片应标注各个特征，并附使用仪器的型号、标尺或放大倍数。色谱鉴别用的对照品和对照药材应符合"中药新药质量标准用对照品研究的技术要求"。重点考察多来源的药材、饮片的色谱行为相同和不同点，说明选择条件的专属性，明确所使用对照药材的植物来源。注重选择专属性和重现性好的鉴别方法。

The basis of each identification should be clarified and all research data should be provided. Such as tissue or powder microscopic features should be provided with color photographs. Each feature in the photographs should be marked, and the type, scale and magnification of the used instrument should also be marked. Focus on the method's specificity and reproducibility. The reference substances used for chromatographic identification should meet the 'technical requirements for reference substance research for quality standards of new Chinese medicines'. The same and different points of chromatographic behavior of medicinal material and decoction pieces from multiple sources should be focally investigated. The specificity of the selected conditions should be explained, and the plant source of the reference substance used should be clarified. Pay attention to the selection of methods, which have good specificity and reproducibility.

（五）检查

## 5. Test

说明选定各检查项目的理由及试验数据。根据药材和饮片的具体情况规定检查项目，制定切实可行的指标和限度，阐明制定该检查项目限度指标的意义及依据。所测成分为毒性成分时，规定上限。

Explain the reasons for selecting each test item and the test data. According to the specific conditions of medicinal material and decoction pieces, the test items, practical indicators and limits are stipulated. The meaning and basis for confirming the limits of the test items should be clarified. The upper limit is specified when the tested component is a toxic component.

（六）浸出物

## 6. Extractives

说明测定浸出物的理由，提供所用浸出溶剂的依据及测定方法的研究资料，确定该浸出物限量指标的依据（至少应有 10 批样品 20 个数据）。有下列情况的药材和饮片应尽量选择浸出物测定：尚无含量测定；所测定成分含量低于万分之一；有效成分不明确。

Explain the reasons for measuring the extractive. Provide the basis of the used extractive solvent and the research data of the determination method, and the basis for defining the limit of extractive (there should be at least 20 data from 10 batches of samples). The medicinal material and decoction pieces in the following cases should be selected for extractive determination as far as possible: No the content determination; the content of the measured component is less than one ten-thousandths; the effective component is not clear.

（七）特征图谱或指纹图谱

## 7. Characteristic Chromatography or Fingerprint

说明选用特征图谱或指纹图谱的依据，并提供全部试验资料，包括测试条件的选择、供试品溶液制备、图谱建立和辨识、方法验证、数据处理和分析等，并附相应图谱。

Explain the basis for selecting characteristic chromatography or fingerprint, and provide all test data, including the selection of test conditions, test solution preparation, establishment and identification, of chromatography method verification, data processing and analysis. Attached corresponding chromatography.

（八）含量测定

## 8. Assay

根据药材功效、样品特点和有关化学成分的性质，选定测定成分和相应测定方法。应阐明所选含量测定项目的理由及测定方法和含量限度的依据，并提供相应试验数据资料。含量测定用对照品如为非现行国家药品标准收载者，应按照现行版《中国药典》"国家药品标准物质制备指导原则"进行验证。

According to the efficacy of the medicinal material, the characteristics of sample and the properties of the relevant chemical components, the determining components and corresponding measuring methods are selected. The reasons for selecting the assay item, and the basis of assay method and content limit should be clarified. The corresponding test data should be provided. If the reference substance for assay is not included in the current national drug standard, it should be verified in accordance with "Guidelines for the Preparation of National Drug Standard Substances" in the current *Chinese Pharmacopoeia*.

1. 测定成分选定　首选有效成分、专属成分或特征成分，应尽量选择与中医用药功能与主治相关的成分。为实现更加全面地控制质量，可采用一测多评；对不能建立有效成分含量测定，或所测定成分与功效相关性差或含量低者，而有效成分类别又清楚的，可测定有效成分类别（总成分），如总黄酮、总生物碱、总皂苷等；含量测定成分的选定应选择其原型成分，不宜选择水解成分；此外，不宜选择非专属性成分或微量成分（含量低于万分之二的成分）。

**(1) Determining Component Selection**　The effective ingredient, specific ingredient and characteristic ingredient should be preferentially selected. The ingredient involved with the action and indication (which used by Chinese medicine) of the drugs tries to be selected. One method can be used to determine the content of multiple ingredients to achieve more comprehensive quality control. Some drugs which a method cannot be establish to assay the effective ingredient, the measured ingredient has a poor correlation with efficacy, and the content of the measured ingredient is low, while the active ingredient category is clear, a type of active ingredients can be determined (total components), such as total flavones, alkaloids and saponins. The determined components should choose their prototypes, and not choose hydrolyzed components. In addition, non-specific ingredients or trace ingredients (the content is less than two ten-thousandths) should not be selected.

2. 测定方法　优选专属性好、测定条件稳定、精准度高的方法，如高效液相色谱法、气相色谱法等。也可采用化学分析法、分光光度法、生物测定法等。对选定的含量测定方法需进行方法学考察。提供方法学考察资料和相关数据与图谱（包括线性、范围、精密度、稳定性、定量限、耐用性及回收率等）。

**(2) Determining Method**　The method with good specificity, stable measurement conditions and high accuracy is preferentially selected, such as high performance liquid chromatography and gas chromatography. Chemical analysis, spectrophotometry and bioassay can also be used. The methodological investigation of the selected determining method is performed. The data of methodological investigation and the related illustrations need to be provided, such as linearity, range, precision, stability, limit of quantitation, robustness and recovery.

3. 含量限（幅）度制定　阐明确定该含量限（幅）度的意义及依据（至少应有 10 批样品 20 个数据）。含量限度规定方式有以下两种：①所测成分为有效成分时，规定下限；②所测成分既为有效成分又为有毒成分时，规定幅度（同时规定上下限）。

**(3) Content Limit (Amplitude) Formulation**　Explain the meaning and basis for the defined content limit (amplitude) (at least 20 data from 10 batches of samples). The content limit is indicated by the following two ways: ① When the effective component is determined, the lower limit is stipulated; ② when the component that have both activity and toxicity is measured, the range is stipulated (i.e. the upper and lower limits are simultaneously stipulated).

（九）炮制

## 9. Processing

说明炮制目的、制定工艺的依据和试验数据。还可简述历代本草对本品的炮制记载，炮制研究情况（文献资料及起草时研究情况）以及全国主要省份炮制规范。

Explain the purpose of processing, basis for craft formulation, and test data. It can also briefly describe the processing records of this product in previous reference, processing research (documentary materials and research at the time of drafting quality standards), and the processing standards of main provinces.

【性味与归经】【功能与主治】【用法与用量】【注意】【贮藏】等项目应根据实际情况提供可能的试验及文献研究资料，并说明相关规定的依据。

Other items, including "Property and Flavor and Meridian Tropism" "Action and Indications" "Administration and Dosage" "Precautions and Warnings" and "Storage" should provide possible experimental and literature research data according to actual situation, and explain the basis of relevant regulations.

### 二、植物油脂和提取物
### 10.3.2 Vegetable Oil, Fats and Extracts

（一）名称
#### 1. Title

说明命名的依据。一般挥发油和油脂名以药材名加"油"构成；粗提物命名以药材名加提取溶剂加"提取物"构成，提取溶剂为水时可省略为药材名加"提取物"构成；有效部位、组分提取物名以药材名加有效部位、组分名构成。

Explain the basis for naming. The name of volatile oils and fats is usually composed of the name of medicinal material and "oil". The name of crude extracts is composed of the name of medicinal material, extractive solvent and "extracts", which can be composed of the name of medicinal material and "extracts" when water is the extractive solvent. The name of extracts containing fractional components is composed of the name of medicinal material and the name of components.

（二）来源
#### 2. Sources

写明油脂和提取物的来源。写出该中药的原植（动）物科名、植（动）物中文名、拉丁学名、药用部位；有效成分应写出分子式、分子量和结构式；挥发油和油脂要简要写出提取方法。多基源药材提取物需固定一种基源，如须用两种以上基源的须写明相互间比例。

Describe the source of vegetable oil and extracts. Write the family name and Chinese name of the original plant (animal), Latin name and the medicinal part of the material. The molecular formula, molecular weight and structural formula should be written for the active chemicals. Extractive method of volatile oil and fats should be written briefly. A certain source of medicinal material should be definited for the extract with multi-sources. If two or more sources are applied, the proportion between them must be indicated.

（三）制法
#### 3. Procedure

说明各项技术指标和要求的含义，写明药材前处理方法（粉碎、切制等），需考察提取工艺所采用溶剂、提取方法、提取次数等主要条件，浓缩干燥方法与指标（如相对密度），分离纯化方法与主要条件，并提供研究过程中全部数据资料。

The detailed preparation process should be listed. The meanings of various technical indicators and requirements should be listed. The pre-treatment methods of medicinal materials, such as crushing and cutting, should be stated. The main conditions for the extractive process, including solvent, extractive method and extractive number, methods and indicators for concentration and drying (e.g. relative density), and methods and main conditions for separation and purification, should be investigated, and all data during the research should be provided.

（四）性状

## 4. Description

说明性状描述的依据及其他需要说明的问题。

Explain the basis for characterization and other issues that need to be explained.

（五）鉴别

## 5. Identification

说明各项鉴别的理由，提供相应数据和图片，要求同药材和饮片。

Explain the reason for each identification, and provide the corresponding data and pictures. The requirements are same as the medicinal material and pieces.

（六）检查

## 6. Test

说明各检查项目的理由及依据，要求同药材和饮片。还应根据原料药材中可能存在的有毒成分、生产过程中可能造成的污染情况、贮藏条件等建立检查项目。对于有效成分提取物，应对主成分以外的其他成分进行研究，并设有关物质检查项。作为注射剂原料的提取物，检查项除一般检查项外，还需对其安全性等检查项进行研究，包括酸碱度、蛋白质、鞣质、树脂、草酸盐、钾离子、重金属、砷盐、溶剂残留量等项目，按照相应注射剂品种项下的规定选择检查项目，并列出控制限度。

Explain the reason and basis for each test item, and the requirements are same as those of medicinal material and decoction pieces. In addition, the test items should be developed according to the possible toxic components in raw materials, pollution during production and storage conditions. For the active substance, other substances coexisted in the active substance should be studied, and the test items of the related substances should be established, which is required as the materials of chemical drugs. For the extract used for the material of injection, in addition to the general test items, other items (e.g. safety) should also be studied, including pH, protein, tannin, resin, oxalate, potassium ions, heavy metal, arsenic salt and solvent residues. The test items are selected according to the regulations under the corresponding injection category, and the control limits should be also listed.

（七）特征图谱或指纹图谱

## 7. Characteristic Chromatography or Fingerprint

要求同药材和饮片。此外，还要求在建立提取物特征或指纹图谱的同时建立原药材饮片的相应图谱，并要求药材饮片与提取物特征或指纹图谱具有相关性，提取物图谱中的特征或指纹峰在药材饮片的图谱上应能指认。提取物图谱建立应重点考察主要工艺过程中谱图的变化；油脂和提取物图谱需采用对照品、对照提取物或参照物作对照。

The requirements are same as the medicinal materials and decoction pieces. Additionally, The fingerprints of original decoction pieces should also be developed, when the characteristic chromatography or chromatography of vegetable oil and extracts is developed. A correlation of the characteristic chromatography or fingerprint between extracts and decoction pieces is required. The characteristics or fingerprint peaks in the chromatography of extracts should be able to be assigned in the chromatography of decoction pieces. The changes of chromatography in the main process should be emphatically investigated in the establishment of chromatography of extracts. The reference substance, reference extracts or reference object should be used as the comparison for the chromatography of oil, fats and extracts.

（八）含量测定

### 8. Assay

要求同药材和饮片。

The requirements are same as the medicinal materials and pieces.

（九）贮藏

### 9. Storage

说明贮藏的要求及理由。需考察光照、温度、湿度等因素对提取物稳定性的影响，可按照现行版《中国药典》通则"原料药物与制剂稳定性试验指导原则"进行，并提供研究资料。

Explain requirements and reasons for the storage. The influence of light, temperature, humidity and other factors on the stability of extracts should be investigated, which can refer to 'Guidelines for Stability Test of Raw Materials and Preparations' in the General Principles of current edition of *Chinese Pharmacopoeia*, and the research data should be provided.

（十）制剂

### 10. Preparation

有明确制剂的油脂和提取物需列出可制成的制剂。

The produced preparations should be listed for the oil, fats and extracts that are used for specific preparation.

## 三、中药制剂

### 10.3.3 Preparation of Traditional Chinese Medicine

（一）名称

### 1. Title

说明命名的依据和理由。应简短、科学、明确，不宜用人名、地名、企业名称，不应与已有的药品名称重复。此外，药品应一方一名，如九味羌活丸、九味羌活颗粒。同时应注意不宜中西医不同理论功效混杂命名。

Explain the basis and reason for the naming. It should be short, scientific and clear. It is not appropriate to use names of people, places and companies, and it should not duplicate the existing drug names. In addition, one prescription should have only one name. such as Jiuwei Qianghuo Pills and Jiuwei Qianghuo Granules. Additionally, it should be noted that the mixed naming using different theoretical efficacies of Chinese and western medicine should not be adopted.

1. **单味制剂** 采用原料（药材、饮片）名与剂型名结合。

**(1) Preparation Comprised of One Medicinal Material** Combine name of raw materials (crude drug and decoction pieces) with medicament name to naming.

2. **复方制剂** 根据处方组成可采用以下命名方式：①方内主要药味缩写加剂型，如参芍片、银黄口服液、参苓白术颗粒；②方内主要药味缩写加功效加剂型，如木香顺气丸、银翘解毒颗粒、牛黄解毒片；③君药前加复方加剂型，如复方丹参注射液、复方龙血竭胶囊；④功效加剂型，如妇炎康复片、镇脑宁胶囊；⑤方内药物剂量比例或服用剂量加剂型，如七厘散、九分散、六一散；⑥药味数与主要药名或功效加剂型，如六味地黄丸、十全大补丸；⑦主要药材和药引加剂型，如川芎茶调散，以茶水调服；⑧形象比喻加剂型，如玉屏风散、泰山磐石散；⑨单一成分或一类成分的复方制剂，成分加剂型，如黄杨宁片；⑩源于古方的品种，不违反命名原则，可用古方名加剂型，如血府逐瘀胶囊、九味羌活丸。

**(2) Compound Preparation** According to composition of prescription, the following naming methods can be applied: ① The abbreviation of main materials in the prescription plus medicament, such as Shen Shao Tablet, Yinhuang Oral Liquid, and Shenling Baizhu Granule; ② The abbreviation of main materials in the prescription plus efficacy and medicament, such as Muxiang Shunqi Pill, Yinqiao Jiedu Granule and Niuhuang Jiedu Tablet; ③ "Fufang" plus name of "Junyao"(the most important material in prescription) and medicament, such as Fufang Danshen Injection and Fufang Longxuejie Capsule; ④ Efficacy plus medicament, such as Fuyan Kangfu Tablet and Zhennaoning Capsule; ⑤ Dose proportion of materials in the prescriptions or dosage plus medicament, such as Qili San, Jiufen San and Liuyi San; ⑥ Number of materials in the prescriptions plus main drug name or efficacy and medicament, such as Liuwei Dihuang Pill and Shiquan Dabu Pill; ⑦ Main material and medicinal usher plus medicament, such as Chuanxiong Chatiao San which is administrated with tea; ⑧ Image and metaphor plus medicament, such as Yupingfeng San, Taishan Panshi San; ⑨ Compound preparation comprised of single ingredients or a type of ingredients is named as 'ingredients plus medicament', such as Huangyangning tablet; ⑩ The drug origin from ancient prescription can be named as 'prescription name plus medicament', which do not violate the naming principle, such as Xuefu Zhuyu Capsule and Jiuwei Qianghuo Pill.

### （二）处方

### 2. Prescription

列出处方详细药味和用量，包括主要辅料，并说明该药处方来源与方解（君、臣、佐、使）。处方中如有药典未收载的炮制品，应详细说明炮制方法和炮制品的质量要求。

List the medicinal materials and their dosage in prescription, including the main auxiliary materials, and explain the source and principle of composition (Jun, Chen, Zuo and Shi) of the prescription. If there are processing products that are not recorded in the *Pharmacopoeia* in the prescription, the processing methods and quality requirements of the processing products should be explained in detail.

### （三）制法

### 3. Procedure

列出详细的工艺流程，包括全部工艺参数和技术指标、关键半成品的质量标准及确定最终制备工艺与技术条件的依据。一般需确定提取溶剂、时间、提取方法、分离、浓缩、干燥的方法与主要参数。另外，要说明主要辅料标准收载情况，药典未收载的辅料应附执行标准。

List the detailed process flow, including all process parameters and technical indicators, quality standards of key semi-finished products, and the basis for defining the final preparation process and its technical conditions. Generally, extraction solvent, time and method, separation, concentration and drying method and those main parameters need to be determined. In addition, the record situation of the standard of main excipients needs to be explained, and the implementation standards of main excipients that are not recorded in the *Pharmacopoeia* need to be accompanied.

### （四）性状

### 4. Description

说明性状拟定的依据。至少观察 3~5 批中试或大生产的样品，根据制剂在贮藏期间颜色实际观察情况规定色度范围。

Explain the basis for drafting the characterization. The standard establishment should be based on pre-produced or mass-produced products, and at least 3-5 batches of samples should be observed. The chromaticity range is stipulated according to the actual observations of color of the preparation during storage.

（五）鉴别

## 5. Identification

说明制剂各鉴别项目和鉴别方法选定的依据，并提供完整研究资料，要求同药材和饮片。

Explain the basis for the selection of identification items and methods of preparations, and provide complete research data. The corresponding requirements are similar with the medicinal materials and decoction pieces.

1. 鉴别项目　根据处方组成及研究资料确定相应的鉴别项目，原则上处方各药味均应进行鉴别，首选君药、贵重药、毒性药列入标准中，再选其他药味，未列入标准的药味应说明理由。

**(1) Identification Item**　The identification items are determined according to the composition of prescription and the related research data. In principle, all medicinal materials in the prescription should be identified. "Junyao", valuable drug and toxic drug are preferentially listed in the standard. After that, the other materials in the prescription can also be selectively listed. Reasons for not listing materials in the standard should be provided.

2. 鉴别方法　薄层色谱鉴别是复方制剂中最常用的鉴别方法，提供的资料包括前处理选择的依据、数据，实验条件、指标的选择依据，对照品和对照药材的来源，阴性对照的制备方法等，随资料附相关图谱，至少包含3批样品和阴性样品TLC的结果。经饮片粉末直接制成的制剂或添加有部分饮片粉末的制剂，可选用显微鉴别，附上粉末特征墨线图或照片。

**(2) Identification Methods**　Thin layer chromatography is the most commonly used identification method in compound preparations. The information provided includes the basis and data for the selection of pretreatment, the selection of the experimental conditions and indicators, the source of the reference substance and the reference medicinal material, the preparation method of the negative reference solution, etc., attached the relevant dates , at least the TLC result of 3 batches of samples and negative sample. For the preparations prepared directly by piece powder or added with some piece powder, microscopic identification can be used, and the ink diagram or photo of the powder characteristic is attached.

（六）检查

## 6. Test

主要检查制剂中可能引入的杂质及与质量有关的项目。说明各检查项目的制订理由及限度，并提供完整研究资料。

Mainly check the possible impurities and quality-related items in the preparation. Explain the reasons and limits for each test item, and provide complete research data.

1. 参照现行版《中国药典》通则规定各剂型需检查的项目及限度值。如与通则中检查要求不同的，需说明理由并列出具体数据；对药典通则规定以外的检查项目需说明制订依据及其限度拟定的理由；药典未收载的剂型则根据剂型和用药需求制定相应的检查项目。

(1) Refer to the current version of the "General Chapters" of the *Chinese Pharmacopoeia* to stipulate the test items and limit values of each medicament. If it is different from the test requirements in the General Chapters, the reasons and specific data should be stated. For the test items that are not stipulated in the *Pharmacopoeia*, the reasons for formulating the items and their limits should be stated. The test items of medicament that is not recorded in the *Pharmacopoeia* are formulated according to the requirements of medicament and usage.

2. 单一成分制剂或中西药复方制剂中的化学药需检查含量均匀度。

(2) Content uniformity of single-component preparation and western medicines in the compound preparation comprised of Chinese and western medicines should be tested.

3. 含有毒性药材的制剂，需制定毒性成分的检查项及限度。

(3) For the preparations containing toxic medicinal materials, the test items and limits of toxic components need to be formulated.

4. 需进行重金属和砷盐限量检查，必要时纳入标准。

(4) Testing methods and the limits of heavy metals and arsenic salts need to be formulated.

5. 使用有机溶剂萃取、分离、重结晶等制成的制剂需检查溶剂残留量，规定残留溶剂限量。检查方法按现行版《中国药典》通则"残留溶剂测定法"检查。

(5) For the preparations prepared using organic solvents (such as extraction, separation and recrystallization), the residual solvent amount should be tested and the limit is stipulated. The test method is accordance with the 'Residual Solvents Determination' in the General Chapters of current *Chinese Pharmacopoeia*.

6. 所用对照品含量限度应与含量测定用对照品基本相同。

(6) The content limit of the reference substance used should be basically consistent with that of the reference substance for assay.

（七）浸出物

## 7. Extractive

根据剂型和品种的需要，选择适当溶剂和方法测定。要求及方法同药材和饮片。

Appropriate solvents and methods are selected for determination according to the needs of medicament and sample type. The requirements and methods are same as those of medicinal materials and decoction pieces.

（八）特征图谱或指纹图谱

## 8. Characteristic Chromatography or Fingerprint

方法及要求同药材和饮片。还应建立饮片及中间体的相应图谱，并对制剂与饮片及中间体之间的相关性进行分析，饮片图谱中的特征或指纹峰在中间体和制剂的图谱上应能指认。

The methods and requirements are same as those of medicinal materials and decoction pieces. The chromatography of decoction pieces and intermediates should also be developed, and the correlation between the preparations and decoction pieces and intermediates should be analyzed. The characteristics or fingerprint peaks in the chromatography of decoction pieces should be able to be assigned in the chromatography of intermediates and preparations.

（九）含量测定

## 9. Assay

说明含量测定药味、测定成分及测定方法选定的理由，提供完整研究资料。

Explain the reasons for the selection of medicinal materials, ingredients and assay method, and provide complete research data.

1. 药味选定　以中医理论为指导，首选方中的君药、贵重药、毒性药作为含量测定药味。如上述药味无法进行测定时，可选臣药及其他药味进行测定，但需具有代表性，保证临床用药的安全、有效和质量可控。制剂中进行含量测定的药其原料药必须有含量限度。

(1) **Determining Material Selection** Under the theory of traditional Chinese medicine, and 'Junyao', precious medicine and toxic medicine are preferentially selected. If the above-mentioned drugs

cannot be measured, the 'Chenyao' and other drugs in preparation can be selected for measurement, but it must be representative to ensure the safety, effectiveness and quality controllability of clinical administration. Only the materials that already have the content limit can be selected as the assayed goals in the preparation.

2. 测定成分选定　一般遵循以下几项原则。

（1）测定有效成分，并尽量与该药味的药理作用和功能主治一致。

（2）测定毒性成分，保障用药安全，如九分散中的士的宁。

（3）测定总成分，有效部分或成分类型清楚的，可测定总成分，如总黄酮、总皂苷、总多糖等。

（4）测定易损失的成分，在制剂的制备、储藏过程中易损失的成分，如挥发性成分。

（5）测定指标性成分，有效成分不明确的制剂，可测定专属性强的指标性成分，其含量高低可代表药物在制剂中的量。

（6）测定专属性成分，若为两味或两味以上药物共有的成分，则不宜选定为定量指标，如处方中同时含有黄连、黄柏，最好不选小檗碱为测定指标。

（7）处方中如含有化学药成分应进行测定。

**(2) Determining Component Selection**　The principle of assayed ingredients as follows: ① Assay of effective ingredients, try to be consistent with the pharmacological effects and "actional and indications" of the drug; ② Assay of toxic ingredients to ensure the safety of medicines, such as strychnine in Jiufen San; ③ Assay of total components, if the effective part or type of the ingredient is clear, the total composition can be determined, such as total flavonoids, total saponins, total polysaccharides, etc.; ④ Determination of easily lost ingredients, which are lost during preparation and storage of the preparation. Such as volatile components; ⑤ Determination of index component, preparations with unclear active ingredients, can determine index components with strong specificity, and their content can represent the amount of drugs in the preparation; ⑥ The determination of specific ingredients, if it is a component shared by two Chinese crude drugs or more than two Chinese crude drugs, it should not be selected as a quantitative indicator. If the prescription contains both Phellodendri Chinensis Cortex and Coptidis Rhizoma, it is best not to select berberine as the measurement indicator; ⑦ Western medicine in the prescription should be measured.

3. 测定方法选定　应参考有关质量标准或文献及相关资料，结合制备工艺和剂型的特点及被测成分的性质等综合考虑测定方法，选择的方法需有专属性、重现性、稳定性、先进性、适用性等，一般优选色谱法进行含量测定，并进行方法学考察。

**(3) Determining Method Selection**　Reference the relevant quality standards or literature , combined with the preparation process and the characteristics of the dosage form and the nature of the tested ingredients, to comprehensively considered the measurement method. Generally, chromatographic method is preferentially used to perform assay, which is validated by methodological investigation.

4. 含量限度　根据多批样品（至少10批）的测定数据，结合原料药饮片的含量及工艺收率情况确定，制定含量限度。有毒性的有效成分及中西药复方制剂中化学药品的含量必须规定上下限幅度。

**(4) Content Limit**　Content limit is defined according to the measured data of preparations, the content of the material (decoction pieces) and the process yield. it should be defined based on the data from at least 10 batches of preparation samples. The upper and lower limits must be stipulated for the content of toxic ingredients and the chemical drugs in compound preparation comprised of Chinese and western medicines.

### （十）功能与主治
### 10. Action and Indication

根据药理试验及临床试验研究结果，说明制定理由。

Based on the research results from pharmacological tests and clinical trials, the reasons for the formulation should be explained.

### （十一）用法与用量
### 11. Administration and Dosage

根据实际情况提供可能的试验及文献资料，说明制定理由。

According to the actual situation, provide possible test and literature data, and explain the reason for the establishment.

### （十二）注意
### 12. Precautions and Warnings

说明制定注意项的理由。

Explain the reasons for the precautions and warning.

### （十三）规格
### 13. Specifications

规格要考虑与常用剂量相衔接，方便临床使用。

Specifications should be considered to coordinate with commonly-used doses, which facilitates clinical usage.

### （十四）贮藏
### 14. Storage

根据成分稳定性研究说明贮藏要求和理由。需特殊贮存条件的应有数据说明。

The requirements and reasons of storage are explained based on the ingredient stability studies. Data should be explained for special storage conditions.

## 第四节　中药的稳定性研究
## 10.4　Study on the Stability of Traditional Chinese Medicine

中药的稳定性是指中药的化学、物理及生物学特性发生变化的程度。通过稳定性试验，考察中药在温度、湿度、光线的影响下随时间变化的规律，为药品的生产、包装、贮存、运输条件和有效期的建立提供科学依据。

The stability of traditional Chinese medicine is the degree of changes in the chemical, physical and biological characteristics of traditional Chinese medicine. Through the stability test, the rhythms of change of traditional Chinese medicine with time under the influence of temperature, humidity and light is investigated, which provides scientific basis for the conditions of production, packaging, storage, transportation and set validity period of drugs.

**一、稳定性研究实验设计**

### 10.4.1 Experimental Design for Stability Study

应根据研究目的，结合原料药的理化性质、剂型的特点和处方及工艺条件进行设计。

The design should be based on the research purpose, physical and chemical properties of the raw material, characteristics of medicament and conditions of prescription and processing craft.

**样品的批次与规模** 影响因素试验可采用 1 批样品，如果试验结果不明确，则应加试 2 个批次样品；加速试验和长期试验可采用 3 批样品。若供试品为原料药应是一定规模生产的。若是制剂应是放大实验的样品，处方工艺与大生产一致。

***Batch and Scale of Samples*** One batch of samples with a certain scale can be used for influencing factor test, if the test result is not clear, two batches of samples should be tested; three batches of samples with a certain scale can be used for accelerated test and long-term test. if the test product is an Chinese crude drug, it should be produced on a certain scale. If the preparation is a sample for scale-up experiment, the prescription process is consistent with mass production.

**包装与贮藏条件** 加速试验和长期试验所用包装材料和封装条件应与拟上市包装一致。稳定性试验要求在一定的温度、湿度、光照等条件下进行，这些放置条件的设置应充分考虑到药品在贮存、运输及使用过程中可能遇到的环境因素。

***Packaging and storage conditions*** The packaging materials and conditions used for accelerated test and long-term test should be consistent with the packaging that will be marketed. Stability test is required to be performed under a certain condition, such as temperature, humidity and light. The setting of these conditions should fully consider the environmental factors that may be encountered during the storage, transportation and usage of drugs.

**二、中药稳定性考察内容**

### 10.4.2 Investigative Contents of Stability of Traditional Chinese Medicine

（一）考察项目

### 1. Investigative Items

稳定性研究的考察项目应根据所含成分和（或）制剂特性，选择在药品保存期间易于变化、可能会影响到药品安全性和有效性的项目，以便客观、全面地评价药品的稳定性。重点考察项目参照"原料药物与制剂稳定性试验指导则原则"（《中国药典》通则 9001）。

The investigative items should be set according to the ingredients in the drug and/or characteristics and quality requirements of the medicament. The items that are easy to be changed during the storage and may affect the safety and effectiveness of drugs should be selected to objectively and comprehensively evaluate the drug stability. The stability is usually systematically investigated according to the 'Key Investigative Items in *Chinese Pharmacopoeia* (General Chapters 9001).

（二）考察时间

### 2. Investigative Time

稳定性研究中需设置多个考察时间点。时间点应基于对药品理化性质的认识、稳定性变化趋势而设置。如长期试验中，总考察时间应涵盖所预期的有效期，中间取样点的设置应考虑药品的稳定特性和剂型特点。

In stability study, multiple time points that need to be investigated should be set, which should be based on the understanding of physical and chemical properties of the drug and the trend of stability change. For example, in a long-term test, the total investigative time should cover the expected period of validity, and the setting of the intermediate sampling point should consider the characteristics of stability and medicament of the drug.

### 三、稳定性研究实验方法
### 10.4.3　Experimental Methods for Stability Study

稳定性试验包括影响因素试验、加速试验与长期试验。

**（一）影响因素试验**

#### 1. Influencing factor test

影响因素试验一般包括高温、高湿、强光照射试验。将原料置适宜容器中（如称量瓶或培养皿），分散放置，厚度不超过 3mm（疏松原料药厚度可略高些）；对于固体制剂产品，除去外包，并根据试验目的和产品特性考虑是否除去内包装，置适宜的开口容器中，进行高温试验、高湿度试验和强光照试验。当试验结果发现降解产物有明显变化，应考虑其潜在的危害性，必要时应对降解产物进行定性或定量分析。

Influencing factor test is generally included by high temperature, high humidity, and strong light irradiation test. The raw materials are put into a suitable container (such as weighing bottle and culture dish) and then scattered, thickness of ≤3mm (loose raw materials thickness can be slightly higher) for testing. For solid preparation, the preparation with smallest unit except the outer packaging is placed in a suitable open container for high temperature test, high humidity test and strong light test. When the test results show significant changes of degradation products, their potential hazards should be considered and qualitative or quantitative analysis of degradation products should be performed if necessary.

高温试验、高湿度试验及强光照试验的试验条件、方法、取样时间及重点考察项目参照 2020 年版《中国药典》通则 9001 "原料药物与制剂稳定性试验指导原则"中相关规定。

The high temperature, high humidity and strong light exposure test methods and requirements can refer to *Chinese Pharmacopoeia* General Chapters 9001 Guidelines for the Stability Testing of Drug Substances and Preparations..

**（二）加速试验**

#### 2. Accelerated Test

一般在 40℃±2℃、相对湿度 75%±5% 条件下放置 6 个月。稳定性研究中所用设备应能控制温度 ±2℃、相对湿度 ±5%，并能对真实的温度与湿度监测。检测至少包括初始和末次的 3 个时间点（如 0、3、6 月）。如在 25℃±2℃、相对湿度 60%±5% 条件下进行长期试验，当加速 6 个月中任何时间点的质量发生了显著变化，则应进行中间条件试验。中间条件为 30℃±2℃、相对湿度 60%±5%，建议的考察时间为 12 个月，应包括所有的考察项目，检测至少包括初始和末次的 4 个时间点（如 0、6、9、12 月）。

Generally, sample with market packages should be placed at 40℃±2℃, relative humidity 75%±5% for 6 months. The equipment must be capable of monitoring the actual temperature and humidity and keeping the variation of temperature within a range of ±2℃ and that of relative humidity within ±5%RH. The testing includes at least the initial and last 3 time points (eg. 0, 3, 6 months). If the long-term testing is carried out at 25℃±2℃ and relative humidity 60%±5%, if the quality of sample occurs significant changes at any time point within 6 months of acceleration testing, the intermediate condition testing shall be carried out. an intermediate condition are at 30°C ± 2°C and relative humidity of 65% ± 5%, the recommended inspection time is 12 months, all inspection items should be included, and the test includes at least the initial and last 4 time points (such as 0, 6, 9, 12 months).

溶液剂、混悬剂、乳剂、注射液等含有水性介质的制剂可不要求相对湿度。对于包装在半透性容器中的药物制剂，如低密度聚乙烯制备的输液袋、塑料安瓿、眼用制剂容器等，则应在 40℃±2℃、相对湿度 25%±5% 的条件下进行试验。

Relative humidity is not required for the preparation containing aqueous medium, such as solution, suspension, emulsion and injection. For the preparation packaged in semi-permeable container, such as infusion bag made of low-density polyethylene, plastic ampoules and ophthalmic preparation container, the test should be performed at 40°C ± 2°C and relative humidity of 25% ± 5%.

对乳剂、混悬剂、软膏剂、乳膏剂、糊剂、凝胶剂、眼膏剂、栓剂、气雾剂、泡腾片及泡腾颗粒宜直接采用温度 30℃ ± 2℃、相对湿度 65%±5% 的条件进行试验。

Some preparations, such as plaster, gum, ointment, gel, eye ointment, suppository and aerosol, can be directly tested under the conditions of 30°C ± 2°C and relative humidity of 65% ±5%.

对温度特别敏感药物或者药物制剂，预计在冰箱 2~8℃ 内保存使用，加速试验可在 25℃±2℃、相对湿度 60%±5% 条件下进行 6 个月。

The drugs that are particularly sensitive to temperature need to be stored in a refrigerator (2-8°C). The accelerated test of these drugs can be performed at 25°C ± 2°C and relative humidity of 60% ± 5% for 6 months.

对拟冷冻贮藏的药物或者药物制剂，应对一批样品在温度如 5℃ ± 3℃ 或 25℃ ± 2℃ 下放置适当的时间进行试验，以了解短期偏离标签贮藏条件（如运输或搬运）对药物或者药物制剂的影响。

For drugs or pharmaceutical preparations to be stored frozen, a batch of samples should be tested at a temperature (eg 5°C±3°C or 25°C±2°C) for an appropriate period of time to understand the short-term deviation from the label storage conditions (eg transportation or move) the impact on drugs or pharmaceutical preparations.

（三）长期试验

### 3. Long-term Testing

长期试验是在接近药品的实际贮存条件下进行，在 25℃±2℃、相对湿度 60%±5% 的条件下放置 12 个月，或在 30℃±2℃、相对湿度 65%±5% 的条件下放置 12 个月，每 3 个月取样一次，按稳定性重点考察项目检测。12 个月以后，仍需继续考察，根据产品特性，分别于 18 个月、24 个月、36 个月等，取样检测。将结果与 0 个月比较，确定药物有效期。

The long-term test is performed under the conditions that are close to the actual storage of the drug, at 25°C±2°C and relative humidity of 60% ± 5% for 12 months, or at 30°C±2°C and relative humidity of 65% ± 5% for 12 months, sampling once every 3 months, according to the stability of key inspection project testing. After 12 months, still need to continue to inspect, according to product characteristics, respectively, 18 months, 24 months, 36 months, etc., sampling test. Compare the results with 0 months to determine the expiration date of the drug.

对温度特别敏感的药物或药物制剂，长期试验可在温度 5℃±3℃ 条件下放置 12 个月，按上述时间要求检查，12 个月以后，仍需继续考察，确定低温储存条件下的有效期。

For drugs or pharmaceutical preparations that are particularly sensitive to temperature, the long-term testing can be placed at a temperature of 5°C±3°C for 12 months, check according to the above time requirements, after 12 months, continue to investigate and determine the validity period under low temperature storage conditions.

对拟冷冻贮藏的药物或药物制剂，长期试验在温度 –20℃ ± 5℃的条件下至少放置 12 个月。

For drugs or pharmaceutical preparations to be stored frozen, the long-term testing should be allowed to stand for at least 12 months at a temperature of -20°C ± 5°C.

### （四）药品上市后的稳定性考察
### 4. Stability Test of Drug after Marketing

药品注册申请单位应在药品获准生产上市后，采用实际生产规模的药品进行留样观察，以考察上市药品的稳定性。根据考察结果，对包装、贮存条件进行进一步的确认或改进，并确定有效期。

After the drug has been approved for production and marketing, the corporation of drug registration and application should reserve and observe the drug samples with actual production scale to investigate the stability of the marketed drug. According to the testing results, the packaging and storage conditions are further confirmed and improved, and the validity period is also defined.

### 四、稳定性研究结果评价
### 10.4.4　Evaluation of Stability Research Results

稳定性试验的研究结果为药品生产、包装、贮存、运输条件提供科学依据，同时通过试验建立药品的有效期。

The research results of the stability test provide a scientific basis for the conditions of drug production, packaging, storage, and transportation.

## 第五节　中药质量标准实例
## 10.5　Examples for Quality Standard of Traditional Chinese

PPT

### 一、质量标准
### 10.5.1　Quality Standard

### 荆芥穗（Jingjiesui）

Schizonepetae Spica
Schizonepeta Spike

本品为唇形科植物荆芥 *Schizonepeta tenuisfolia* Briq. 的干燥花穗。夏、秋二季花开到顶、穗绿时采摘，除去杂质，晒干。

Schizonepeta Spike is the dried fruit-spike of *Schizonepeta tenuifolia* Briq.. The drug is collected in summer and autumn when the spike becomes green, removed from foreign matter, and dried in the sun.

【性状】本品穗状轮伞花序呈圆柱形，长 3~15cm，直径约 7mm。花冠多脱落，宿萼黄绿色，钟形，质脆易碎，内有棕黑色小坚果。气芳香，味微涩而辛凉。

**Description**　Spike cylindrical-shaped, 3-15cm long, about 7mm in diameter. Corolla often fallen off, persistent calyx yellowish-green, campanulate, fragile, easily broken, with small brownish-black nutlets. Odour, aromatic; taste, pungent, and slightly astringent.

【鉴别】（1）本品粉末黄棕色。宿萼表皮细胞垂周壁深波状弯曲。腺鳞头部 8 细胞，直径 95~110μm，柄单细胞，棕黄色。小腺毛头部 1~2 个细胞，柄单细胞。非腺毛 1~6 细胞，大多具壁疣。外果皮细胞表面观多角形，壁黏液化，胞腔含棕色物；断面观细胞类方形或类长方形，胞腔小。内果皮石细胞淡棕色，表面观垂周壁深波状弯曲，密具纹孔。纤维成束，壁平直或微波状。

**Identification**　(1) Powder: Yellowish-brown. Epidermal cells of persistent calyx with deeply sinuous anticlinal walls. The glandular scales head with 8-celled, 95-110μm in diameter, and an unicellular stalk, brownish-yellow. Small glandular head with 1-2 celled and an unicellular stalk. Non-glandular hair 1-6 celled, mostly with warty walls. Cells of exocarp polygonal in surface view, with mucilaginous walls, and containing brown contents. Subsquare and oblong in section view, lumina small. Stone cells of endocarp pale brown, with deeply sinuous anticlinal walls, and densely pitted. Fibre bundles with straight or slight sinuous walls.

（2）取本品粗粉 0.8g，加石油醚（60~90℃）20ml，密塞，时时振摇，放置过夜，滤过，滤液挥至约 1ml，作为供试品溶液。另取荆芥穗对照药材 0.8g，同法制成对照药材溶液。再取胡薄荷酮对照品，加石油醚（60~90℃）制成每 1ml 含 4mg 的溶液，作为对照品溶液。照薄层色谱法（通则 0502）试验，吸取供试品溶液 3μl、对照药材溶液和对照品溶液各 10μl 分别点于同一硅胶 G 薄层板上，以石油醚（60~90℃）乙酸乙酯（37：3）为展开剂，展开，取出，晾干，喷以 1% 香草醛硫酸溶液，加热至斑点显色清晰。供试品色谱中，在与对照药材色谱和对照品色谱相应的位置上，显相同颜色的斑点。

(2) To 0.8g of the coarse powder, add 20ml of petroleum ether (60-90℃), stopper tightly, shake frequently, and allow to stand overnight. Filter and evaporate the filtrate to 1ml as the test solution. Prepare a solution of 0.8g of Schizonepetae Spica reference drug as the reference drug solution in the same manner. Dissolve 1-pulegone CRS in petroleum ether (60-90℃) to produce a solution containing 4mg per ml as the reference solution. Carry out the method for thin layer chromatography, using silica gel G as the coating substance and a mixture of petroleum ether (60-90℃) and ethyl acetate (37：3) as the mobile phase. Apply separately 3μl of the test solution, 10μl of each of the reference solution and reference drug solution to the plate. After developing and removal of the plate, dry in air. Spray with a 1% solution of vanillin in sulfuric acid, and heat to spots clear. The spots in the chromatogram obtained with the test solution correspond in position and colour to the spots in the chromatogram obtained with the reference solution the reference drugs solution.

【检查】水分　不得过 12.0%。

**Test**　*Water*　No more than 12.0 percent.

总灰分　不得过 12.0%。

*Total ash*　No more than 12.0 percent.

酸不溶性灰分　不得过 3.0%。

*Acide-insoluble ash*　No more than 3.0 percent.

【浸出物】照醇溶性浸出物测定法项下的冷浸法测定，用乙醇作溶剂，不得少于 8.0%。

**Extractives**　Carry out the cold maceration method for determination of ethanol-soluble extractives, using ethanol as the solvent, not less than 8.0 percent.

【含量测定】挥发油　照挥发油测定法测定。

**Assay** *Volatile oil* Carry out the method for determination of volatile oil.

本品含挥发油不得少于 0.40%（ml/g）。

It contains not less than 0.4 percent (ml/g) of volatile oil.

**胡薄荷酮**　照高效液相色谱法测定。

*l-pulegone* Carry out the method for high performance liquid chromatography.

色谱条件与系统适用性试验　以十八烷基硅烷键合硅胶为填充剂；以甲醇 - 水（80∶20）为流动相；检测波长 252nm。理论板数按胡薄荷酮峰计算应不低于 3000。

*Chromatographic system and system suitability* Use octadecylsilane bonded silica gel as the stationary phase, a mixture of methanol and water (80:20) as the mobile phase. As detector a spectrophotometer set at 252nm. The number of theoretical plates of the column is not less than 3000, calculated with the reference to the peak of l-pulegone.

对照品溶液的制备　取胡薄荷酮对照品适量，精密称定，加甲醇制成每 1ml 含 20μg 的溶液，即得。

*Reference solution* Weigh accurately a quantity of l-pulegone CRS, dissolve in methanol to produce a solution containing 20μg of l-pulegone per ml as the reference solution.

供试品溶液的制备　取本品粉末（过二号筛）约 0.5g，精密称定，置具塞锥形瓶中，加入甲醇 10ml，超声处理（功率 250W，频率 50kHz）20 分钟，滤过，滤渣和滤纸再加甲醇 10ml，再超声处理一次，滤过，加适量甲醇洗涤 2 次，合并滤液和洗液，转移至 25ml 量瓶中，加甲醇至刻度，摇匀，即得。

*Test solution* Weigh accurately 0.5g of the coarse powder (through No.2 sieve) to a stoppered conical flask, add 10ml of methanol, ultrasonication for 20 minutes (power 250W, frequency 50kHZ), filter, add 10ml of methanol to the residue, extract again for one time as the same manner. Transfer the filtrate to a 25ml volumetric flask, wash the container with a quantity of methanol twice, filter the washings to the same flash, dilute with methanol to volume. Mix well.

测定法　分别精密吸取对照品溶液与供试品溶液各 10μl，注入液相色谱仪，测定，即得。

*Procedure* Inject accurately 10μl of the reference solution and the test solution into the column respectively, and calculate the content.

本品按干燥品计算，含胡薄荷酮（$C_{10}H_{16}O$）不得少于 0.080%。

It contains not less than 0.080 percent of l-pulegone ($C_{10}H_{16}O$), calculated with reference to the dried drug.

【性味与归经】辛，微温。归肺、肝经。

**Property and Flavor** Mild warm; pungent.

【功能与主治】解表散风，透疹，消疮。用于感冒，头痛，麻疹，风疹，疮疡初起。

**Meridian tropism** Lung and liver meridians.

**Actions** To release the exterior, disperse wind, promote eruption, and relieve sore.

**Indications** Common cold, headache, measles, rubella, and early onset of sore and ulcer.

【用法与用量】5~10g。

**Administration and dosage** 5-10g.

【贮藏】置阴凉干燥处。

**Storage** Preserve in a cool and dry place.

**二、起草说明**

## 10.5.2　Drafting Instruction

Schizonepetae Spica

Jingjiesui

Schizonepeta Spike

**名称**　中药材名加药用部位命名。

**Title**　It is named as 'medicinal material name plus of medicinal part name'.

**来源**　拉丁学名：SCHIZONEPETAE SPICA

**Sources**　Latin name: SCHIZONEPETAE SPICA.

中药荆芥始载于《神农本草经》，具有祛风，解表，止血作用，中医临床使用历史悠久，为最常用的解表药物之一。应夏、秋二季花开到顶、穗绿时采摘，除去杂质，晒干。荆芥在我国分布广泛，安徽、江西、湖北、四川等地都有野生。江苏、扬州等地亦有种植。

Schizonepetae Herba was first recorded in *Shennong's Herbal Classic*. It has the functions of dispelling wind-evil, diaphoresis and hemostasis. It has a long history of clinical usage and is one of the most commonly used medicines for diaphoresis. It should be picked when the spikes bloom to the top and turn green in summer and autumn, and then be separated with impurities and dried in the sun. Schizonepetae Herba is widely distributed in China. Historically, It wild in Anhui, Jiangxi, Hubei, Sichuan etc. It is planted in many regions, such as Jiangsu, Yangzhou etc.

**性状**　根据荆芥穗药材实际形态描述。本品穗状轮伞花序呈圆柱形，长 3~15cm，直径约 7mm。花冠多脱落，宿萼黄绿色，钟形，质脆易碎，内有棕黑色小坚果。气芳香，味微涩而辛凉。

**Description**　It is described according to the actual morphology of Schizonepetae Spica. The spike is a cylindrical shape with a length of 3-15cm and a diameter of about 7mm. Corolla is often shed, and the persistent calyx is yellowish green, bell-shaped, brittle and fragile, with brownish black small nuts inside. The smell is fragrant, and the taste is slightly astringent and spicy cold.

**鉴别**　（1）粉末显微鉴别　取药材细粉（过5号筛），显微镜下观察，确定显微特征。图谱见《中华人民共和国药典中药材显微鉴别彩色图鉴》。

**Identification**　① Microscopic identification of powder can pass through No. 5 sieve) is taken and observed under a microscope to determine the microscopic characteristics. The picture is shown in the *Color Pictures of Microscopic Identification of Chinese Medicinal Materials in the Pharmacopoeia of the People's Republic of China.*

（2）薄层鉴别　荆芥穗主要成分为挥发油，而胡薄荷酮为挥发油中主要成分，所以采用以荆芥穗对照药材和胡薄荷酮对照品双对照的薄层色谱法对荆芥穗药材进行鉴别。由于本品挥发油为脂溶性成分，故采用石油醚为提取溶剂，以石油醚（60~90℃）- 乙酸乙酯（37：3）为展开剂，效果较好。见图10-1。

② TLC identification　The main component of Schizonepetae Spica is volatile oil, and l-pulegone is the

The powder of medicinal materials (which

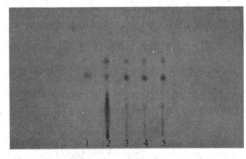

图10-1　荆芥穗药材 TLC 图

Fig. 10-1　TLC of Schizonepeta Spike

1. 胡薄荷酮；2. 荆芥穗对照药材；3，4，5. 三批荆芥穗药材

1. 1-pulegone; 2. Schizonepetae Spica reference drug; 3，4，5. Samples

main component in volatile oil. Therefore, TLC with double control of reference herb of Schizonepetae Spica and l-pulegone reference is used to identify this material. As the volatile oil of this product is a fat soluble component, it is better to use petroleum ether as extraction solvent, and petroleum ether (60-90℃) - ethyl acetate (37 : 3) as developing agent, as Fig. 10-1.

**检查** 按《中国药典》水分测定法（通则 0832 第四法）、总灰分测定法（通则 2302）、酸不溶性灰分测定法（通则 2302），测定 10 批荆芥穗药材水分、灰分、酸不溶性灰分的含量。根据测定结果及贮藏要求，制定荆芥穗药材水分不得过 12.0%，总灰分不得过 12.0%，酸不溶灰分不得过 3.0%。

**Test** According to the water content determination method, total ash content determination method and acid insoluble ash content determination method in *Chinese Pharmacopoeia*, the water, ash and acid insoluble ash content of 10 batches of Schizonepetae Spica were determined. According to the test results and storage requirements, the water, total ash and acid insoluble ash content of Schizonepetae Spica were not more than 12.0%, 12.0% and 3.0%, respectively.

**浸出物** 由于荆芥穗主要成分挥发油为脂溶性成分，故以乙醇为溶剂，用冷浸法提取。根据 10 批荆芥穗药材测定结果制定荆芥穗药材浸出物不得少于 8.0%。

**Extractives** As the volatile oil that is the main ingredient of Schizonepetae Spica is fat-soluble, it is extracted by cold soak with ethanol as solvent. According to the determination results of 10 batches of Schizonepetae Spica, the extractives of the materials should not be less than 8.0%.

**含量测定** 由于荆芥穗主要成分为挥发油，胡薄荷酮为挥发油中主要成分，故含量测定指标选择挥发油和胡薄荷酮。

**Assay** The main component of Schizonepetae Spica is volatile oil, and l-pulegone is the main component in volatile oil. Thus, the volatile oil and l-pulegone are selected as the assay indexes.

（1）挥发油 照《中国药典》挥发油测定法（通则 2204）测定 10 批次荆芥穗药材，根据测定结果制定荆芥穗挥发油限度为不得少于 0.40%（ml/g）。

① *Volatile oil* According to the volatile oil determination method of *Chinese Pharmacopoeia* 10 batches of materials were determined. According to the determination results, the content limit of volatile oil of Schizonepetae Spica was determined to be no less than 0.40% (ml/g).

（2）胡薄荷酮 文献中胡薄荷酮的测定方法有 GC 和 HPLC。根据胡薄荷酮在 252nm 处有较强紫外吸收，且 HPLC 法具有灵敏度高、选择性好的特点，采用 HPLC 法测定荆芥穗药材中胡薄荷酮含量。实验中比较了提取方法、提取溶剂、提取次数、提取时间等因素，根据实验结果确定最佳供试品制备方法。

② *l-pulegone* Methods for the determination of l-pulegone in the literatures contain gas chromatography and high performance liquid chromatography. Considering the strong UV absorption of l-pulegone at 252nm and the characteristics of high sensitivity, selectivity and universality of HPLC, HPLC was used to determine the content of l-pulegone in Schizonepetae Spica. In the experiment, several factors, such as extraction method, extraction solvent, extraction times and extraction time, were compared, which determined the optimal preparation method of the analyzed samples.

**方法学验证** 胡薄荷酮在 117~1872ng 之间呈良好线性关系（$Y=0.002254+7.407X$，$r=0.9999$）；对照品精密度试验结果 RSD 为 0.42%（$n=6$）；供试液中胡薄荷酮在 8 小时内稳定，RSD 为 0.26%；重复性试验的平均含量为 1.028mg/g，RSD=1.07%（$n=6$）；平均回收率为 98.85%，RSD=1.29%（$n=9$）；定量限为 9.36ng。

*Methodological validation* l-pulegone with 117-1872ng showed a good linear relationship ($Y =$

0.002254 + 7.407$X$, $r$ = 0.9999). The RSD of the precision test of reference substance was 0.42% ($n$ = 6). l-pulegone in the tested sample was stable within 8 hours, with RSD 0.26%. The average content of repeatability test was 1.028mg/g, with RSD 1.07% ($n$ = 6). The average recovery was 98.85% with RSD 1.29 % ($n$ = 9). Limit of quantification was 9.36ng.

含量限度　根据10批药材中胡薄荷酮的含量，考虑产地、采收季节、存放条件和时间等因素的影响，将含量限度定为以干燥品计，含胡薄荷酮（$C_{10}H_{16}O$）不得少于0.080%。

*Content limit*　According to the l-pulegone content in 10 batches of materials and considering the quality of the materials affected by some factors such as producing region, harvest season, storage conditions and time, the content limit of l-pulegone is determined to no less than 0.080% (which was calculated as drying products).

# 岗 位 对 接
# Post Docking

本章为中药学相关专业学生必须掌握的内容，为成为合格的中药学服务人员奠定坚实的基础。

This task must be mastered by students majoring in traditional Chinese medicine, traditional Chinese medicine pharmacy and traditional Chinese medicine resources, and lay a solid foundation for becoming qualified Chinese medicine service personnel.

本章内容对应岗位包括中药学服务及药品质量监督管理的相关工种。

The corresponding positions of this task include Chinese medicine service and drug quality supervision and management.

上述从事中药学服务及药品质量监督管理相关所有岗位的从业人员均需要掌握中药质量标准和制定方法，学会应用本章所学知识开展中药学服务工作。

The above-mentioned practitioners in all positions related to traditional Chinese medicine service need to master Chinese medicine quality standards and formulation methods, and learn to apply this task to carry out traditional Chinese medicine analysis services.

# 重 点 小 结
# Summary of Key Points

中药质量标准的主要内容包括：品名、来源或处方、制法、性状、鉴别、检查、浸出物、特征图谱或指纹图谱、含量测定、炮制、性味与归经、功能与主治、用法与用量、规格、贮藏等项目，中药材、中药饮片、中药提取物和中药制剂的质量标准内容依据各自特点又稍有差异。起草说明是对制定的质量标准的详细注释，充分反映标准制定的全过程。起草说明包括理论性解释和全部实践工作中的经验、数据总结。

The main contents of Chinese medicine quality standards include: Title, Sources or Ingredients, Procedure, Description, Identification, Test, Extractives, Characteristic Chromatography or Fingerprint, Assay, Processing, Property and Flavor and Meridian Tropism, Function and Indications, Usage and Dosage, Precautions and Warning, Storage and other items, the quality standards of Chinese Medicinal Materials (Decoction Pieces), Chinese medicine extracts and Chinese medicine preparations are slightly different according to their characteristics. The drafting instructions are detailed notes on the established quality standards, which fully reflect the entire process of standard setting. Drafting instructions include theoretical explanations and experience and data summaries of all practical work.

稳定性试验的目的是考察原料药物或制剂在温度、湿度、光线影响下随时间变化的规律，为药品生产、包装、贮存、运输条件提供科学依据，同时通过试验建立药品的有效期。

The purpose of the stability test is to investigate the laws of raw materials or preparations that change with time under the influence of temperature and wet light, to provide a scientific basis for the conditions of drug production, packaging, storage, and transportation, and to establish the validity period of the drug through the test.

题库

# 目 标 检 测

## 一、选择题

### （一）单项选择题

1. 中药制剂质量标准的主要内容中处方量一般制备成剂型单位数是
   A. 100 个　　　　B. 500 个　　　　C. 1000 个　　　　D. 10000 个

2. 下列不属于测定成分选择原则的是
   A. 有效成分　　　B. 毒性成分　　　C. 易损成分　　　D. 含量最大成分

3. 属于测定成分选择原则的是
   A. 有效成分　　　B. 已知成分　　　C. 含量高的成分　　　D. 含量最大成分

4. 不属于分析方法选择原则的是
   A. 准确　　　　　B. 先进　　　　　C. 灵敏　　　　　D. 简便

5. 建立含量测定项目需要测定的样品批次和提供的数据分别为
   A. 5 批、10 个数据　　　　　　　　B. 10 批、10 个数据
   C. 5 批、20 个数据　　　　　　　　D. 10 批、20 个数据

6. 经检验符合规定的药材制成制剂后，一般不再做
   A. 砷盐　　　　　B. 重金属　　　　C. 甲醇量　　　　D. 总灰分

### （二）多项选择题

1. 制定质量标准的前提条件包括
   A. 处方组成固定　　　　B. 原辅料稳定　　　　C. 工艺稳定
   D. 制定试验方案　　　　E. 查阅文献

2. 制定中药质量标准的原则包括
   A. 处方组成固定　　　　B. 原辅料稳定　　　　C. 工艺稳定
   D. 制定试验方案　　　　E. 查阅文献

3. 中药含量测定中，测定成分选择原则包括有
   A. 测定有效成分　　　　B. 测定毒性成分　　　　C. 测定专属性成分
   D. 测定总成分　　　　　E. 测定指标性成分

4. 下列属于方法学考察项目的是
   A. 提取方法的选择　　　B. 净化方法的选择　　　C. 测定条件的选择
   D. 重复性试验　　　　　E. 专属性试验

5. 中药复方命名时采用主要药味缩写加剂型方法的有
   A. 生脉注射液　　　　　B. 银黄口服液　　　　　C. 川芎茶调散

医药大学堂
WWW.YIYAODXT.COM

　　D. 香连丸　　　　　　　　　E. 十全大补丸

6. 检测有效成分不明确的中药，可测定的指标有

　　A. 浸出物　　　　　　　　　B. 指标性成分　　　　　　C. 物理常数

　　D. 灰分　　　　　　　　　　E. 炽灼残渣

## 二、思考题

**戊己丸的质量标准**

处方：黄连 300g、白芍（炒）300g、吴茱萸（制）50g

制法：以上三味，粉碎成细粉，过筛，混匀，用水泛丸，干燥，即得。

性状：本品为棕黄色的水丸；味苦，稍有麻辣感。

鉴别：取本品，置显微镜下观察：纤维束鲜黄色，壁稍厚，纹孔明显。草酸钙簇晶直径 18~32μm，存在于薄壁细胞中，常排列成行，或一个细胞中含有数个簇晶。非腺毛 2~6 细胞，胞腔内有的充满红棕色物；腺毛头部多细胞，椭圆形，含棕黄色至棕红色物，柄 2~5 细胞。

1. 该制剂的命名方式是什么？

2. 制剂性状描述中"味苦"主要原因是什么？"稍有麻舌感"主要原因是什么？

3. 为何该制剂采用显微鉴别法？标准中描述的鉴别特征都分别是鉴别何种药物的？在采用显微鉴别法鉴别复方制剂时，应注意哪些事项？

# 参 考 答 案

**第一章**

**一、选择题**

（一）单项选择题
| 1. D | 2. B | 3. B | 4. C | 5. A |
| 6. C | 7. C | 8. B | 9. C | 10. A |
| 11. C | 12. B | 13. D | | |

（二）多项选择题
| 1. ABCDE | 2. ABCDE | 3. ABD | 4. ABCDE | 5. ABCDE |
| 6. ABCDE | 7. ABC | 8. ABCDE | 9. ABCDE | 10. ABCDE |

**第二章**

**一、选择题**

（一）单项选择题
| 1. D | 2. C | 3. A | 4. B | 5. D |

（二）多项选择题
| 1. ABCDE | 2. ABD | 3. ABC | 4. ABCDE | 5. ABCD |

**第三章**

**一、选择题**

（一）单项选择题
| 1. A | 2. C | 3. A | 4. D | 5. B |
| 6. D | 7. D | 8. A | 9. B | 10. D |
| 11. A | 12. B | | | |

（二）多项选择题
| 1. ABC | 2. ABCD | 3. ABCDE | 4. ABCDE | 5. ABDE |

**第四章**

（一）单项选择题
| 1. C | 2. A | 3. D | 4. B | 5. D |
| 6. C | 7. C | 8. B | 9. C | 10. D |
| 11. A | | | | |

（二）多项选择题

CD

## 第五章

### 一、选择题

（一）单项选择题

| | | | | |
|---|---|---|---|---|
| 1. A | 2. B | 3. C | 4. D | 5. A |

（二）多项选择题

| | | | | |
|---|---|---|---|---|
| 1. ABD | 2. BD | 3. CDE | 4. ABCDE | 5. AB |

## 第六章

### 一、选择题

（一）单项选择题

| | | | | |
|---|---|---|---|---|
| 1. A | 2. B | 3. A | 4. C | 5. D |
| 6. D | 7. B | 8. B | 9. A | 10. D |

（二）多项选择题

| | | | | |
|---|---|---|---|---|
| 1. ABCDE | 2. ABCD | 3. BCE | 4. ABCDE | 5. ABCDE |
| 6. ABCD | 7. ACDE | 8. ABC | 9. ABCDE | 10. AB |

## 第七章

### 一、选择题

（一）单项选择题

| | | | | |
|---|---|---|---|---|
| 1. A | 2. D | 3. C | 4. B | 5. C |
| 6. A | 7. C | 8. C | 9. A | 10. D |
| 11. B | | | | |

（二）多项选择题

| | | | | |
|---|---|---|---|---|
| 1. ABD | 2. BD | 3. AC | 4. ACD | 5. ABE |
| 6. AC | | | | |

## 第八章

### 一、选择题

（一）单项选择题

| | | | | |
|---|---|---|---|---|
| 1. A | 2. B | 3. B | 4. D | 5. A |
| 6. C | 7. D | 8. C | 9. C | 10. D |
| 11. C | 12. A | 13. A | 14. B | 15. D |

（二）多项选择题

| | | | | |
|---|---|---|---|---|
| 1. ABCE | 2. ABCD | 3. ABC | 4. BDE | 5. BCDE |
| 6. ADE | 7. ABC | 8. AE | 9. BCDE | 10. ACDE |
| 11. BE | 12. ABCDE | | | |

## 第九章

### 一、选择题

（一）单项选择题

1. D      2. A      3. C      4. C

（二）多项选择题

1. ABCD      2. ABC      3. ABCD      4. ABCDE

## 第十章

### 一、选择题

（一）单项选择题

1. D      2. B      3. D      4. D

5. D      6. D

（二）多项选择题

1. ABCDE      2. ABCDE      3. BD      4. ABC

5. BD      6. ABC

# 参 考 文 献

［1］张丽，尹华．中药分析学［M］．北京：中国医药科技出版社，2018.

［2］梁生旺，贡济宇．中药分析［M］．北京：中国中医药出版社，2016.

［3］贡济宇，张丽．中药分析学［M］．北京：人民卫生出版社，2019.

［4］中国食品药品检定研究院．中国药品检验标准操作规范（2019年版）［M］．北京：中国医药科技出版社，2019.

［5］李政，孟勤，尹建元，等．天然熊胆粉与人工合成熊胆粉的红外吸收特征比较［J］．中草药，2009，40（05）：713-714.

［6］李文龙，邢丽红，薛东升，等．一种基于近红外光谱技术的熊胆粉鉴别方法［J］．光谱学与光谱分析，2011，31（03）：673-676.

［7］郑岸冰，杨天鸣，孙晓露．板蓝根颗粒的X-射线衍射Fourier指纹图谱分析［J］．化学与生物工程，2007（06）：75-78.

［8］陈广云，吴启南，沈蓓，等．中药龙齿与龙骨X-射线衍射鉴别研究［J］．中药材，2012，35（04）：553-557.